Contemporary Drug Information:
An Evidence-Based Approach

Claude J. Gaebelein, PhD
Associate Professor of Biostatistics
St. Louis College of Pharmacy
St. Louis, Missouri

Brenda L. Gleason, PharmD
Associate Professor of Pharmacy Practice
St. Louis College of Pharmacy
St. Louis, Missouri

Acquisitions Editor: David Troy
Managing Editor: Meredith Brittain
Marketing Manager: Marisa O'Brien
Production Editor: Gina Aiello
Designer: Doug Smock
Compositor: Nesbitt Graphics

9 8 7 6 5 4 3 2 1

Library of Congress Cataloging-in-Publication Data

Gaebelein, Claude J.
  Contemporary drug information : an evidence-based approach / Claude J. Gaebelein, Brenda L. Gleason.
    p. ; cm.
  ISBN-13: 978-0-7817-8280-7
  ISBN-10: 0-7817-8280-5
  1. Chemotherapy. 2. Biometry. 3. Medical literature. 4. Evidence-based medicine. 5. Pharmacy. I. Gleason, Brenda L. II. Title.

  [DNLM: 1. Drug Therapy. 2. Biomedical Research. 3. Biometry. 4. Evidence-Based Medicine. 5. Review Literature. WB 330 G127c 2008]
  RM263.G32 2008
  615.5'8--dc22
                              2007013835

DISCLAIMER

Care has been taken to confirm the accuracy of the information present and to describe generally accepted practices. However, the authors, editors, and publisher are not responsible for errors or omissions or for any consequences from application of the information in this book and make no warranty, expressed or implied, with respect to the currency, completeness, or accuracy of the contents of the publication. Application of this information in a particular situation remains the professional responsibility of the practitioner; the clinical treatments described and recommended may not be considered absolute and universal recommendations.

The authors, editors, and publisher have exerted every effort to ensure that drug selection and dosage set forth in this text are in accordance with the current recommendations and practice at the time of publication. However, in view of ongoing research, changes in government regulations, and the constant flow of information relating to drug therapy and drug reactions, the reader is urged to check the package insert for each drug for any change in indications and dosage and for added warnings and precautions. This is particularly important when the recommended agent is a new or infrequently employed drug.

Some drugs and medical devices presented in this publication have Food and Drug Administration (FDA) clearance for limited use in restricted research settings. It is the responsibility of the health care provider to ascertain the FDA status of each drug or device planned for use in their clinical practice.

To purchase additional copies of this book, call our customer service department at **(800) 638-3030** or fax orders to (301) 223-2320. International customers should call **(301) 223-2300**.

Visit Lippincott Williams & Wilkins on the Internet: http://www.lww.com. Lippincott Williams & Wilkins customer service representatives are available from 8:30 am to 6:00 pm, EST.

To our parents and families

Contributors

Chapter 9:

Kem P. Krueger, PharmD, PhD
Associate Professor
Pharmacoeconomics and Health Outcomes Research
University of Wyoming School of Pharmacy
Laramie,Wyoming

Linda Gore Martin, PharmD, MBA, BCPS
Assistant Professor
Social and Administrative Pharmacy
University of Wyoming School of Pharmacy
Laramie, Wyoming

Reviewers

Cydreese Aebi PhD, RPh
Assistant Professor
Oregon State University
Corvallis, Oregon, USA

Zubin Austin, PhD
Assistant Professor
University of Toronto
Toronto, Ontario, Canada

Allison Bernknopf, PharmD
Assistant Professor
Ferris State University
Kalamazoo, Michigan, USA

Brenda Swanson-Biearman, MPH, RN
Assistant Professor
Chatham College
Pittsburgh, Pennsylvania, USA

Matthew Blommel, PharmD
Assistant Clinical Professor
West Virginia University
Morgantown, West Virginia, USA

Karen Beth Bohan, PharmD
Assistant Professor
Wilkes University
Wilkes-Barre, Pennsylvania, USA

Rachel A. Bongiorno, PharmD
Assistant Professor
University of Maryland
Baltimore, Maryland, USA

Sherrill Brown, PharmD
Director, Drug Information
Service
Assistant Professor, Pharmacy
Practice
University of Montana
Missoula, Montana, USA

Loraine Cicero, BA, BS, MS, PharmD
Associate Professor of
Pharmacy Practice
Long Island University
Brooklyn, New York, USA

Gary Cochran, PharmD, SM
Assistant Professor
University of Nebraska Medical
Center
Omaha, Nebraska, USA

John Foxworth, PharmD
Professor of Medicine and
Pharmacology
Associate Program Director for
Research, Internal Medicine
Residency Program
Department of Medicine,
Truman Medical Center-
Hospital Hill
University of Missouri-Kansas
City School of Medicine
Kansas City, Missouri, USA

Terri Levien, PharmD
Assistant Professor
Washington State University
Spokane, Washington, USA

Wesley Lindsey, PharmD
Director of Drug Information
Assistant Professor
Palm Beach Atlantic University
West Palm Beach, Florida, USA

Bernie Olin, PharmD
Clinical Associate Professor
Auburn University School of
Pharmacy
Auburn, Alabama, USA

Teresa O'Sullivan, PharmD, BCPS
University of Washington
Seattle, Washington, USA

Pat Parteleno RPh, PharmD
Director of Experiential
Education
Associate Professor
Ohio Northern University
Raabe College of Pharmacy
Ada, Ohio, USA

Evan Robinson, PhD
Assistant Dean
University of Charleston
Charleston, West Virginia, USA

Yvonne Shevchuk, BSP, PharmD
Professor of Pharmacy
University of Saskatchewan
Saskatoon, Saskatchewan,
Canada

Meera Thadani, BSc(Pharm), MSc
Assistant Professor
University of Manitoba
Winnipeg, Manitoba, Canada

Lee Vermeulen, RPh, MS, FCCP
Director, Center for Drug Policy
University of Wisconsin
Hospital and Clinics
Clinical Associate Professor
University of Wisconsin
Madison, Wisconsin, USA

Kristina E. Ward, PharmD, BCPS
Clinical Assistant Professor
Director, Drug Information
Services
University of Rhode Island
College of Pharmacy
Kingston, Rhode Island, USA

Preface

Contemporary Drug Information: An Evidence-Based Approach provides a practical, up-to-date introduction to the acquisition, evaluation, and application of healthcare information to clinical settings. The book integrates information on drug data, biostatistics, and biomedical literature review into a synthetic whole, united by the principles of evidence-based medicine. Thus the reader is exposed to an integrated approach to examining healthcare literature and making decisions about its applicability to patient care.

The content is intended for pharmacy students, professional pharmacists, and other healthcare students as well as practitioners who must conduct critical evaluations of healthcare literature as part of their professional duties. This text meets the needs of contemporary students and practitioners in acquiring both the skill set and the strategic approach necessary to search, identify, analyze, synthesize, and apply healthcare information in a variety of clinical settings. *Contemporary Drug Information* can also serve as a resource for research methods, biostatistics, therapeutics, and epidemiology courses as well as provide a launching point for literature searches and literature evaluations.

This book is not intended to be a how-to guide to data analysis. Rather its purpose is to guide those who will use the products of healthcare research—primary, secondary, and tertiary literature—in making decisions regarding the assessment and treatment of their patients. To this end, the authors stress information regarding the acquisition of appropriate material, its critical evaluation, and its application, enumerating biostatistical principles as they are needed to understand the fundamentals of research methods and presenting major statistical tests used to evaluate and report healthcare information.

Specifically, *Contemporary Drug Information* helps readers:

- Appreciate the role of drug information, biostatistics, and biomedical literature evaluation in the healthcare profession
- Understand the rationale for using evidence-based medicine as a clinical decision-making paradigm
- Evaluate critically the appropriateness of research reports in the healthcare literature
- Critically evaluate conclusions presented in the healthcare literature, communicate that knowledge to professional and nonprofessional audiences, and apply that knowledge in professional settings

Organizational Philosophy

Contemporary Drug Information begins at the very beginning. From a foundation of basic concepts, the reader is transported through a process that progressively teaches new principles, infuses novel skill sets, and develops new capabilities. The manner of presentation is narrative, examples are drawn from the current healthcare literature, and study problems foster the application of the relevant principles and concepts in clinical settings. The arrangement of the text permits the presentation of the material in distinct units, allowing for the flexible presentation by different instructors or in different courses.

Section 1, "A Framework for Evaluating Contemporary Healthcare Information," presents a comprehensive structure for understanding the use of healthcare information. An introductory discussion explains the need for pharmacists to possess drug information skills along with an understanding of how biostatistics are appropriately employed as one aspect of critically evaluating biomedical literature. In addition, the text describes the interrelationship of these skills in the provision of pharmaceutical care and presents practical examples of how this triad of skills is integrated into routine clinical practice. This part emphasizes the importance of developing such skills as part of a life-long learning strategy to maintain professional competency. Ethical issues surrounding the provision of pharmaceutical care are also addressed, including the fiduciary responsibility to patients and professional responsibility to the healthcare team, along with beneficence and negligence.

Section 2, "Tools for Evaluating Contemporary Healthcare Information," presents an overview of clinical research and conclusions from research based on particular study designs. A discussion of observational and interventional study designs, with an overview and examples drawn from the biomedical literature, is followed by a detailed treatment of both descriptive statistics and inferential statistical principles. These topics are embedded in a discussion of observational and experimental research paradigms, which provide a context for the specific statistical tests presented. Multivariable statistical tests, meta-analyses, active and placebo controlled randomized trials, and pharmacoeconomics evaluations receive comprehensive treatment.

Section 3, "Clinical Decision Making Using Contemporary Healthcare Information," details the clinical decision-making process, including evaluating the evidence in accordance with clinical practice guidelines and using primary literature to make evidence-based recommendations. The text presents barriers to implementing clinical practice guidelines and strategies for their successful implementation. The part concludes with essential plans to becoming an information master by keeping current with the literature, including valuable advice on electronic information management and literature foraging and hunting tools.

For the serious learner, more detailed information is provided in the appendices. Appendix A presents useful drug information tools, including a schema for classifying drug information questions that students or practitioners can either use as is or easily modify to meet their specific needs. The appendix also contains a list, with detailed descriptions, of commonly used secondary resources and a list of commonly used tertiary resources.

No treatment of biostatistics would be complete without tables of critical values for the statistical tests emphasized in the text. These tables appear in Appendix B, which includes values of z in the standard normal distribution, as well as critical values of t, F, and χ^2.

To facilitate the principles involved in the critique of drug information sources, Appendix C contains reprints of many of the studies that are reviewed in detail in this text. (Unfortunately, the policies of several journals precluded the inclusion of their articles in this section, so those papers must be obtained from the journals themselves.)

Finally, a glossary maximizes the acquisition of novel terms and concepts. These terms appear in boldface at their first use in each chapter. Each glossary entry includes a chapter number, so readers can find that term in use.

Features of this Book

The chapters of *Contemporary Drug Information* contain the following elements to maximize learning:

- **Chapter goals:** This list of competencies appears at the beginning of each chapter, and the items should be mastered upon the completion of the chapter.
- **Key terms:** Students must know these basic vocabulary words to attain a full understanding of the material. Key terms, which are set in boldface at first use in each chapter, are defined in the glossary.
- **Literature critiques:** Students are exposed to critical evaluations of published healthcare literature, including both line-by-line commentary on the contents of the research report and an overall evaluation of the internal and external validity of the paper.
- **Perspectives:** These sections provide a historical basis for a better understanding of the context of contemporary drug information, including an appreciation of the contribution of other disciplines, notably epidemiology, to the treasury of healthcare information. In addition, the Perspectives offer further discussion and details on chapter topics or highlight current controversies pertaining to the topic.
- **Extra-credit:** These features offer either a more detailed or a different approach to the topic under discussion. Although students not looking for an in-depth explanation might choose to skip over these sections, they will interest and benefit most students.
- **Chapter summary:** Each chapter contains a summary section that provides a synopsis of the information presented; this is a handy study aid and quick reference guide.
- **Study problems:** Each chapter concludes with several practice problems that reinforce the concepts covered in that chapter.
- **Figures:** Illustrations encapsulate and clarify important concepts.
- **Tables:** Tables synthesize useful information in an easy-to-reference format.

As mentioned, Appendix A contains drug information tables, Appendix B contains statistical tables, and Appendix C contains reprints of some of the articles critiqued in this text.

Student and Instructor Resources

STUDENT RESOURCES

A Student Resource Center at http://thePoint.lww.com/gaebelein includes the following materials:

- Additional practice with evaluating recently published research reports
- Links to literature evaluation and statistics resources
- An Image Bank that contains the figures and tables from the textbook.

INSTRUCTOR RESOURCES

We understand the demand on an instructor's time, so to help make your job easier, you will have access to Instructor Resources upon adoption of *Contemporary Drug Information: An Evidence-Based Approach*. In addition to the student resources just listed, an Instructor's Resource Center at http://thePoint.lww.com/gaebelein includes the following:

- Active learning strategies and activities
- Answer keys for assessing students' evaluations of recently published research reports
- Answers to select study problems found in the text.

Acknowledgments

DR. GAEBELEIN

I am indebted to two teachers, Roy S. Lilly and Robert Moran, who introduced me to statistics during my graduate studies at Kent State University; to many other mentors during my career, and to the students at St. Louis College of Pharmacy for their patience during the evolution of these ideas. I am particularly grateful for the collaboration of Brenda Gleason, who lent a clinical perspective to a dry biostatistics tome, transforming it into an exciting exposition of evidence-based medicine. Last, I am grateful for the patience and support of my wife, Debra, during this project.

DR. GLEASON

I would like to thank Claude Gaebelein for his encouragement and guidance throughout the process of writing this textbook. It has been a real pleasure to collaborate with Claude on this text. In addition, I would like to thank Sheldon Holstad, Michael Maddux, and Thomas Zlatic for their mentorship throughout my academic career. Finally, I would like to thank my husband, Aaron, and son, Carter, who have been so supportive and understanding of my many hours at the computer during the development of this text.

JOINTLY

We acknowledge the support, encouragement, patience, and intervention of those at Lippincott Williams & Wilkins who made this work possible: David Troy, our developmental editor, and Meredith Brittain, our principal managing editor. In addition, we would like to thank Kem Krueger and Linda Gore Martin, who lent their expertise in pharmacoeconomics literature evaluation by writing Chapter 9. Finally, we thank family, friends, colleagues, and students for their encouragement and support during this project.

Contents

SECTION 3: Clinical Decision Making Using Contemporary Healthcare Information

A Framework for Evaluating Contemporary Healthcare Information

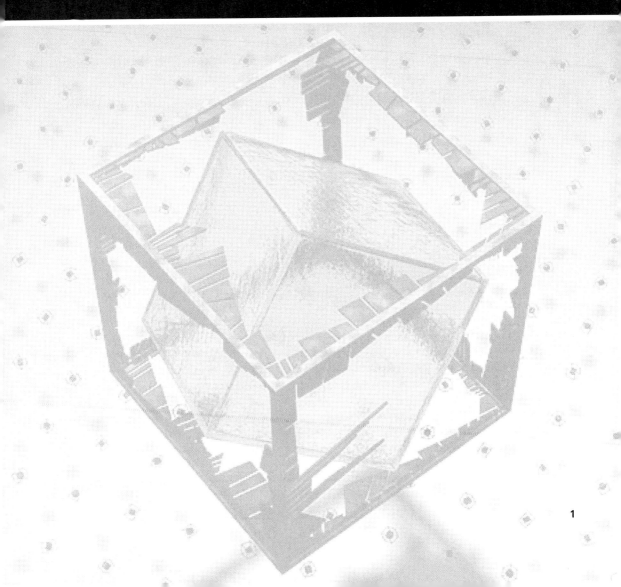

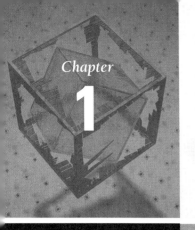

Chapter

1

Integrating Drug Information, Literature Evaluation and Biostatistics to Provide Evidence-Based Pharmaceutical Care

CHAPTER GOALS

After studying this chapter, the student should be able to:

1. Explain the need for pharmacists to possess knowledge and skills in drug information, biostatistics, and literature evaluation to provide pharmaceutical care.

2. Describe how drug information, biostatistics, and literature evaluation skills interrelate to provide pharmaceutical care.

3. Describe the evidence-based medicine paradigm and discuss how pharmaceutical care is delivered within this model.

4. Explain the information mastery concept and its relationship to providing pharmaceutical care within the evidence-based medicine environment.

5. Justify the necessity of drug information, biostatistics, and literature evaluation skills to foster life-long learning and ongoing professional competency.

Pharmacists are key members of the multidisciplinary healthcare team both in managing individual patients and populations as a whole. The provision of **pharmaceutical care**—the current mission of the profession and the academy[1]—requires integration of sound therapeutic principles and evidence-based data to render preeminent, patient-centered care. Specifically, pharmacists must be able to retrieve, analyze, and interpret professional, lay, and scientific literature to provide drug information to patients, their families, and other healthcare providers. Furthermore, as indoctrinated in the Oath of a Pharmacist[2] (Table 1-1), it is paramount that pharmacists keep abreast of new and emerging therapeutics, scientific theories, and medical practices to not only maintain professional competency and foster life-long learning but also to ensure optimal drug therapy outcomes for patients. This cannot be accomplished successfully without possessing drug information, biostatistics, and literature evaluation skills. Fortunately, each element of this triad of skills effectively and efficiently interrelates with the others, allowing the professional to provide pharmaceutical care within the evidence-based model of medicine.

Beginning in the early 1990s a new paradigm emerged in medicine. **Evidence-based medicine (EBM)**, defined as the conscientious, explicit, and judicious use of current best evidence along with clinical expertise and patient values in making clinical decisions about the care of individual patients,[3] became a new focus for many clinicians in the United States and abroad. The EBM approach was in contrast to the previous model of

TABLE 1-1	**The Oath of a Pharmacist**

At this time, I vow to devote my professional life to the service of all humankind through the profession of pharmacy.

I will consider the welfare of humanity and relief of human suffering my primary concerns.

I will apply my knowledge, experience, and skills to the best of my ability to assure optimal drug therapy outcomes for the patients I serve.

I will keep abreast of developments and maintain professional competency in my profession of pharmacy.

I will maintain the highest principles of moral, ethical and legal conduct.

I will embrace and advocate change in the profession of pharmacy that improves patient care.

I take these vows voluntarily with the full realization of the responsibility with which I am entrusted by the public.

Reprinted with permission from American Pharmaceutical Association Academy of Student Pharmacists/American Association of Colleges of Pharmacy—Council of Deans (APhA-ASP/AACP-COD) Task Force on Professionalism. Oath of a pharmacist. June 26, 1994. Available at: www.aphanet.org/students/leadership/professionalism/oath.htm. Accessed June 2006.

practice, called opinion-based medicine-in which decisions regarding patient care were based mainly on the clinician's own preferences, opinions, experiences, and habits and not necessarily on scientific, clinical evidence that is pertinent to the patient. For example, in the opinion-based model, a clinician might routinely recommend clonidine for blood pressure reduction and use his or her previous successful experience with clonidine to justify its use regardless of the patient.

The EBM approach to practicing medicine compels the clinician to go beyond his or her own clinical experience and expertise (Fig. 1-1). Using the EBM paradigm, the healthcare provider must seek and critically evaluate evidence from the biomedical literature (i.e., clinical trials and research) that specifically pertains to the patient and use that evidence in conjunction with his or her clinical judgment and the patient's values to make a recommendation regarding the patient's care. So, using the EBM model, a clinician would not routinely recommend clonidine for treating hypertension but instead would consider the patient's comorbidities and preferences (e.g., the patient may be newly married and may be concerned about an antihypertensive medication that is likely to cause sexual dysfunction). Using the patient's comorbidities and preferences, the clinician looks to the biomedical literature and uses scientific research along with personal expertise to justify any recommendation of a blood pressure-lowering therapy.

Since the mid-1990s, the development and implementation of EBM has been enhanced by education, dissemination of information, and information technologies and has been endorsed by governments and various private sectors, including academic institutions and managed-care organizations. The pharmacy profession has followed suit. Three key components of practicing EBM are conducting comprehensive yet efficient searches of the professional, lay, and scientific literature; critically appraising the evidence obtained; and applying that evidence to individual patients and populations. This is where drug information, biostatistics, and literature evaluation skills come into play. A pharmacist must become an information master to be an integral member of a healthcare team working under the EBM paradigm.

What is **information mastery**? In today's fast-paced world, clinicians continually struggle to keep up with the wealth of information available. They are constantly bombarded with new information from medical journals, pharmaceutical representatives, colleagues,

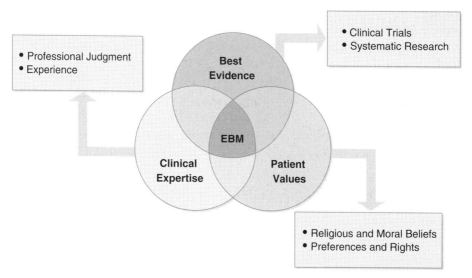

FIGURE 1-1   The Evidence-Based Medicine Paradigm. Best evidence from the healthcare literature is combined with clinical experience and the patient's value system to reach clinical decisions.

practice guidelines, and the media. But most clinicians are never formally trained to develop effective and efficient ways of identifying, critically evaluating, and using new information.[4]

The ability to efficiently forage through vast amounts of available information, find and critically assess the best and most pertinent pieces of information, and apply information to the clinical situation is a skill that pharmacists—the information masters—can and should bring to the multidisciplinary medical team. Possessing drug information, biostatistics, and literature evaluation skills is imperative to becoming an information master working under the EBM paradigm. The remainder of this book focuses on honing these skills. The concept of information mastery will be further explored in Chapter 12.

The Triad of Skills

As noted earlier, using the EBM model to achieve information mastery requires expertise in a triad of areas: drug information, biostatistics, and literature evaluation.

DRUG INFORMATION

Drug information involves the provision of data as they relate to any area of pharmacotherapy or pharmacy practice. At its best, drug information should be cogent, reliable, impartial, well referenced, and critically appraised before being disseminated to other healthcare providers or the lay public.

The concept of drug information began with the establishment of the first official drug information center at the University of Kentucky in 1962.[5] The ensuing decades have seen an expansion of drug information centers across the country. As of 2005, more than 100 pharmacist-managed drug information centers were currently operating in 35 states, the District of Columbia, and Puerto Rico.[6,7] Many of these centers are affiliated with hospitals, medical centers, and colleges or schools of pharmacy.[5] Although many pharmacists practicing in such institutions received advanced training through residency or fellowship programs, providing credible drug information is an important skill for all pharmacists, regardless of their practice setting, as the profession becomes more integrated in direct patient care within the medical team.

This book is not geared toward developing drug information specialists but instead is focused on drug information generalists, those pharmacists who will practice and provide drug information in a broad range of settings from community to hospital to industry to clinics. Drug information skills are further explored in Chapter 2 and are revisited throughout the remaining text.

BIOSTATISTICS

Pharmacists use **biostatistics** to classify, measure, analyze, and interpret health-related data generated through scientific research. Evidence-based clinical decisions and recommendations thus depend, at least in part, on biostatistics. Specifically, biostatistics is the application of statistical techniques to scientific research in health-related fields such as medicine, biology, and public health and to the development of new tools to study these areas.

Since the beginning of the 20th century, biostatistics has become an important tool in improving health and reducing illness. Biostatisticians play a crucial role in designing clinical trials, analyzing data, and creating methods for addressing a diversity of research queries such as determining major risk factors for heart disease and cancer, testing of new drugs to combat HIV/AIDS, and evaluating potential environmental factors harmful to human health such as cigarette smoking and exposure to asbestos or pollutants.

Although most pharmacists are not expected to expertly manipulate data from scientific discovery for statistical purposes (although some do), knowledge of biostatistics and its appropriate application in research paradigms is key to avoiding the use of invalid biostatistical findings. Biostatistics is further elucidated in Chapters 3–5 and is revisited throughout the remaining text.

LITERATURE EVALUATION

To make evidence-based clinical decisions and recommendations on pharmaceutical care issues, the final skill in the triad that pharmacists must master is **literature evaluation**.

Pharmacists must be able to analyze and interpret information from a variety of sources to apply that data to a clinical situation. The community pharmacist might be asked to evaluate claims for a herbal supplement that a patient obtained from a TV commercial. A hospital pharmacist might be required to dissect and critically evaluate the exact methodology and results of a clinical trial to surmise the efficacy of a novel, but expensive, drug and to apply those findings to a patient in the intensive care unit.

Literature evaluation skills do not come automatically. They must be honed and practiced and are improved with experience. Pharmacists must also integrate their clinical judgment along with literature evaluation principles to make evidence-based clinical decisions. The student can sharpen these skills by working through the following chapters, which focus on critically evaluating the most common types of clinical trials.

The interdependence of this triad of skills—drug information, biostatistics, and literature evaluation—is given in Figure 1-2. Drug information, the provision of credible data on pharmacy-related issues, integrates both biostatistics and literature evaluation into the process. Biostatistics and literature evaluation are key to critically appraising information before it is disseminated so valid recommendations regarding patient care can be made. The next section presents examples of this process.

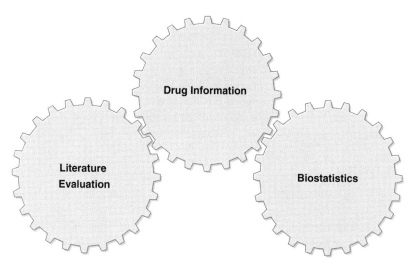

FIGURE 1-2 Integration of Drug Information, Biostatistics, and Literature Evaluation. Drug information, the provision of credible data on pharmacy-related issues, integrates biostatistics and literature evaluation.

Integrating the Skill Triad into Routine Clinical Situations

In July 2004, the Adult Treatment Panel III (ATP III) of the National Cholesterol Education Program (NCEP) issued a report to update their evidence-based treatment guidelines in light of recently published clinical trials that had new implications for cholesterol management, particularly in high-risk patients.[8–13] Evidence from these clinical trials raised new questions for the ATP III group, such as the optimal time to initiate 3-hydroxy-3-methylglutaryl-coenzyme A (HMG-CoA) reductase inhibitor (or statin) therapy after an acute coronary event and for the optimal treatment goal for low-density lipoprotein (LDL) cholesterol levels in high-risk patients. Unfortunately, the evidence did not provide clear answers to these questions. Based on the evidence it had, the ATP III group issued the following treatment recommendations (Table 1-2).[9–13]

The revised recommendation of an optional goal of LDL cholesterol levels to less than 70 mg/dL leaves clinicians in a somewhat nebulous state when trying to determine how to best treat very high risk patients. Should we treat these patients to obtain an LDL cholesterol level < 70 mg/dL? There is much debate surrounding this question and evidence continues to accumulate. Imagine the following clinical scenario.

A pharmacist consulting with a medical team in a community hospital is asked to provide pharmacotherapy recommendations for a 68-year-old man who was admitted 2 days earlier for pneumonia. His medical history includes treatment-controlled hypertension, stable coronary heart disease (CHD) (the patient experienced a myocardial infarction 2 years earlier), and type 2 diabetes (controlled with oral hypoglycemic agents). The medical team is successfully treating the patient's pneumonia. The man is now afebrile, has been switched from intravenous antibiotics to oral antibiotics, and is scheduled for discharge the next day.

The medical team ordered a fasting lipid profile for the patient, which revealed an LDL cholesterol level of 98 mg/dL while on simvastatin 20 mg daily. (The patient has been taking this statin for 6 months.) Because the ATP III-NCEP updated recommendations are ambiguous and because this patient has stable CHD and thus is not considered to be very high risk, the medical team looks to the pharmacist for an evidence-based recommendation on whether the patient should be treated with the goal of lowering his LDL levels to

TABLE 1-2	Adult Treatment Panel III: Goals for Drug Therapy Based on Recent Clinical Trial Evidence	
RISK CATEGORY	**LDL GOAL**	**CONSIDER DRUG THERAPY**
High risk: CHD[a] or CHD risk equivalents[b] (10-year risk > 20%)	< 100 mg/dL (optional goal: < 70 mg/dL)[c]	> 100 mg/dL[d] (< 100 mg/dL consider drug options)[e]

[a]Coronary heart disease (CHD) includes history of myocardial infarction, unstable angina, stable angina, coronary artery procedures (angioplasty or bypass surgery), or evidence of clinically significant myocardial ischemia.

[b]CHD risk equivalents include clinical manifestations of noncoronary forms of atherosclerotic disease (peripheral arterial disease, abdominal aortic aneurysm, and carotid artery disease [transient ischemic attacks or stroke of carotid origin or > 50% obstruction of a carotid artery]), diabetes, and at least two risk factors with a 10-year risk for hard CHD > 20%.

[c]Very high risk favors the optional LDL cholesterol goal of < 70 mg/dL, and in patients with high triglycerides, non-HDL cholesterol < 100 mg/dL.

[d]If the baseline low-density lipoprotein (LDL) cholesterol is < 100 mg/dL, institution of an LDL-lowering drug is a therapeutic option on the basis of available clinical trial results. If a high-risk patient has high triglycerides or low HDL levels, combining a fibrate or nicotinic acid with an LDL-lowering drug can be considered.

[e]When LDL-lowering drug therapy is employed, it is advised that intensity of therapy be sufficient to achieve at least a 30–40% reduction in LDL cholesterol levels.

Adapted with permission from Grundy SM, Cleeman JI, Bairey, et al. Implications of recent clinical trials for the National Cholesterol Education Program Adult Treatment Panel III guidelines. Circulation 2004;110:227–239.

< 70 mg/dL or whether he should stay with his current therapy, which maintains the LDL level at < 100 mg/dL.

Knowing the guideline recommendations, the pharmacist sees if any new evidence has been published to help shed light on this clinical dilemma. She searches through the medical literature and finds a newly published trial—the Treating to New Targets (TNT) Study,[14] which investigates the targeting of an LDL cholesterol level of ~ 70 mg/dL in patients with stable CHD. Approximately 10,000 patients aged 35–75 years with stable CHD were randomly assigned to receive either atorvastatin 10 mg daily or atorvastatin 80 mg daily for almost 5 years. The TNT Study investigators primarily compared the occurrence of a first major cardiovascular event—death from CHD, fatal or nonfatal stroke, nonfatal or nonprocedure-related myocardial infarction, and resuscitation after cardiac arrest—between the treatment groups.

The investigators found that the atorvastatin 80 mg daily group reached an average LDL cholesterol of 77 mg/dL and experienced a statistically significant reduction in a first major cardiovascular event compared to the atorvastatin 10 mg daily group, which reached an average LDL cholesterol of 101 mg/dL. This decrease in cardiovascular events came at the expense of a 1% increase in the number of patients with persistently elevated liver enzymes in the atorvastatin 80 mg daily group compared to the atorvastatin 10 mg daily group, but no differences were noted between treatment groups in regard to rhabdomyolysis or myalgias. Furthermore, no differences were found in overall mortality between the patient groups.

Before the pharmacist makes a recommendation to the medical team regarding the treatment for the 68-year-old patient, she must ask herself, How compelling is the evidence from the TNT Study? Is it convincing enough to lower the LDL cholesterol goal for this patient? Is the potential reduction in cardiovascular events worth the potential increased risk of elevated liver enzymes? To reach a conclusion, the pharmacist must critically evaluate the TNT Study, including its statistical methods.

The pharmacist deems that the TNT Study was well designed and executed and her patient is similar to the subjects studied in the trial. She contemplates that, although atorvastatin 80 mg daily further reduced cardiovascular risk compared to atorvastatin 10 mg daily, the higher dose did not further reduce overall mortality, an important clinical end point. However, the trial was not designed to detect statistically significant differences in overall mortality.

A closer look at the data from the trial reveals that while deaths from cardiovascular causes decreased in the atorvastatin 80 mg daily group, the number of non-cardiovascular-related deaths increased compared to the atorvastatin 10 mg daily group. The pharmacist notes that this could have been a chance finding; however, it is still a matter of concern, especially because the outcome was death related.

Finally, when evaluating the adverse effects reported in the trial, the pharmacist concludes that the increased risk of elevated liver enzymes is not substantial enough to withhold a recommendation of atorvastatin 80 mg daily. Because adverse events, such as myalgias and rhabdomyolysis, were similar in the two treatment groups, the pharmacist is further compelled to recommend the higher atorvastatin dose.

The pharmacist then explains the pros and cons of atorvastatin 80 mg daily to the patient, who decides to adopt the higher daily dose. Because he has already experienced one heart attack, the patient wants to do all he can to avoid dying from a second heart attack and is not as concerned about dying from noncardiovascular causes.

Thus, based on a critical evaluation of the evidence, clinical expertise, and the patient's values, the pharmacist recommends the patient's prescription be changed to atorvastatin 80 mg daily to reach a goal LDL cholesterol level of < 70 mg/dL and a repeat fasting lipid panel be performed in 4–6 weeks.

PERSPECTIVE 1-1

Although it is clear in the example how the pharmacist used her literature evaluation and biostatistics skills to provide evidence-based drug information to the patient and the medical team, a different recommendation could have been derived from the same report. For example, it could be argued that the increase in non-cardiovascular-related deaths in the atorvastatin 80 mg daily group merits further study before it is safe to recommend the higher dose. Also, the atorvastatin 80 mg daily treatment group did not meet the LDL goal of <70 mg/dL. Thus what should the LDL goal for this patient be: 77 mg/dL or 70 mg/dL? Finally, is more evidence needed to be certain that benefits of atorvastatin 80 mg daily outweigh the risks in patients with stable CHD?

Some of questions that remain unanswered regarding the use of statins and lowering LDL levels to <70 mg/dL in high-risk patients are

- *Is cardiovascular protection a function of the LDL-lowering effect and not specifically tied to the statin used? Can statins other than atorvastatin 80 mg daily afford similar protection as long as an LDL of <70 mg/dL is reached?*
- *Are pleiotropic effects (i.e., properties other than cholesterol reduction such as anti-inflammatory effects) of high-dose atorvastatin responsible in part for the cardiovascular protection?*

In addition, a question remains concerning the current ATP III-NCEP guideline recommendations on LDL goals in high-risk patients. Should the guideline's statement that it is optional to target an LDL level of <70 mg/dL in high-risk patients be changed to the more definitive statement of recommending a target of LDL <70 mg/dL?

To be sure, medical decision making is complex. Many times more than one appropriate recommendation can be made based on the same evidence. Practicing in the evidence-based model of medicine requires not only critical evaluation of the literature but also clinical expertise and judgment paired with the patient's values. What would you have recommended to the medical team for this patient?

Drug information, biostatistics, and literature evaluation skills are not only used in hospital environments but in community pharmacies as well. Consider the following scenario.

A pharmacist is filling prescriptions at his local community pharmacy when a long-standing customer approaches the counter with a worried look on her face. It's Mrs. Johnson, a pleasant 70-year-old who suffers from obesity, osteoporosis, arthritis, and hypertension and is a longtime smoker. She is somewhat concerned because she saw a report from a morning TV news show that stated, based on a new study, women should not take aspirin for protection against heart disease. The report contradicted the recommendation from her doctor that she should take a baby aspirin daily. Unfortunately, she can't get in contact with her doctor to discuss this issue.

The pharmacist informs Mrs. Johnson that the American Heart Association (AHA) currently recommends a daily low-dose aspirin for all adults whose 10-year risk for a first CHD event is at least 10% and that she has such a risk.[15] Although the pharmacist is unaware of any newly published evidence on this matter, he reassures Mrs. Johnson that he'll look into the report and get back to her by the next morning.

The pharmacist searches the medical literature and finds the new study, the Women's Health Study,[16] a large, 10-year, randomized controlled trial of low-dose aspirin for primary prevention of cardiovascular disease among almost 40,000 women aged 45 years or older (average age of subjects = 54.6 years).

The Women's Health Study showed that aspirin 100 mg every other day provided no further statistically significant reduction in fatal or nonfatal myocardial infarction, death from cardiovascular causes, or death from any cause when compared to placebo. Low-dose aspirin did significantly decrease the risk of stroke, including ischemic stroke, and transient ischemic attacks compared to placebo.

A closer examination of the evidence revealed that the most consistent benefit of low-dose aspirin was found among women aged 65 years or older. In a prespecified subgroup analysis, low-dose aspirin significantly reduced the overall risk for cardiovascular events by 26%, ischemic stroke by 30%, and myocardial infarction by 34% when compared to placebo. However, side effects were significantly more common in the low-dose aspirin group. For example, women in the aspirin group were 1.4 times more likely to experience gastrointestinal bleeding than those taking placebo.[16]

The pharmacist critically assesses the Women's Health Study and deems it to be well designed with a sound methodology. However, he noted one problem with applying the study in practice: A dosing schedule of one aspirin every other day was used in the study, but that schedule is not widely used in clinical practice and is not the low-dose aspirin regimen recommended by the AHA guidelines.[15]

Thus the pharmacist cannot rule out the possibility that the lack of benefit in reducing the risk for myocardial infarction in women was owing to inadequate dosing of aspirin. However, despite the inadequate dosing, Mrs. Johnson at 70 years of age fits the subgroup of women in the trial for which aspirin still proved beneficial. Furthermore, although the risk for gastrointestinal bleeding is increased with aspirin use, and Mrs. Johnson's smoking habit further increases that risk, the benefits of aspirin in lowering her risk for myocardial infarction and stroke outweigh the potential risks of bleeding.

So although this study raises questions about the efficacy of low-dose aspirin for some women, for Mrs. Johnson the benefits of aspirin still outweigh the risks of side effects based on the current evidence, especially because Mrs. Johnson has major risk factors for heart disease (smoking, hypertension, and age).

The pharmacist calls Mrs. Johnson and tells her of his evaluation of the Women's Health Study,[16] discussing how it applies to her specifically, and recommends that she continue her daily low-dose aspirin until she can reach her physician to get his or her input as well. The pharmacist documents his conversation and recommendations in Mrs. Johnson's pharmacy records.

PERSPECTIVE 1-2

Would your recommendation for Mrs. Johnson have differed from the pharmacist's? What if Mrs. Johnson were 45 years old?

The Women's Health Study[16] raises a puzzling question: Are sex-based differences present in regard to aspirin efficacy? Previous studies documented aspirin efficacy for reducing cardiovascular events,[17–20] but women were not well represented in those trials. In fact, the results of the Women's Health Study were the opposite of those from the Physician's Health Study[20]—a randomized controlled study of >22,000 healthy men (average age of subjects = 53.2 years). The Physician's Health Study sought to determine the efficacy of aspirin 325 mg given every other day for reducing cardiovascular events over a 5-year period. While the Women's Health Study showed no benefit in reducing myocardial infarction in women <65 years, the Physician's Health Study showed a 44% reduction in the risk of myocardial infarction in men ≥50 years of age. The inverse was true for stroke–aspirin provided a benefit for women but no benefit for men.[16,20]

Although researchers continue to look for explanations for such sex-based differences, current recommendations for daily low-dose aspirin remain unclear and debatable for women based on the evidence from the Women's Health Study. Depending on how the study is critically appraised and judged by the clinician, it may be reasonable to shun the use of low-dose aspirin for primary prevention of coronary heart disease in women. On the other hand, if the clinician believes that no benefit was seen because an inadequate aspirin dose was used, then the AHA's low-dose aspirin recommendations could remain intact. What do you think?

Summary

Pharmacists, no matter what facet of pharmacy they practice in, take on a fiduciary responsibility to provide the best possible care for their patients. Patients trust that the pharmacist will do whatever is in the best interest of the patient. Patients also expect their pharmacist to maintain his or her professional competency. To do this well, pharmacists must be life-long learners—they must be intellectually curious, be able to adapt to inevitable changes, and take responsibility for learning and providing skilled pharmaceutical care.

Because medicine, pharmacy, technology, and science are constantly evolving, pharmacists must stay abreast of new and emerging therapeutics, advances in medicine and science, and novel practice theories to maintain professional competency and engage in a trusting relationship with patients. Most often, the premier source for new information comes from articles published in medical journals. Pharmacists need to be information masters—possessing the ability to search out reliable information, critically appraise the information, and apply the information to the situation at hand. Drug information, literature evaluation, and biostatistics skills are imperative if the pharmacist is to become an information master. The subsequent chapters of this book are devoted to honing these skills.

STUDY PROBLEMS

1. Describe how drug information, biostatistics, and literature evaluation interrelate to help the professional provide pharmaceutical care in the evidence-based medicine model.

2. Elucidate the strengths of the evidence-based medicine model of clinical practice.

3. Formulate a basic plan to become an information master. How might you keep current with the medical literature? Include a list of the knowledge, skills, and attitudes needed to be a successful information master. Discuss why being an information master is so important to practicing evidence-based pharmaceutical care.

4. Discuss how you might use the triad of skills to ensure life-long learning and professional competency. Why would your patients want you to possess this triad of skills?

5. Contact a pharmacist and ask how he or she uses drug information, biostatistics, and literature evaluation skills in his or her work. Seek out examples.

6. Reconsider the first clinical scenario outlined in this chapter of the hospitalized 68-year-old man with stable CHD. The pharmacist was asked to provide an evidence-based recommendation regarding the patient's cholesterol-lowering therapy. Find and read the Pedersen et al.[21] article describing the Incremental Decrease in End Points through Aggressive Lipid Lowering (IDEAL) Study. Discuss whether and how the findings from this study could potentially change the recommendation made by the pharmacist in the clinical scenario. Could the IDEAL Study affect current NCEP-ATP III treatment guidelines for goal LDL cholesterol levels in high-risk patients?

REFERENCES

1. 2004 CAPE Advisory Panel on Educational Outcomes. Educational outcomes 2004. American Association of Colleges of Pharmacy Center for the Advancement of Pharmaceutical Education. Available at: www.aacp.org. Accessed June 2006.
2. American Pharmaceutical Association Academy of Student Pharmacists/American Association of Colleges of Pharmacy—Council of Deans (APhA-ASP/AACP-COD) Task Force on Professionalism. Oath of a pharmacist. June 26, 1994. Available at: www.aphanet.org/students/leadership/professionalism/oath.htm. Accessed June 2006.
3. Sackett DL, Straus SE, Richardson WS, et al. Evidence-Based Medicine: How to Practice and Teach EBM. 2nd ed. Edinburgh, UK: Churchill Livingstone, 2000.
4. Center for Information Mastery at the University of Virginia Health System. Mission of the Center for Information Mastery. Available at: www.healthsystem.virginia.edu/internet/familymed/docs/info_mastery.cfm. Accessed June 2006.
5. Rosenberg JM, Koumis T, Nathan JP, et al. Current status of pharmacist-operated drug information centers in the United States. Am J Health Sys Pharm 2004;61:2023-2032.
6. Koumis T, Cicero LA, Nathan JP, et al. Directory of pharmacist-operated drug information centers in the United States—2003. Am J Health Sys Pharm 2004;61:2033-2042.

7. Koumis T, Rosenberg JM. Update of directory of drug information centers. Am J Health Sys Pharm 2005; 62:1348.

8. Grundy SM, Cleeman JI, Bairey, et al. Implications of recent clinical trials for the National Cholesterol Education Program Adult Treatment Panel III guidelines. Circulation 2004;110:227-239.

9. Heart Protection Study Collaborative Group. MRC/BHF Heart Protection Study of cholesterol lowering with simvastatin in 20,536 high-risk individuals: A randomised placebo-controlled trial. Lancet 2002;360:7–22.

10. Shepherd J, Blauw GJ, Murphy MB, et al. Pravastatin in elderly individuals at risk of vascular disease (PROSPER): A randomised controlled trial. Prospective Study of Pravastatin in the Elderly at Risk. Lancet 2002;360:1623-1630.

11. ALLHAT Officers and Coordinators for the ALLHAT Collaborative Research Group. The Antihypertensive and Lipid-Lowering Treatment to Prevent Heart Attack Trial. Major outcomes in moderately hypercholesterolemic, hypertensive patients randomized to pravastatin vs usual care: The Antihypertensive and Lipid-Lowering Treatment to Prevent Heart Attack Trial (ALLHAT-LLT). JAMA 2002;288:2998–3007.

12. Sever PS, Dahlof B, Poulter NR, et al. Prevention of coronary and stroke events with atorvastatin in hypertensive patients who have average to lower-than-average cholesterol concentrations, in the Anglo-Scandinavian Cardiac Outcomes Trial-Lipid Lowering Arm (ASCOT-LLA): A multicentre randomized controlled trial. Lancet 2003;361:1149–1158.

13. Cannon CP, Braunwald E, McCabe CH, et al. Intensive versus moderate lipid lowering with statins after acute coronary syndromes. N Engl J Med 2004;350:1495–1504.

14. LaRosa JC, Grundy SM, Waters DD, et al. Intensive lipid lowering with atorvastatin in patients with stable coronary disease. N Engl J Med 2005;352:1425–1435.

15. Pearson TA, Blair SN, Daniels SR, et al. AHA guidelines for primary prevention of cardiovascular disease and stroke: 2002 update: Consensus panel guide to comprehensive risk reduction for adult patients without coronary or other atherosclerotic vascular diseases. Circulation 2002;106:388–391.

16. Ridker PM, Cook NR, Lee IM, et al. A randomized trial of low-dose aspirin in the primary prevention of cardiovascular disease in women. N Engl J Med 2005;352:1293–1304.

17. Peto R, Gray R, Collins R, et al. Randomised trial of prophylactic daily aspirin in British male doctors. Br Med J 1988;296:313–316.

18. Hansson L, Zanchetti A, Carruthers SG, et al. Effects of intensive blood pressure lowering and low-dose aspirin in patients with hypertension: Principal results of the Hypertension Optional Treatment (HOT) randomised trial. Lancet 1998;351:1755–1762.

19. Collaborative Group of the Primary Prevention Project. Low-dose aspirin and vitamin E in people at cardiovascular risk: A randomized trial in general practice. Lancet 2001;357:89–95.

20. Steering Committee of the Physician's Health Study Research Group. Final report on the aspirin component of the ongoing Physician's Health Study. N Engl J Med 1989;321:129–135.

21. Pedersen TR, Faergeman O, Kastelein JJ, et al. High-dose atorvastatin vs usual-dose simvastatin for secondary prevention after myocardial infarction: The IDEAL study: A randomized controlled trial. JAMA 2005; 294:2437–2445.

Asking and Answering Drug Information Questions

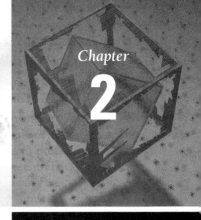

CHAPTER GOALS

After studying this chapter, the student should be able to:

1. Explain why drug information questions are asked and how they are answered.

2. Use a systematic approach to answer drug information questions.

3. Employ efficient and effective search strategies for finding an answer to drug information questions.

4. Briefly discuss ethical and legal issues surrounding the provision of pharmaceutical care in the evidence-based model via drug information queries.

Pharmacists are the drug information experts. Healthcare providers and patients continually look to pharmacists for unbiased, evidence-based, accurate information regarding drug therapies and pharmaceutical issues. But why are drug information questions asked? The answer is simple. Questions are asked because medicine is constantly evolving. Everything is not known or fully understood and likely never will be. We are always searching for a better understanding of health and disease and for truth in the universe.

Healthcare providers seek insight into health and disease and how medications can palliate, treat, cure, heal, or sometimes even cause disease. Scientists strive to further our knowledge of pharmacotherapeutic principles and medical theories. Particularly in the evidence-based model of medicine, researchers incessantly ask and answer scientific and clinical questions, hoping to improve healthcare and patient outcomes. Because pharmacotherapies are integral to improving healthcare and patient outcomes and because pharmacists are the experts in pharmacotherapy, it stands to reason that providing drug information is a prime role for pharmacists to fill.

As discussed in Chapter 1, part of providing pharmaceutical care involves provision of information related to drug therapies and the practice of pharmacy. This information can be disseminated to a variety of audiences from healthcare providers to the lay public. To do this well, pharmacists need to hone their drug information skills, including literature evaluation and biostatistics skills. This chapter focuses on methods used to best provide drug information.

A Systematic Approach to Providing Drug Information

Although relying on intuition, gut instinct, and practice experience to answer drug information questions will work in some instances, in most occasions it will not. If pharmacists responded to drug information queries with simple off-the-cuff replies, the information provided would often be inappropriate and/or lacking in quality. Without some sort of stepwise approach, communication could be impaired, important information could be overlooked, and evidence supporting the response could be deficient. Thus in the mid-1970s Watanabe et al.[1] developed a systematic approach to answering drug information requests. Today, many practicing pharmacists use Watanabe's systematic approach or some modification thereof to provide drug information. The benefits of using a systematic approach are threefold. A systematic approach

- Improves efficiency (e.g., decreases literature searching time)
- Improves effectiveness (e.g., helps avoid overlooking significant information or facts)
- Improves value (e.g., helps ensure the requester finds the information useful)

Watanabe's systematic approach can be used by pharmacists practicing in a wide variety of environments. The approach involves five basic steps (Table 2-1).[1]

Watanabe's five-step approach has been adapted and modified over the years.[2–4] Although it is important to use some sort of systematic method when answering drug information questions, the exact approach taken depends on personal preferences and what works best in the pharmacist's practice environment. Keep in mind that the overall goals of using a systematic approach are to improve efficiency and effectiveness and to enhance the overall value of the information provided. The systematic approach employed should routinely be assessed to make certain it is meeting these goals. One such systematic approach is presented here. This eight-step approach is outlined in Figure 2-1 and detailed in the following sections.[2]

STEP 1: RECEIVE

Although step 1, receive, seems obvious—of course the pharmacist must *receive* a question to answer it—the drug information provision process begins here. Critical elements within this step should be considered and practiced. The first element is *from where or from whom the question is coming*. Pharmacists receive drug information questions from a variety of people, but the demographics of drug information requesters can generally be categorized into two main groups: healthcare providers and the lay public. Following this initial classification, further clarification is required. Healthcare providers include physicians, nurses, occupational and physical therapists, medical technologists, social

TABLE 2-1	Five-Step Approach to Answering Drug Information Questions
STEP	DESCRIPTION
1	Classification of request
2	Obtaining background information
3	Systematic search
4	Response
5	Reclassification

Adapted from Watanabe AS, McCart G, Shimomura S, et al. Systematic approach to drug information requests. Am J Hosp Pharm 1975;32:1282–1285.

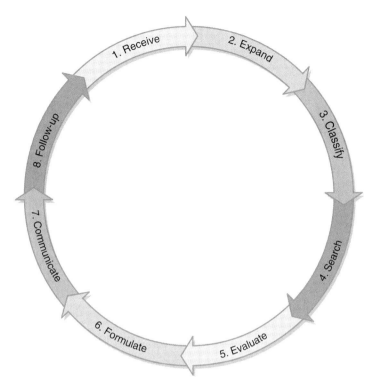

FIGURE 2-1 A Systematic Approach to Answering Drug Information Questions. To use this approach, follow the eight steps in order. (Adapted with permission from Butler CD. Modified systematic approach. Presented at St. Louis College of Pharmacy, drug information course, 1981.)

workers, psychologists, and medical informatics specialists. Each of these professionals possesses a unique constellation of knowledge and expertise, level of training, clinical focus, and experience. Lay people also present a broad spectrum of characteristics—for example, in terms of education level, ethnic and religious background, cultural beliefs, value system, and personality. Thus, once it has been determined who the requester is—healthcare provider or layperson—the next step is to classify the requester further within the main category.

By looking at the received information request in this manner, the pharmacist can determine the *level of information complexity* the requester can likely manage or want and the *demeanor* needed interact successfully with the requester. For example, if asked about the interaction between warfarin and St. John's wort, the level of sophistication and the extent of information provided may be widely different for a dietician and a cardiothoracic surgeon. This same idea holds true when assessing the information complexity level of the lay public. An electrical engineer may (although not always) be able to understand more sophisticated drug information than an elderly grandmother who left school after the sixth grade.

The pharmacist's demeanor while providing the answer to the question may also depend on the person making the drug information request. Although a pharmacist always maintains professional conduct, regardless of the audience, the manner of interaction between the pharmacist and requester depends on the requester's background and the pharmacist's practice environment. For example, a pharmacist is expected to take a concise, pointed approach when receiving a drug information question from a busy attending physician who is in the middle of his or her patient rounds. In contrast, a less formal intercourse may occur with a diabetes educator who casually stops the pharmacist in passing. Likewise, the pharmacist needs to adapt his or her approach to the layperson's background and frame of reference. The pharmacist's demeanor may be different for a harried young mother sporting a crying 2-year-old than for a middle-aged lawyer requesting drug information in the early evening.

Determining the *urgency* of the request and the *mode of communication for the response* are the final details of step 1 of the systematic approach. Does the requester need the response immediately, later that day, or by some other specified time? How would the requester prefer to receive the response—via e-mail, telephone, letter, or in person? Be certain to obtain contact information from the requester, because it will be difficult to deliver the response if such information is unknown.

In summary, the main points of step 1, receive, are to determine the requester's background and how to deliver the response. The remaining steps of the systematic approach can then be adapted accordingly. Figure 2-2 is an algorithm to assist the pharmacist in completing step 1.

STEP 2: EXPAND

In addition to the fundamental process of asking questions to obtain background information about the requester, step 2, expand, also involves determining the focus and scope of the needed information. It is surprising how often the original question does not address the actual needs of the requester. The requester may not know exactly what information he or she is seeking. That others consult with a pharmacist is objective evidence that the pharmacist has drug-related expertise. Thus the pharmacist must help requesters clarify the information they need so the question can be satisfactory answered.

Expanding the received question is an art; it's where true drug information skills are needed and must be practiced to mastery. So what does it mean to *expand* a question? To expand a question properly, a dialog must be started with the requester to determine the *true* question being asked. In this way, broad questions can be narrowed, vague questions can be clarified, and the efficiency of the overall process can be improved.

Because each dialog is unique, the first detail in the expand step is to consider the requester. The expansion information requested from a healthcare provider is different from that requested from a layperson, not only in the terminology used but also in the type and extent of information needed. For example, the pharmacist receives the following question: Is there an interaction between warfarin and St. John's wort? When expanding this question, the pharmacist should consider that a physician might need more than just a yes or no response. Details to be provided might include how this natural

PERSPECTIVE 2-1

During step 2, expand, the pharmacist should remember not to inundate the requester with unnecessary questions. For the busy attending physician who asked a drug information question in the middle of patient rounds, the expand step needs to be concise and pointed and should include only pertinent and needed information to allow for continuation of the systematic approach. Asking inappropriate questions may make the pharmacist appear incompetent and inefficient and may affect the ongoing relationship with the requester.

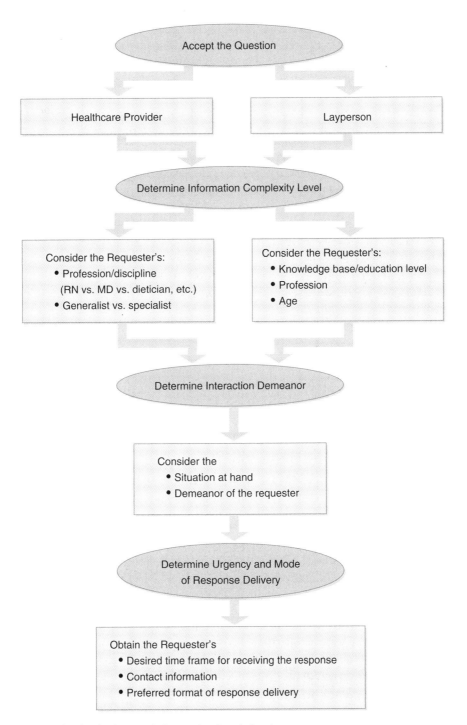

FIGURE 2-2 Algorithm for the Systematic Approach— Step 1: Receive.

supplement interacts with warfarin mechanistically and how well this interaction might be clinically managed. A patient, on the other hand, may not be concerned with understanding exactly how warfarin and St. John's wort interact but may only wish to learn if it's safe to take St. John's wort while taking warfarin. So different expansion questions might be used for the layperson. Regardless of the requester, appropriate information

TABLE 2-2	Example Expansion Questions[a]	
FOR THE HEALTHCARE PROVIDER		**FOR THE LAYPERSON**
• Is this for general or academic purposes?		• Who is the question concerning: self or family member?
• Is this for a specific patient? If so, the pharmacist may need some or all of the following information about that patient:		• What are the person's current and past medical problems, medications, and allergies?
• Age, gender, height, weight, pertinent labs, etc.		• Has the person discussed the question with his or her primary healthcare provider? If so, what information was obtained?
• Diagnoses and past medical history		
• Current and/or past medications		• Where has the person previously searched for the requested information?
• Drug and/or food allergies		
• Were previous search strategies employed to find the requested information? If so, what were those?		• Has the person previously tried anything to resolve the problem?

[a]The example questions are not meant to be inclusive. The originally received question will, in part, help determine what expansion questions to ask. The main goal of the expand step is to clarify the originally received question or to arrive at the true question. *Note:* After the question has been properly expanded, the pharmacist must restate the question to the requester to ensure proper understanding.

should be gathered to arrive effectively at the true question being asked and to execute the remainder of the systematic approach.

Examples of expansion questions geared toward the healthcare provider and toward the layperson are given in Table 2-2. The original question helps determine, in part, how to proceed with the expand step. The specific approach taken by the pharmacist depends on the original question asked.

The expand step of the systematic approach is one of the most critical because a correct response cannot be provided if the pharmacist is unsure of the nature of the information being requested. As mentioned, expanding the original question is an art, and the ability to do this improves with continued practice and experience. Expansion questions usually depend on the original question received. The question received will help trigger what additional information is needed. Keep in mind that not all questions need to be expanded. Some questions are clear and specific, requiring minimal to no expansion. But, most often, at least some expansion will be required. The main goal of step 2, expand, is to ask questions to clarify the originally received question to determine the *true* question being asked.

After the original question has been properly expanded, the final action for the pharmacist is to repeat the question, rephrased in his or her own words, incorporating new or additional information gathered during the expand step. Restating the question is important; this way the pharmacist can verify that he or she understands the true question. Most important, by concurring with this restatement, both pharmacist and requester signify their agreement with respect to the information that will be provided.

STEP 3: CLASSIFY

Once the true question is identified, the next step in the systematic approach is to classify the query. Questions can be categorized based on numerous factors, such as urgency (now or later), source (healthcare provider, layperson), and setting (clinic, hospital rounds, community pharmacy). However, these classifications are mainly used for administrative purposes—for example, to discover a drug information center's main source of questions (hospital interns, community physicians, or the lay public) or to report the number of urgent questions received per month.

But most often, and most important to the systematic approach, the question needs to be classified according to the type of information requested—for example, whether the question pertains to a drug interaction, pediatric dosing, adverse drug reaction, or pharmacokinetics. Classifying the question according to the type of information requested allows for a more efficient search of the literature to find an answer. In effect, then, step 3, classify, determines the scope of the search.

Some questions can be classified by only one characteristic; others can be classified by more than one. Ultimately, as noted, classifying the question helps lead the pharmacist to the most efficient and effective search strategy. After the question is properly classified according to type of information requested, the next step of the systematic approach can begin. One method of classifying drug information questions is given in Table A-1 (Appendix A). Suppose an elderly lady asks a question concerning the safe use of St. John's wort and warfarin. The pharmacist may find the following classifications to be appropriate: (1) drug—natural product interactions and (2) adverse drug reactions.

In summary, categorizing the question by type of information requested serves to determine the scope of the literature search and to focus on the critical information to be obtained during the search. Remember, however, to use the categorization step judiciously. Too few categories will not provide enough information, whereas too many may make an inefficient search process.

STEP 4: SEARCH

Once the question has been properly classified, the next step is to search for an answer. With the vast amount of biomedical literature available, where is the best place to begin the search? The answer is, it depends. It depends in large part on the question. Judgment, experience, and personal preferences will help determine the best and most efficient search strategy. However, some general guidelines can be followed to help the pharmacist search the literature efficiently and effectively.

First, pharmacists need to be familiar with the different types of literature available. Generally, biomedical literature can be classified into three main categories: primary, secondary, and tertiary (Fig. 2-3).

Primary Literature

Primary literature refers to original scientific investigations or clinical studies. These original research papers are the building blocks of biomedical information and are generally considered to be the most current source of information. Original research information is obtained by using specific experimental designs, statistical analyses, and rules for decision making. These include randomized controlled trials (RCTs); epidemiologic designs, such as case-control trials; and individual investigations, such as case reports. These research designs are introduced in Chapter 3 and are discussed in greater detail in subsequent chapters of this text.

Primary literature of interest to pharmacists may appear in pharmacy-related journals such as *Annals of Pharmacotherapy* and *Pharmacotherapy* or in more general medical journals such as the *New England Journal of Medicine, Journal of the American Medical Association (JAMA), Lancet,* and the *British Medical Journal.* But, with more than 20,000 journals published annually and each containing many studies, how does the pharmacist go about finding the exact article or articles needed to answer the requester's question? The next category of literature may help.

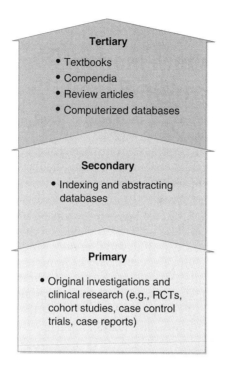

FIGURE 2-3 Three Categories of Biomedical Literature. Primary literature (or original investigations) is the building block of literature. Secondary literature consists of indexes and abstracts of the primary literature. Tertiary literature (or general literature) provides an overview the primary literature. *RCT*, randomized controlled trial.

Secondary Literature

Secondary literature includes resources that index and abstract primary literature. Indexing is a process of using specific terms to categorize a primary research study. This process includes basic bibliographic information, such as the authors' names, study title, and publication citation (journal—including volume, issue, and page numbers—in which the study was published). Research reports are also indexed with respect to, for example, type of drug used, patients treated, and major outcome measures.

Abstracting primary literature consists of providing a brief synopsis of the research report, including the purpose of the study, major variables studied, results obtained, and conclusions reached (Table 2-3).

Multiple secondary resources are available, and many have specific focus areas. Some of the most useful and frequently used secondary sources are MEDLINE, International Pharmaceutical Abstracts (IPA), and EMBASE, which are described in detail in Table A-2 (Appendix A). MEDLINE is the most accessible and widely used general medicine and sciences database. IPA focuses on indexing and abstracting literature pertaining to the practice of pharmacy. EMBASE is a general medicine and sciences database that covers more international journals. MEDLINE is freely available and accessible via the World Wide Web. IPA and EMBASE are available by subscription only. Each secondary source has its own searching system. MEDLINE and EMBASE contain tutorials to help the user learn how to navigate the database to find information of interest. The best way to learn how to search secondary sources is to take a hands-on approach—that is, actually use them.

Regardless of the secondary resource used, however, the pharmacist should follow some general searching guidelines. For example, to perform a thorough search, it is best to search for articles using at least two secondary sources. Choose secondary sources

TABLE 2-3	Example Abstract[a]

PubMed search of MEDLINE using the following limiters

- Clinical trial
- Randomized controlled trial

Bibliographic information and abstract

Br J Clin Pharmacol. 2004 May; 57(5): 592–9.

Erratum in:

Br J Clin Pharmacol. 2004 Jul;58(1):102.

Effect of St John's wort and ginseng on the pharmacokinetics and pharmacodynamics of warfarin in healthy subjects.

Jiang X, Williams KM, Liauw WS, Ammit AJ, Roufogalis BD, Duke CC, Day RO, McLachlan AJ.

Faculty of Pharmacy, The University of Sydney, NSW 2006, Australia.

M: The aim of this study was to investigate the effect of St John's wort and ginseng on the pharmacokinetics and pharmacodynamics of warfarin. METHODS: This was an open-label, three-way crossover randomized study in 12 healthy male subjects, who received a single 25-mg dose of warfarin alone or after 14 days' pretreatment with St John's wort, or 7 days' pretreatment with ginseng. Dosing with St John's wort or ginseng was continued for 7 days after administration of the warfarin dose. Platelet aggregation, international normalized ratio (INR) of prothrombin time, warfarin enantiomer protein binding, warfarin enantiomer concentrations in plasma and S-7-hydroxywarfarin concentration in urine were measured. Statistical comparisons were made using anova and 90% confidence intervals are reported. RESULTS: INR and platelet aggregation were not affected by treatment with St John's wort or ginseng. The apparent clearances of S-warfarin after warfarin alone or with St John's wort or ginseng were, respectively, 198 +/− 38 ml h(−1), 270 +/− 44 ml h(−1) and 220 +/− 29 ml h(−1). The respective apparent clearances of R-warfarin were 110 +/− 25 ml h(−1), 142 +/− 29 ml h(−1) and 119 +/− 20 ml h(−1) [corrected]. The mean ratio and 90% confidence interval (CI) of apparent clearance for S-warfarin was 1.29 (1.16, 1.46) and for R-warfarin it was 1.23 (1.11, 1.37) when St John's wort was coadministered. The mean ratio and 90% CI of AUC(0–168) of INR was 0.79 (0.70, 0.95) when St John's wort was coadministered. St John's wort and ginseng did not affect the apparent volumes of distribution or protein binding of warfarin enantiomers. CONCLUSIONS: St John's wort significantly induced the apparent clearance of both S-warfarin and R-warfarin, which in turn resulted in a significant reduction in the pharmacological effect of rac-warfarin. Coadministration of warfarin with ginseng did not affect the pharmacokinetics or pharmacodynamics of either S-warfarin or R-warfarin.

PMID: 15089812 [PubMed – indexed for MEDLINE]

that focus on the content area of the question. For example, suppose the pharmacist is asked, What are the effects of clean room dress codes and laminar flow hoods on contamination rates of intravenous admixtures? Because this question pertains to the practice of pharmacy, IPA would be good database to search. In addition, multiple **search terms**, including terms from the content of the actual question (e.g., drug names, disease names) and terms found in the question classification (e.g., pharmacokinetics, adverse drug reactions, drug interactions) should be used. Various combinations of search terms, linked by Boolean operators (e.g., AND, OR, NOT), should also be tried. Finally, searches should be properly built.

Assume the following drug information question was received from a physician: Is Zyban given in combination with nicotine-replacement therapy (NRT) more effective than NRT alone for smoking cessation in teenagers? Using the general searching guidelines

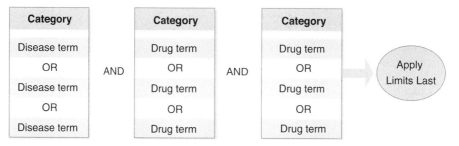

FIGURE 2-4   Framework for Building a Search Using a Secondary Source. Framework for the drug information question, Is Zyban, given in combination with nicotine-replacement therapy (NRT) more effective than NRT alone for smoking cessation in teenagers? The Boolean operator *OR* is used to link terms within a disease or drug category. The Boolean operator *AND* is used to link disease terms to drug terms. Three terms are listed for each category; the number of terms depends on the drug information question received. If the question pertains to only one disease category and one drug category, then build the search on the first two categories only. Limits (if available in the secondary source) should be applied last. (Adapted with permission from Seaton T. Framework for building a search in a secondary source. St. Louis College of Pharmacy, evidence-based medicine course. 2006.)

discussed in the previous paragraph, the pharmacist should search two secondary sources. Because MEDLINE and EMBASE contain primary literature records that pertain to general medicine, these are appropriate databases for this question.

The pharmacist should use multiple search terms such as "bupropion SR" (the generic name for Zyban), "nicotine-replacement therapy," "nicotine polacrilex," "transdermal nicotine," "nicotine patch," "nicotine lozenge," "smoking cessation," "tobacco abuse," and "tobacco use disorder." The pharmacist should also perform searches using Boolean operators to combine the search terms; here are two examples:

- "smoking cessation" OR "tobacco use disorder" AND "nicotine-replacement therapy" OR "nicotine transdermal" AND "bupropion SR"
- "nicotine lozenge" OR "nicotine polacrilex" AND "bupropion SR" AND "tobacco abuse" OR "smoking cessation"

A framework for building searches is given in Figure 2-4.

PERSPECTIVE 2-2

Because MEDLINE is widely accessible via PubMed (www.pubmed.gov) and is often used by pharmacists to answer drug information questions, knowing how to search this database effectively and efficiently is of paramount importance. There are several methods for searching MEDLINE via PubMed, including by text word, author, journal, single citation, and **medical subject heading (MeSH)***.*

Text word searches are performed by simply entering the desired word into the search query box and clicking the go button to start the search. Multiple text words can be linked by using Boolean operators. The computer will search for the term or the combination of terms contained in the MEDLINE records. In addition, PubMed will also use term mapping, a process that maps or links the text word terms to a MeSH term.

MeSH terms make up a controlled vocabulary used to index article records in the MEDLINE database. MeSH terms provide a consistent framework that can be used to identify information expressed in various terminologies.[5] For example, if the pharmacist wishes to find information on the efficacy of zinc for treating a cold, a MeSH search might help target the search. If the word "cold" were entered into the PubMed search box, many citation records would appear that are not related to a cold. However, searching the MeSH database for the word "cold" obtains the following list of terms and definitions:

- *Cold: An absence of warmth or heat or a temperature notably below an accustomed norm.*
- *Common cold: A catarrhal disorder of the upper respiratory tract, which may be viral, a mixed infection, or an allergic reaction. It is marked by acute coryza, slight rise in temperature, chilly sensations, and general indisposition.*[6]

The pharmacist could then choose which term he or she is referring to—the common cold, in this case—and further narrow the search by choosing subheadings within the MeSH database that pertain to the drug information question.

The classification of the question might help in choosing MeSH subheadings. Because the pharmacist is looking for zinc as a treatment for the common cold, he or she might choose the MeSH subheading "drug therapy" or "therapy." The computer would then search the MeSH database for "common cold/drug therapy" or "common cold/therapy."[5] *The pharmacist could also search for "zinc" as a MeSH term and then build a search using Boolean operators to link the disease term(s) with the drug term(s) (Fig. 2-4).*

For thorough searching, it is best to perform both a text word search and a MeSH database search in MEDLINE. Another tip: Once an article of interest is found, the pharmacist should view the full citation to see which MeSH terms are assigned to the article. The article may be associated with additional MeSH terms in the MEDLINE database.

Article citations can also be found based on the author's name. If the author of the particular article is known, the author's name can be entered into the PubMed search box in multiple ways, including the last name followed by first and middle initial (if known) with no punctuation, such as "Cannon CP." If only the last name is known, "Cannon [au]" can be entered. Adding the author tag, "[au]," tells the computer to search only in the author field for the word "Cannon." MEDLINE records published from 2002 forward can be searched by entering the author's full name, in natural or inverted order, in the search box, such as "Christopher P. Cannon" or "Cannon, Christopher P."

PubMed offers a journals database and a single citation matcher, which can be used if the journal is known or if a specific citation record is being sought. The PubMed Web site also includes tutorials for the various ways of searching the MEDLINE database.[5]

Once the search has been properly built, the pharmacist can apply limits to weed out irrelevant articles. PubMed allows users to apply **limiters**, *or criteria by which the user can narrow the focus of the search. For example, the user can choose to limit the search based on date of publication (e.g., search records that were published only in the last 5 years), language (e.g., search for only English-language records), type of study (e.g., search for only randomized controlled trials), and age group of subjects (e.g., search for records that pertain only to adolescents who are 13–18 years of age).*

Let's return to the question about Zyban plus NRT versus NRT alone for smoking cessation in teenagers and assume the basic MEDLINE search was "smoking cessation" OR "tobacco use disorder" AND "nicotine-replacement therapy" OR "nicotine transdermal" AND "bupropion SR." Now let's apply the example limits given in the last paragraph. Such a search provides the following citation record:

> Killen JD, Robinson TN, Ammerman S, et al. Randomized clinical trial of the efficacy of bupropion combined with nicotine patch in the treatment of adolescent smokers. J Consult Clin Psychol 2004 Aug;72(4):729–735.

It takes practice to become an efficient and effective forager of secondary sources. To hone these skills, begin by completing the tutorials offered by secondary sources. Keep notes on the search terms that are particularly productive and those that are not. Also, be on the alert for secondary databases that are not discussed in this chapter—for example, the CINAHL (Cumulative Index to Nursing and Allied Health Literature) database,[7] which focuses on nursing and allied health literature, and the IBIDS (International Bibliographic Information on Dietary Supplements) database,[8] which covers international scientific literature on dietary supplements, including vitamins, minerals, and botanicals.

Tertiary Literature

Tertiary literature is sometimes referred to as *general literature*. It consists of media that summarize, integrate, and evaluate original research reports. Examples of tertiary literature are textbooks, compendia, computer databases, and personal digital assistant (PDA) databases such as Micromedex and Clinical Pharmacology (not to be confused with secondary sources, which are also electronic databases), Internet sources, and review articles. Other electronic sources, such as Stat!Ref (www.statref.com) and UpToDate (www.uptodate.com), provide clinicians with easy access to multiple tertiary sources.

Although review articles are typically published in biomedical journals alongside original research studies, they are not considered original investigations and thus are not classified as primary literature. Review articles are classified as tertiary literature. These articles may evaluate information from original scientific and clinical investigations quantitatively or qualitatively. Quantitative reviews, also known as *meta-analyses*, are discussed in Chapter 10.

Qualitative review articles are sometimes called *narrative reviews*. A narrative review article often attempts to integrate information from a variety of research areas to provide a state-of-the-art vision of the research or clinical area. Typically, the review reflects the perspective of the author. The article "Drug Therapy: Effectiveness of Antimalarial Drugs" by J. K. Baird[9] is one example. The author discusses the risk of malaria worldwide, antimalarial drug activity, and drug resistance. Although Baird evaluates data from original investigations on antimalarial drug resistance, this qualitative review contains no original research.

Because review articles are published in biomedical journals, they can be found by searching the secondary literature indexing and abstracting resources described earlier in this chapter. In fact, one of the limiters in PubMed can narrow a search to review articles only.

PERSPECTIVE 2-3

Drug information today can easily be found on the Internet and the World Wide Web. Thousands of Web sites are dedicated to providing drug and health information. Not all Web sites are created equal, however; you must use caution and evaluate the credibility of everything you read on the Web. Here are a few tips:[10,11]

- *Who created or maintains the Web site? One of the initial indicators of reliability is the Web site's domain (the last three letters at the end of the Web site address). Government (.gov) or university-run (.edu) Web sites are among the best free sources for scientifically sound drug information. Associations or nonprofit organizations (.org) may also offer high-quality information. Commercial Web sites (.com) may have hidden marketing or sales agenda that can influence their content. Although many commercial Web sites offer trust-worthy drug information, these sites should be examined closely to ensure their reliability. All sponsorship, advertising, and funding (such as from pharmaceutical companies) should be clearly stated and separated from the actual drug information to avoid bias or influence.*

- **Is there an editorial board or a list of the names and credentials of those responsible for preparing and reviewing the Web site's content?** *Find out who is writing or reviewing the drug information on the Web site, and evaluate their authority to do so. Trustworthy sites will clearly provide this information. Look for trained medical professionals—physicians, pharmacists, nurses—and their credentials. The best Web sites are set up to allow users to contact the authors or reviewers if questions arise about the site's content or if the user wants additional information.*

- **Are there links from the Web site to other sources of drug and health information?** *Be leery of sites that claim to be the sole source of information on a topic or that show disre-spect for other sources of knowledge. A reputable site will not claim to be the only authority on a particular health or drug topic. On the other hand, links to other Web sites do not auto-matically guarantee credibility and do not mean mutual endorsement. Don't be misled by a long list of links to well-recognized Web sites.*

- **When was the content last updated?** *Medical knowledge is continually evolving. Advances in medicine are made on a daily basis. Look to see that the site is keeping up with new dis-coveries. To provide timely information, health and drug information Web sites should be updated weekly or at least monthly. Reputable and up-to-date Web sites show the date on which the site was last revised; this is typically found at the bottom of each Web page.*

- **What about graphics and multimedia files?** *Although graphics, videos, and audio clips can enhance the appeal of a Web site and help explain or clarify medical concepts, these bells and whistles are not a substitute for sound medical information. Be cautious of drug information sites that provide elaborate multimedia but don't provide scientifically sound information.*

- **Does the Web site charge an access fee?** *Many reputable health and drug information Web sites provide their information for free. If a site does charge a fee, make sure that it offers value for the money. Continue to browse the Internet to see if the same information can be found for free at another site.*

- **Is there a list of resources or references that were used to create the Web site's content?** *When appropriate, information contained on a drug information Web site should be sup-ported by clear references to the sources or origin of the information. Look for a bibliogra-phy or list of references.*

- **Does the site have HONcode accreditation?** *Health on the Net Foundation's HON Code of Conduct (HONcode)[12] is the most-used ethical and trustworthy guide for evaluating medical and health information available on the Internet. HONcode specifies eight principles intended to hold Web site developers to basic ethical standards and to make sure users always know the source and purpose of the data they are presented. Although participation is voluntary, sites dis-playing the HONcode symbol are generally considered credible sources of information.*

Search Strategies

Once the three main categories of biomedical literature—primary, secondary, and tertiary—are understood, the pharmacist must decide how these are best used when searching for an answer to a drug information query. Generally, the most efficient and effective searches begin with tertiary literature. Even if the answer cannot be found in the tertiary literature, consulting tertiary references may help provide the pharmacist with general background information on the subject and point out information that may help when formulating searches of other information sources.

The choice of tertiary reference depends on the question classification. For example, suppose a physician inquires about the proper dose of loratadine for a 6-year-old child who has seasonal allergies. This query could be classified as a pediatric dosing question (see Table A-1, Appendix A). Consulting tertiary references that specialize in providing pediatric dosing recommendations, such as the *Harriet Lane Handbook*[13] and the *Pediatric Dosing Handbook*,[14] would be the best search strategy to use. Likewise, if the question pertains to use of fluoxetine during pregnancy, consult tertiary references that specialize in drug use in pregnancy, such as *Drugs in Pregnancy and Lactation*[15] and the REPRORISK System.

Table A-3 (Appendix A) provides a list of commonly used tertiary resources for various types of question classifications.[16] Depending on the practice setting, the pharmacist may not have access to every tertiary reference listed in the table. However, all pharmacists should be aware of the wide array of these sources and should determine which references are best and most efficient for their personal use.

The 1990 Omnibus Budget Reconciliation Act (OBRA) requires that certain tertiary references, including *AHFS Drug Information*,[17] and *U.S. Pharmacopoeia Dispensing Information (USP DI)*,[18] be available in pharmacies for drug evaluation activities such as patient counseling. However, these sources will not answer all drug information questions. Thus it is imperative that pharmacists develop broader reference libraries in their practices to help ensure that drug information questions can be answered efficiently, completely, and correctly.

One final note about searching tertiary literature: To verify that a search yields valid results, it is best to consult at least two reputable references. If the two references offer inconsistent information (e.g., different dosing recommendations), then a third reference and maybe even a fourth reference need to be consulted. In addition, even if the answer is easily found in the tertiary literature, it is good practice to search for pertinent primary literature to be certain that more recent data are not available.

Often answers will not be found in the tertiary literature. When this happens, the next step of the search strategy is to refer to secondary sources to find pertinent primary literature. While the choice of a secondary source will depend on the question, in general, most searches can begin with MEDLINE because it is widely available and covers a broad range of biomedical journals and science and medicine topics.

When using a secondary source, search for primary literature that addresses issues related directly to the expanded question. Choose studies that evaluate subjects who are similar to the patient(s) in the drug information question received. Select studies that measure clinical outcomes that pertain to the question and use similar criteria for determination of diagnosis, course of therapy, and cure. For example, if a physician inquires about the efficacy of metformin for lowering fasting blood glucose levels in elderly patients, the pharmacist would want to search for a study involving elderly subjects who were administered metformin and in whom fasting blood glucose levels were measured.

When providing recommendations on pharmacotherapy, large randomized controlled trials are the best to consult. However, RCTs may not be available to answer all questions; thus other types of studies will need to be consulted. Chapter 3 provides an overview of the various types of study designs and how they are used to provide drug information.

Figure 2-5 provides a general strategy for searching the tertiary, secondary, and primary literature. Exceptions to this search strategy include instances in which the question pertains to a drug, medical theory, or topic that is too new to be included in tertiary literature. If the pharmacist knows the answer will not be found in tertiary literature because of recent research, secondary resources should be consulted to find the answer in the primary literature. Remember, however, that tertiary sources will still provide useful background information.

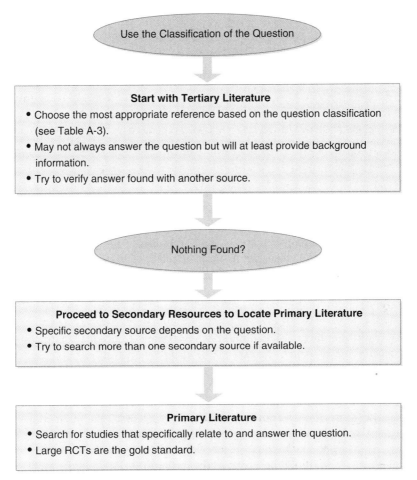

FIGURE 2-5   General Search Strategy for Finding Information. Start with tertiary literature. If nothing is found, proceed to secondary sources to locate pertinent primary literature.

All pharmacists, regardless of their practice environment, need to be effective and efficient foragers of biomedical literature. Search skills develop with practice. Learn by doing. It is useless to merely read about the variety of tertiary references available. Table A-3 offers a guide to the best tertiary references; but ultimately, the pharmacist must practice classifying questions and consulting references to find the answers to the questions he or she receives. Hands-on use of references is the most effective way of learning what each has to offer. The study questions at the end of this chapter begin this process.

STEP 5: EVALUATE

The next step of the systematic approach is to evaluate the literature found from the search. The pharmacist must critically evaluate all information to provide a correct and credible answer to the requester. A pharmacist should question everything he or she reads, and verify every recommendation in the final report. Never take anything at face value. Evaluation of primary literature—the critical assessment of each type of study design, including the biostatistics commonly employed—will be discussed in later chapters. Evaluation of tertiary and secondary literature will be discussed here.

TABLE 2-4	Points of Evaluation for Tertiary Literature[a]

- Relevance of the reference to the question type
- Credibility of the information provided (citing primary literature augments credibility)
- Expertise, training, experience of the authors
- Currency of information (what is the publication date?)
- Ease of use (Is the reference easily accessible and clearly organized; can you quickly find an answer?)

[a] Tertiary literature should be critically evaluated before using the information to construct a response to a drug information question.

Tertiary Literature

Several aspects of the tertiary literature should be assessed to determine the credibility of the information it contains (Table 2-4). First, consider the relevance of the reference to the question asked. As discussed previously, select tertiary references that specialize in the information related to the question classification. For example, for drug interaction questions, consult a reference that specializes in drug interaction information. For a drug compatibility question, consult a reference that specializes in drug compatibility information.

One aspect that increases credibility of a tertiary reference is the citing of primary literature within the reference. To extend the drug interaction example, a well-recognized specialty reference is *Drug Interactions Facts*.[19] This reference provides information concerning the severity, mechanism of action, and management of the interaction. It also provides the sources of the information by citing the primary literature. Thus, if the pharmacist desired, he or she could access the evidence behind the interaction information—the primary literature—to evaluate and determine whether the tertiary reference correctly interpreted the original research.

When using tertiary references, compare information in texts that cite primary literature versus those that do not. Which is more credible? Keep in mind that authors of tertiary references are only human—mistakes are sometimes made when compiling and evaluating data and publishing them in the reference.

Next, consider the reference authors. Are they specialists in the type of information provided in the reference? What is their level of experience or expertise? Authors' opinions and conclusions may reflect their own perspectives or biases. Thus a well-respected expert in the area would lend credibility to the information the resource contains.

Consider the currency of the tertiary reference. Is it the most current publication available? Does it account for new therapies, medical theories, or clinical practices? For textbooks especially, publication time must be considered. Even if the text is brand new, information discussed may be outdated.

The last aspect to evaluate is reference's ease of use. Is the reference easily accessible? Is the information contained clearly organized? Is it quick and easy to find an answer? Ease of use may be more a personal preference.

Secondary Literature

Because secondary literature consists of databases that index and abstract primary and some tertiary literature, secondary literature itself is not explicitly evaluated, except that the pharmacist should consider the lag time for entering articles into the database. Information may be available but not yet accessible via the secondary database if the database managers have not entered the newest articles.

The pharmacist should evaluate his or her *use* of secondary resources. Was the search strategy adequate? Were appropriate secondary sources used? Were multiple databases accessed? Were appropriate search terms and limiters used to find the needed information?

The main point of step 5, evaluate, in the systematic approach is to critically appraise the literature found. Don't just merely accept the written word as fact. Assess the credibility of the information and verify its correctness with another source. The pharmacist should also evaluate his or her own search strategy—was the search efficient and effective?

STEP 6: FORMULATE

Once the answer has been located in an appropriate resource, confirmed with another resource, and critically evaluated, a response must be formulated. When formulating the response, the pharmacist must consider the mode of communication—oral or written—and how to best construct the response to make the information transmission clear, correct, complete, persuasive, and credible.

The first step in formulating the response is to restate the expanded question so that each point included in the query is addressed in the response. The pharmacist should also note the scope of the search, check that the information is applicable to the question or situation, consider any strengths or weaknesses of the information, avoid including personal bias, and provide objective and balanced information. References to the literature used for the response should also be provided. Finally, to foster a continuing relationship with the requester, the pharmacist should invite additional questions or follow up with the requester. Example responses are presented later in this chapter.

STEP 7: COMMUNICATE

The next step of the systematic approach involves communicating with, or relaying the response back to, the requester. Really, though, communication occurs throughout the systematic approach. Communicating effectively is an ability that all pharmacists must master to provide drug information. Communicating effectively involves developing a flexible and sophisticated approach to professional reading, writing, speaking, and listening. The pharmacist must also be mindful of nonverbal communication.

Throughout the systematic approach, the pharmacist must listen closely to the requester, starting with the first two steps, receive and expand. He or she must also employ a flexible and sophisticated approach to classifying the drug information question and searching for and evaluating the literature used to answer the query. When formulating the response, the pharmacist must consider the mode of communication and how to best construct the response to make the information transmission clear, correct, complete, persuasive, and credible. Finally, when actually communicating the response back to the requester, the pharmacist must be flexible and choose a level of communication sophistication that ensures the response is well received by the requester. Tables 2-5 and 2-6 provide tips for oral and written communication, respectively.

STEP 8: FOLLOW-UP

The final step of the systematic approach is to follow up with the requester to verify the desired response was received. This is an important step: It ensures that the question asked was answered appropriately. If the requester is a healthcare provider, the pharmacist

TABLE 2-5	Tips for Oral Communication

- Use clear and specific terminology.
- Use terminology that is appropriate for the requester (lay terms for the layperson; medical terms for the healthcare practitioner).
- Articulate information in an organized and logical manner.
- Be clear and direct.
- Be appropriately concise.
- Provide complete, accurate, and rational information.
- Maintain good voice quality, rate, and tone.
- Maintain eye contact with requester and use notes appropriately.
- Employ appropriate nonverbal communication (i.e., body language).
- Display confidence.
- Be credible and persuasive.
- Be respectful.
- Display tact in the approach.
- Establish rapport with the requester.
- Maintain a professional demeanor throughout the encounter.
- Listen attentively and empathetically to questions/concerns from the layperson or healthcare professional.
- Answer any questions in a thoughtful and professional manner.
- Invite follow-up from the requester.

TABLE 2-6	Tips for Written Communication

- Use clear and specific terminology.
- Use terminology that is appropriate for the requester (lay terms for the layperson; medical terms for the healthcare practitioner).
- Articulate information in an organized and logical manner.
- Be clear and direct.
- Provide complete, accurate, and rational information.
- Provide references and sources of information used to construct the response.
- Be appropriately concise.
- Be credible and persuasive.
- Be respectful.
- Check that response is mechanically correct.
    - Make sure all sentences are clear.
    - Begin each paragraph with a topic sentence.
    - Use effective transitions between paragraphs and ideas.
    - Use correct grammar, spelling, and punctuation.
    - Use a professional style and tone.

might want to confirm that the information was useful. If the requester is a layperson, the pharmacist might want to confirm that the patient responded to the recommendation made or followed through with the instructions provided. In addition, the follow-up step allows the pharmacist to determine whether more information is needed. This step may also help the pharmacist identify any deficiencies in his or her systematic approach and/or communication skills.

Putting It all Together—Practicing the Systematic Approach

The previous sections of this chapter detailed an eight-step systematic approach to answering drug information questions. Such a systematic approach helps the pharmacist work efficiently and effectively to create a quality response. Providing drug information via a systematic approach takes practice, but with experience, the sequence of steps becomes natural.

It is worthwhile to review a couple of examples of this complete process: one involving a healthcare provider (Table 2-7) and the other, a layperson (Table 2-8).

TABLE 2-7	**Pharmacist's Systematic Approach to Providing an Answer to a Healthcare Provider's Drug Information Question**

SETTING

The pharmacist is working in a hospital pharmacy when a physician calls. It's Dr. Holcomb, a family medicine attending physician whose office is in the doctors' building adjacent to the hospital.

STEP 1: RECEIVE

QUESTION: I have a 5-year-old patient who was bitten by a dog. I'd like to start the boy on Augmentin. Can you provide me with a proper dosage recommendation? I need to call a prescription in for him later today.

The pharmacist asks the doctor if he wants to wait on the phone while she looks for the dosing information or if he wants the pharmacist to call him back. The doctor asks the pharmacist to send the recommendation via e-mail within an hour, if possible. The pharmacist records Dr. Holcomb's e-mail address. But, before the pharmacist hangs up the phone, she wants to ask the doctor a few questions to get a better understanding of the received question.

STEP 2: EXPAND

PHARMACIST'S QUESTIONS	DOCTOR'S RESPONSES
How much does the patient weigh?	The boy weighs about 26 kg.
Can the patient swallow tablets?	The boy's mother says he has a hard time with swallowing large pills.
Does the patient have any drug allergies?	The boy has no known drug allergies.
Is the patient currently taking any other medications?	No.
How severe is the dog bite?	It's a fairly large bite on the boy's leg. Some broken skin but no need for stitches. He has a lot of inflammation and redness around the bite wound, so I want to treat him with an antibiotic.

Restatement of the Question

The pharmacist restates the question in her own words to make sure she understands what the doctor is asking.

(continued)

TABLE 2-7	*Continued*

RESTATEMENT: Dr. Holcomb, let me make sure I understand. You have a 26-kg boy who has no drug allergies, is not taking any other medications, has difficulty swallowing large pills, and has a fairly severe dog bite that appears to be infected. You want to know the proper dosage of Augmentin for this patient. Is this correct?

STEP 3: CLASSIFY

The pharmacist classifies the question by type of information requested: pediatric drug dosing/administration" (see Table A-1).

STEP 4: SEARCH

The pharmacist starts her search in the tertiary literature and selects the following references based on the question classification (see Table A-3)

Sources Searched

- *Harriet Lane Handbook,* 17th edition (2005).
- *Lexi-Comp's Pediatric Dosing Handbook,* 12th edition (2005).

The pharmacist did not need to consult secondary sources to search for primary literature because the information was easily found in the tertiary literature. In addition, the tertiary literature found is current.

STEP 5: EVALUATE

SOURCE	JUSTIFICATION
Harriet Lane Handbook	A specialty reference relevant to the question; considered one of the best tertiary resources for pediatric drug dosing; current and easy to use Provides the following information: for infections other than otitis media, give 45 mg/kg/day divided every 12 hr for 7 days
Lexi-Comp's Pediatric Dosing Handbook	Does not cite any primary literature, but is a specialty reference relevant to the question; considered one of the best tertiary resources for pediatric drug dosing; latest edition published in 2005; easy to use Provides the following information: for severe infections, give 45 mg/kg/day divided every 12 hr or 40 mg/kg/day divided every 8 hr. For less severe infections, give 25 mg/kg/day divided every 12 hr or 20 mg/kg/day divided every 8 hr

STEP 6: FORMULATE

The pharmacist thinks about how she will formulate her written response. She decides to begin with the restatement of the doctor's question and then provide her recommendations for the Augmentin dosage and the references for the information. She'll also invite additional questions.

STEP 7: COMMUNICATE

The Pharmacist's e-Mail Response: February 21, 2006.

Dr. Holcomb,

Your question pertains to the proper dosage of Augmentin for a 26-kg boy who is suffering from a severe dog bite. Based on the information that you provided, my review of two well-recognized drug information references on pediatric drug dosing provides the following information.

The proper dosage of Augmentin for this child is 45 mg/kg/day divided every 12 hr for 7 days. Because this patient can't swallow pills, has no allergies, and weighs 26 kg, he should take 1 teaspoonful of Augmentin 600 mg/5 mL suspension every 12 hr for 7 days.

I hope this information has been helpful. If you have any additional questions, please do not hesitate to contact me.

References Used

- Robertson J, Shilkofski N. Harriet Lane Handbook, 17th ed. St. Louis, MO: Mosby, 2005.
- Taketomo CK, Hodding JH, Kraus DM. Pediatric Dosing Handbook, 12th ed. Hudson, OH: Lexi-Comp, 2005.

Sincerely,

Amy Thompson, Pharm.D.

STEP 8: FOLLOW-UP
Later that day, the pharmacist receives a reply e-mail from Dr. Holcomb. The e-mail expressed Dr. Holcomb's appreciation for the pharmacist's prompt and helpful assistance.

TABLE 2-8	**Pharmacist's Systematic Approach to Providing an Answer to a Layperson's Drug Information Question**

SETTING
The pharmacist is working at a community pharmacy. A patient approaches the pharmacy counter to pick up a prescription for her son. While she's waiting for the pharmacy technician to locate the prescription, she motions for the pharmacist to come to the counter.

STEP 1: RECEIVE
QUESTION: I can't get in contact with my doctor. Can you tell me which over-the-counter pain medicine is best to use while breast-feeding?

The patient appears to be in a hurry. The pharmacist surmises that the patient would like a response while she's at the pharmacy counter. His response will be verbal.

STEP 2: EXPAND

PHARMACIST'S QUESTIONS	LAYPERSON'S RESPONSES
Does your question pertain to you or to someone else?	To me. I am currently breast-feeding and need a pain medicine.
What type of pain are you experiencing?	Occasional headaches from stress.
Are you experiencing a headache now?	No. They usually occur in the evening.
On a scale from 0 to 10 with 0 meaning no pain and 10 meaning really severe pain, how would you rate your headache pain when it occurs?	Maybe a 2 or 3.
Have you tried any pain products before?	No, I haven't tried any pain products since my pregnancy, but I have used Tylenol before for my headaches and it worked okay.
Are you allergic to any medications?	No, I'm not allergic to any medications, but I am allergic to peanuts.
Are you currently taking any other medications?	No.
Do you have any health problems or medical conditions?	No.
How old is your baby?	He's 6 months old.

(continued)

TABLE 2-8	*Continued*

Restatement of the Question

The pharmacist restates the question in his own words to make sure he understands what the client is asking.

RESTATEMENT: You want to know what over-the-counter analgesic product, for treating occasional, mild headaches, is safe to use while breast-feeding a 6-month old baby. Is this correct?

STEP 3: CLASSIFY
The pharmacist classifies the question by type of information requested: drug use in pregnancy and lactation (see Table A-1).

STEP 4: SEARCH
The pharmacist starts his search in the tertiary literature and selects the following references based on the question classification (see Table A-3).

Sources Searched

- Micromedex: REPRORISK System (2006).
- *Drugs in Pregnancy and Lactation*, 7th edition (2005).

The pharmacist did not need to consult secondary sources to search for primary literature because the answer to the question was easily found in the tertiary literature. In addition, the tertiary literature found is current.

STEP 5: EVALUATE

SOURCE	JUSTIFICATION
REPRORISK	A specialty reference relevant to the question; considered one of the best tertiary resources for drug use in lactation; reference appears to be credible (primary literature is discussed and cited); current edition; easy to use
Drugs in Pregnancy and Lactation	A specialty reference relevant to the question; considered one of the best tertiary resources for drug use in lactation; information appears credible (primary literature is discussed and cited); latest edition published in 2005; easy to use

STEP 6: FORMULATE
The pharmacist quickly thinks about how he will formulate his response. He decides to begin with his restatement of her question, provide the information to answer her question, confirm that she understands, and provide references for the information. He'll also offer to provide any additional assistance or information.

STEP 7: COMMUNICATE
The Pharmacist's Oral Response:

Your question pertains to an over-the-counter analgesic product for treating occasional, mild headaches that is also safe to use while breast-feeding a 6-month-old baby. Based on the information you provided, I consulted two well-recognized references—*Drugs in Pregnancy and Lactation* and REPRORISK—to confirm my recommendation.

Since Tylenol has effectively relieved your headache pain before, I would recommend that you try it again to relieve your mild, occasional headaches. Tylenol is an effective headache pain reliever and is safe to use while breast-feeding. Tylenol is excreted in the breast milk but only at very low concentrations that do not affect the nursing baby. In fact, Tylenol is routinely used during all stages of pregnancy, and the American Academy of Pediatrics considers Tylenol to be compatible with breast-feeding.

The recommended dosage of Tylenol is 325 to 650 milligrams every 4 to 6 hours as needed for headache pain. You should not use more than 4,000 milligrams of Tylenol per day and take a dose only if you need it. Follow the directions written on the bottle label. If Tylenol does not relieve your headaches, or your headaches become more severe or occur more often, you should contact your doctor.

Finally, you should know that Tylenol is available generically as acetaminophen. Generic versions of Tylenol are less expensive and work the same way as the brand name product. You can take either Tylenol or a generic for your headache pain.

Do you understand my recommendation? [The patient answers yes.] Great. If you have any additional questions please do not hesitate to contact me. Is there anything else I can help you with today?

References Used

- Briggs GG, Freeman RK, Sumner JY. *Drugs in Pregnancy and Lactation*, 7th ed. Baltimore: Lippincott Williams & Wilkins, 2005.
- REPRORISK System. Greenwood Village, CO: Thomson Micromedex, 2006.

STEP 8: FOLLOW-UP
The next day, the pharmacist calls the patient to confirm that she knows how to take Tylenol (or its generic) appropriately, and if the drug provided relief for her headache.

Ethics and Legalities of Providing Drug Information

Not only do pharmacists need to take a systematic approach to answering drug information questions but they need to consider legal and ethical ramifications of providing drug information. The pharmacy profession is governed by legal regulations, licensure, and malpractice rules. The pharmacist must function in accordance with the law when rendering pharmaceutical care, including provision of drug information. Pharmacists can be held liable for providing inaccurate information that harms a patient. Liability can also be found in cases in which the pharmacist is negligent—he or she willfully fails to properly counsel or warn of foreseeable detrimental effects or risks of drug therapies.

Consider this example: A pharmacist dispenses an antibiotic to a teenage girl who is being treated for a sexually transmitted disease. The girl asks the pharmacist if she needs to take any special precautions while using the new antibiotic. The pharmacist fails to properly counsel the girl, who is also taking an oral contraceptive, to use a back-up method of contraception while taking her newly prescribed antibiotic. Should the pharmacist be held liable for an unintended pregnancy that resulted from failure to properly advise the teenager that she needed a back-up method of contraception while taking the antibiotic? Although case law supporting the pharmacist's liability in an instance like this is sparse, it is not unreasonable to argue that the pharmacist should be held accountable, especially as the primary role of pharmacists evolves from medication-dispensing functions to direct patient care functions. Using a systematic approach to providing drug information can help limit the risk of providing misinformation or lack of information.

Another facet of this issue is that the pharmacist may receive drug information questions that raise legal concerns. For example, a pharmacist receives a phone call from a patient who he or she knows quite well. The patient's elderly father has terminal pancreatic cancer and is completely bedridden. The patient calls the pharmacist to ask about the maximum daily dose of morphine. As the pharmacist continues to expand on the patient's question, the pharmacist senses that the patient may be attempting to assist his father in suicide. Should the pharmacist provide the caller with information on morphine dosing if the pharmacist suspects an attempt at suicide? This problem raises both ethical and legal concerns.

Because of legal issues, it is important that pharmacists document their drug information activity. Depending on the practice setting, the pharmacist should document any information provided to a patient. For example, in a hospital setting, the pharmacist may

TABLE 2-9	ASHP Guidelines on Documenting Drug Information Responses[a]

Documentation of drug information responses should include the following:

- Date and time the drug information request was received
- Requester's name, address, method of contact (e.g. telephone or pager) and category (e.g., healthcare discipline, patient)
- Person assessing medication information needs
- Method of delivery (e.g., telephone, personal visit, e-mail or postal mail)
- Classification of the request
- Question asked
- Patient-specific information obtained
- Response provided
- References used
- Date and time response was provided
- Person responding to the request
- Estimated time in preparation and for communication
- Materials sent to requester
- Outcome measures suggested (e.g., effect on patient care, improvements in medication use, and requester satisfaction)

[a]The pharmacists may need to adapt this list to his or her particular practice setting.

Reprinted with permission from the American Society of Health-System Pharmacists. ASHP guidelines on the provision of medication information by pharmacists. Am J Health Syst Pharm 1996;53:1843–1845.

want to provide documentation of drug information provided in the patient's medical record; in a community pharmacy setting, the pharmacist may want to provide documentation in the patient's pharmacy profile. The American Society of Health-System Pharmacists (ASHP) provides guidelines on documenting drug information (Table 2-9).[20] Pharmacists should document requests, responses, and follow-up based on the type and purpose of the resulting documentation. If this documentation contains information that identifies the patient, it should be protected according to Health Insurance Portability and Accountability Act (HIPAA) regulations.

PERSPECTIVE 2-4

What is HIPAA? In 1996, the U.S. Congress enacted the Health Insurance Portability and Accountability Act (HIPAA), which established national standards for electronic healthcare transactions and national identifiers for providers, health plans, and employers. It also addressed the security and privacy of patient health data.[21]

HIPPA's security standards provide for the secure storage and transmission of patient information, including patient demographic information, patient health and medical history, and any information that can be used to identify the patient. HIPPA's privacy standards pertain to the use and disclosure of protected, confidential patient health information. Thus if patient-identifying information is contained in drug information questions, the pharmacist must make certain the information is held securely. If a pharmacist documents drug requests, responses, or follow-up, that information must be secure per HIPAA standards.

In addition, HIPAA regulations affect the provision of drug information responses. For example, even if protected patient information will be divulged, HIPAA standards allow for patient counseling and provision of drug information to individuals other than the patient (e.g., spouse, family member, or friend). However, the pharmacist must exercise good judgment and disclose protected information only when absolutely necessary and in the best interest of the patient.

In conjunction with practicing legally, pharmacists also must provide drug information ethically. Pharmacists must always act in the best interest of the patient. Pharmacists are often faced with very difficult ethical dilemmas. For example, should a pharmacist provide instructions on taking the morning-after pill to terminate a pregnancy if the pharmacist is pro-life? Should a pharmacist provide information that he or she deems important and necessary to a patient but that might be in conflict with recommendations made by the patient's doctor? Should a pharmacist employed by a managed care organization be swayed to make drug formulary decisions that are more heavily weighted on drug costs than on drug efficacy and safety?

Pharmacists take an oath to uphold a fiduciary, or trusting responsibility, to patients (see Table 1–1). The oath involves the following principles:

- **Beneficence**: A duty to promote good and act in the best interest of the patient and the health of society.
- **Nonmaleficence**: A duty to protect and do no harm to patients.

When taking the oath, the pharmacist vows to "maintain the highest principles of moral, ethical and legal conduct."[22]

Patients put their trust in the pharmacist to practice ethically to do what is in patients' best interests. That trusting relationship springs from the pharmacist being not only a competent healthcare provider but also a caring provider (Fig. 2-6). Thus, when providing drug information to patients, the pharmacist needs to demonstrate a caring and compassionate attitude while addressing the drug information question.

Pharmacists must bring empathy, compassion, honesty, integrity, accountability, altruism, competency, trustworthiness, and justice to the drug information encounter. Furthermore,

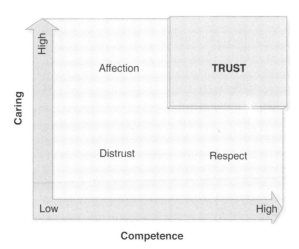

FIGURE 2-6 Competence and Caring in Relation to Building Trust. Patient trust is at its highest when the healthcare provider is highly competent and highly caring. (Adapted with permission from Paling J. Strategies to help patients understand risks. Br Med J 2003;327:745–748.)

TABLE 2-10	**Code of Ethics for Pharmacists**

Preamble

Pharmacists are health professionals who assist individuals in making the best use of medications. This Code, prepared and supported by pharmacists, is intended to state publicly the principles that form the fundamental basis of the roles and responsibilities of pharmacists. These principles, based on moral obligations and virtues, are established to guide pharmacists in relationships with patients, health professionals, and society.

I. A pharmacist respects the covenantal relationship between the patient and pharmacist

Considering the patient-pharmacist relationship as a covenant means that a pharmacist has moral obligations in response to the gift of trust received from society. In return for this gift, a pharmacist promises to help individuals achieve optimum benefit from their medications, to be committed to their welfare, and to maintain their trust.

II. A pharmacist promotes the good of every patient in a caring, compassionate, and confidential manner.

A pharmacist places concern for the well-being of the patient at the center of professional practice. In doing so, a pharmacist considers needs stated by the patient as well as those defined by health science. A pharmacist is dedicated to protecting the dignity of the patient. With a caring attitude and a compassionate spirit, a pharmacist focuses on serving the patient in a private and confidential manner.

III. A pharmacist respects the autonomy and dignity of each patient

A pharmacist promotes the right of self-determination and recognizes individual self-worth by encouraging patients to participate in decisions about their health. A pharmacist communicates with patients in terms that are understandable. In all cases, a pharmacist respects personal and cultural differences among patients.

IV. A pharmacist acts with honesty and integrity in professional relationships

A pharmacist has a duty to tell the truth and to act with conviction of conscience. A pharmacist avoids discriminatory practices, behavior or work conditions that impair professional judgment, and actions that compromise dedication to the best interests of patients.

V. A pharmacist maintains professional competence

A pharmacist has a duty to maintain knowledge and abilities as new medications, devices, and technologies become available and as health information advances.

VI. A pharmacist respects the values and abilities of colleagues and other health professionals

When appropriate, a pharmacist asks for the consultation of colleagues or other health professionals or refers the patient. A pharmacist acknowledges that colleagues and other health professionals may differ in the beliefs and values they apply to the care of the patient.

VII. A pharmacist serves individual, community, and societal needs

The primary obligation of a pharmacist is to individual patients. However, the obligations of a pharmacist may at times extend beyond the individual to the community and society. In these situations, the pharmacist recognizes the responsibilities that accompany these obligations and acts accordingly.

VIII. A pharmacist seeks justice in the distribution of health resources

When health resources are allocated, a pharmacist is fair and equitable, balancing the needs of patients and society.

Reprinted with permission from American Pharmaceutical Association. Code of ethics for pharmacists. Adopted October 27, 1994. Available at: www.aphanet.org/AM/Template.cfm?Section=Pharmacy_Practice_Resources&Template=/CM/HTMLDisplay.cfm&ContentID=2903. Accessed June 2006.

the pharmacist has a duty to respect patient autonomy—to foster a patient's informed, uncoerced choices. The pharmacist must respect the patient's value system. In 1994, the American Pharmacists Association adopted a code of ethics for pharmacists (Table 2-10).[23] That code should serve as a guide for pharmacists when they dispense drug information.

Summary

To be sure, providing drug information is not an easy task. The pharmacist must consider legal and ethical ramifications when rendering drug information as part of providing total pharmaceutical care. All pharmacists, in every conceivable practice setting, will at some point serve as ethical, trusted drug information providers. Some pharmacists will specialize in being drug information experts, but the majority will render drug information as only one part of their daily patient care and professional activities. Regardless of the practice environment, using a systematic approach to providing drug information will improve the professional's efficiency and effectiveness and the quality of the response. A systematic approach will also help the pharmacist avoid overlooking needed pieces of information, which can help eliminate errors and minimize the pharmacist's liability.

The best method for learning the systematic approach to answering drug information questions is by using it. With continued practice, the systematic approach will become inculcated into the routine delivery of drug information.

STUDY PROBLEMS

1. For each of the following pharmacist responses to a question regarding an interaction between simvastatin and grapefruit juice determine the requester: healthcare provider or layperson.
   a. No, it is not okay to eat grapefruit while you are taking simvastatin. Eating grapefruit while taking simvastatin can increase your risk for very serious, even life-threatening, side effects such as damage to your muscles and kidneys. Do not eat any type of grapefruit, including juice or natural supplements that may contain grapefruit juice.
   b. Avoid coadministration of simvastatin and grapefruit juice. Grapefruit juice can inhibit first-pass metabolism via CYP3A4 of simvastatin in the duodenum. This could result in increased serum levels of simvastatin, which could increase the risk for rhabdomyolysis. This interaction is well documented in the scientific literature. You may want to consider fluvastatin or pravastatin because these agents are safer to use with grapefruit ingestion.

2. Expand each the following drug information questions by asking the requester three questions.
   a. Received from a 65-year-old male bus driver at the pharmacy counter: Can you tell me about ginseng?
   b. Received from a registered nurse calling from the intensive care unit: Can I run a heparin drip and ranitidine together?
   c. Received from a 26-year-old mother calling the pharmacy: Can I give my son Benadryl for his cold?
   d. Received from a first-year resident physician in a family medicine clinic: Is ibuprofen or acetaminophen more effective for treating pediatric fever?

3. For each of the following references, determine if it is a primary, secondary, or tertiary source.
   a. Epocrates Rx for personal data assistants
   b. PubMed

    c. DRUGDEX System from Thomson Micromedex

    d. Rich MW. Office management of heart failure in the elderly. Am J Med 2005; 118(4):324–328.

    e. Clinical Pharmacology online from Gold Standard.

    f. Lonn E, Bosch J, Yusuf S, et al. Effects of long-term vitamin E supplementation on cardiovascular events and cancer: A randomized controlled trial. JAMA 2005;293(11):1338–1347.

    g. EMBASE.

4. Answer the following questions using the most appropriate tertiary references for the type of information being requested. Your response should include the question classification, the two best tertiary resources used, a brief comparison of the resources used, and a short answer to the question based on both references. (If references give different answers to the question, you may need to consult additional sources to synthesize a correct response.)

    a. What is the maximum dose of megestrol commonly used for the treatment of cachexia?

    b. How stable is ampicillin in sodium bicarbonate 1.4%?

    c. Name an adverse effect that carbamazepine has on the blood.

    d. What is another name for coletyl?

    e. What should I tell a patient about tamsulosin?

    f. What is the proper dose of calcitriol in a 6-year-old child?

    g. What effects does etodolac have on a nursing infant?

    h. What is the clinical significance of an interaction between bupropion and doxepin?

5. Mr. Johnson is 57 years old with coronary heart disease, hypertension, and hyperlipidemia. He approaches the pharmacy counter. He's confused. He thought it was common knowledge that vitamin E is good for the heart. But last night he heard on the news that vitamin E may not be so good for the heart. He wants a recommendation from you, his trusted pharmacist, on whether or not he should take vitamin E. Use the systematic approach to provide a credible and accurate response to Mr. Johnson's question.

6. Dr. Butler, an attending emergency room physician approaches you regarding secondary prevention of stroke. In general, he would like to know if you recommend the combined use of aspirin and clopidogrel for secondary prevention in adult patients who have experienced a stroke. Use the systematic approach to provide a credible and accurate response to Dr. Butler's question.

7. How would you approach each of the following ethical dilemmas, which you may face when asked to provide drug information?

    a. A frantic mother of a teenage son calls the pharmacy requesting help to identify an unknown tablet that she found in her son's bedroom. Should the pharmacist provide the identifying information to the mother?

    b. A young girl approaches the pharmacy counter with a prescription for the morning-after pill. If the pharmacist does not personally believe in abortion, is he or she required to dispense the medication?

    c. A physician calls in a prescription for Crestor for an 89-year-old patient with stage C prostate cancer. Even though the pharmacist questions the appropriateness of the prescription, the physician insists on treating the patient with Crestor. Knowing that the patient has difficulty affording medications and has a limited life span, should the pharmacist discuss with the patient the pros and cons of using Crestor to treat hyperlipidemia, despite the doctor's insistence that the patient receive the medication?

REFERENCES

1. Watanabe AS, McCart G, Shimomura S, et al. Systematic approach to drug information requests. Am J Hosp Pharm 1975;32:1282–1285.
2. Butler CD. Modified systematic approach. Presented at St. Louis College of Pharmacy, drug information course, 1981.
3. Fischer JM. Modification to the systematic approach to answering drug information requests. Am J Hosp Pharm 1980;37:470,472–476.
4. Holmes SD. Systematic Approach to Responding to Drug Information Inquiries (abstract). American Society of Health-System Pharmacists Midyear Clinical Meeting. New Orleans: 1996, 31:4820.
5. U.S. National Library of Medicine. PubMed Online Training. Available at www.nlm.nih.gov/bsd/disted/pubmed.html. Accessed June 2006.
6. U.S. National Library of Medicine. MeSH Database search page. Available at: www.ncbi.nlm.nih.gov/entrez/query.fcgi?CMD=search&DB=mesh Accessed June 2006.
7. Cumulative Index to Nursing and Allied Health (Cinahl). Available at: www.cinahl.com. Accessed June 2006.
8. Office of Dietary Supplements. International Bibliographic Information on Dietary Supplements (IBIDS) Database. Available at: ods.od.nih.gov/Health_Information/IBIDS.aspx. Accessed June 2006.
9. Baird JK. Drug Therapy: Effectiveness of antimalarial drugs. N Engl J Med 2005;352:1565–1577.
10. Medical Library Association. A user's guide to finding and evaluating health information on the web. Available at: www.mlanet.org/resources/userguide.html. Accessed June 2006.
11. Internet Healthcare Coalition. Tips for healthy surfing online: Finding quality health information on the Internet. Available at: www.ihealthcoalition.org/content/tips.html. Accessed June 2006.
12. Health on the Net Foundation. HON Code of Conduct (HONcode) for medical and health Web sites. Available at: www.hon.ch/HONcode/Conduct.html. Accessed June 2006.
13. Robertson J, Shilkofski N. Harriet Lane Handbook, 17th ed. St. Louis, MO: Mosby, 2005.
14. Taketomo CK, Hodding JH, Kraus DM. Pediatric Dosing Handbook, 12th ed. Hudson, OH: Lexi-Comp, 2005.
15. Briggs GG, Freeman RK, Sumner JY. *Drugs in Pregnancy and Lactation*, 17th ed. Baltimore: Lippincott Williams & Wilkins, 2005.
16. Rosenburg JM, Koumis T, Nathan JP, et al. Current status of pharmacist-operated drug information centers in the United States. Am J Health Syst Pharm 2004;61:2023–2032.
17. AHFS Drug Information. American Society of Health-System Pharmacists. Bethesda: 2007.
18. Drug Information for the Health Care Professional 2007 (Usp Di Vol 1: Drug Information for the Health Care Professional) Edition 27. Greenwood Village, CO: Thomson Micromedex; 2007.
19. Drug Interactions Facts. St. Louis: Facts and Comparisons Publishing Group (part of Wolters Kluwer Health, Inc.); 2007.
20. American Society of Health-System Pharmacists. ASHP guidelines on the provision of medication information by pharmacists. Am J Health Syst Pharm 1996;53:1843–1845.
21. U.S. Department of Health and Human Services. Centers for Medicare and Medicaid Services. HIPPA—General information. Available at: www.cms.hhs.gov/HIPAAGenInfo/01_Overview.asp#TopOfPage. Accessed June 2006.
22. American Pharmaceutical Association Academy of Student Pharmacists/American Association of Colleges of Pharmacy—Council of Deans (APhA-ASP/AACP-COD) Task Force on Professionalism. Oath of a pharmacist. June 26, 1994. Available at: www.aphanet.org/students/leadership/professionalism/oath.htm. Accessed June 2006.
23. American Pharmaceutical Association. Code of ethics for pharmacists. Adopted October 27, 1994. Available at: www.aphanet.org/AM/Template.cfm?Section=Pharmacy_Practice_Resources&Template=/CM/HTMLDisplay.cfm&ContentID=2903. Accessed June 2006.

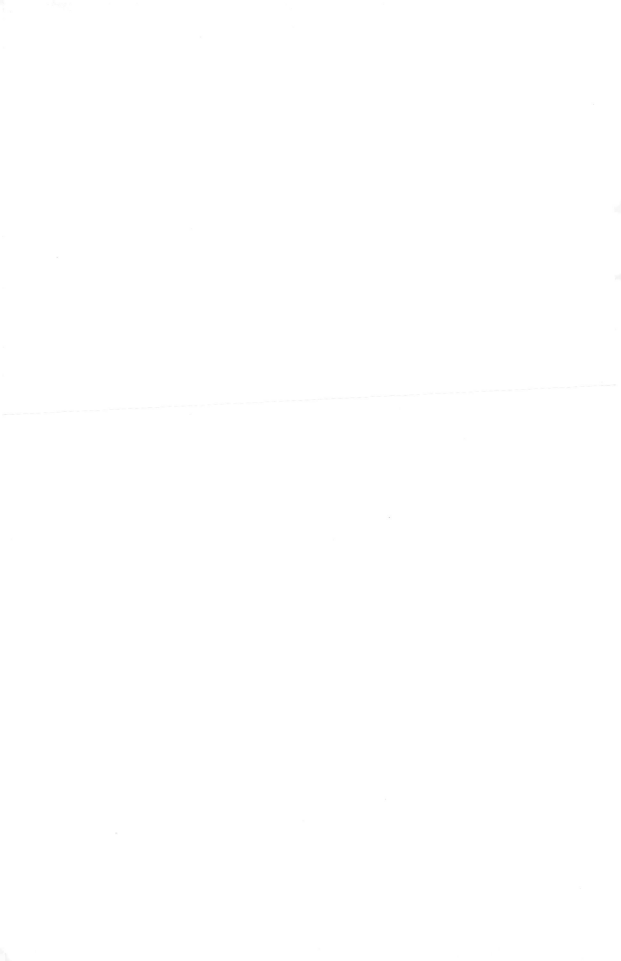

Section

2

Tools for Evaluating Contemporary Healthcare Information

43

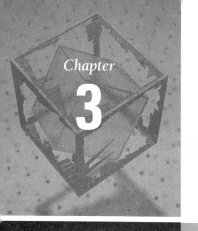

3

Overview of Research Designs Used to Answer Drug Information Questions

CHAPTER GOALS

After studying this chapter, the student should be able to:

1. Explain the general principles of research designs used to gather and provide drug information.

2. Indicate the value of research designs used in healthcare research.

3. Enumerate the kinds of research designs used in healthcare research.

4. Describe the advantages and disadvantages of each research design.

5. Identify published examples of research designs that have shaped the nature of contemporary healthcare.

6. Evaluate in context the results derived from healthcare research designs.

As previously defined, **evidence-based medicine (EBM)** is the conscientious, explicit, and judicious use of current best evidence in making clinical decisions about the care of individual patients. It involves integrating the clinician's expertise with the best available external clinical evidence derived from systematic research to maximize the benefit for the patient.[1] The adoption of the EBM model as the premier method of evaluating and providing clinical drug information has had a profound effect on the manner in which research studies are conducted and the findings reported. The purpose of this chapter is to provide an overview of research designs commonly used to obtain and provide drug information. Each of these study designs receives more detailed treatment in subsequent chapters.

Although several research designs are used in the health sciences, all have several features in common, such as a consideration of one or more **independent variables, dependent variables**, and **extraneous variables**. Independent variables (also termed exposures, antecedent events, treatments, or interventions) are selected by the experimenter, who determines their association with dependent variables (also termed outcomes or results). Extraneous variables are controlled to minimize their influence on the association under study. The conduct of the study is guided by a **research hypothesis**, a proposed relationship between the independent and the dependent variables and whose veracity is tested during the experiment.

The independent variable is the variable that is manipulated. It is explicitly and precisely defined or controlled. Its effect is assumed to be the same in all who exhibit, receive, or are exposed to it. Often, more than one level of the independent variable (e.g., the dose of a drug) is examined to characterize the form of its effect on the dependent variable.

In addition, the effects of several independent variables may be examined in a single research study. Examples of independent variables are drug type and dose, medical history, and level of physiologic function.

Dependent variables reflect objective and measurable effects of the independent variable. In the health sciences, investigators may distinguish between **primary outcomes**, findings the investigators are most interested in examining because they provide the most pertinent evidence, and **secondary outcomes**, research results of less interest that might provide supporting evidence. Examples of dependent variables include mortality or morbidity rates, changes in enzyme function, and the length of survival after the treatment of cancer patients.

All other variables or conditions (i.e., extraneous variables) that could affect the relationship between the independent variable and the dependent variable are controlled so that their effects are minimized. For example, differences in study subjects may be reduced by matching individuals on known factors such as age and gender or by assigning subjects to experimental conditions randomly. This matching is often, though not always, achieved by including a **control group**, whose members receive the same attention as the **treatment group**, except for the independent variable.

Another strategy used to minimize the role of extraneous variables is to standardize the methods by which data are obtained, stored, analyzed, and reported. This is the function of the research designs reviewed in this chapter. By standardizing the process of research, the study designs ensure that the findings obtained will make a contribution to the research community.

In general, research designs used in healthcare may be designated as descriptive, observational, or experimental. **Descriptive research designs** focus on novel or unusual signs, symptoms, or events. **Observational research designs** involve examining participants expressly because they exhibit either a specific characteristic or a specific outcome. **Experimental research designs** involve the random assignment of participants to experimental conditions. The most prominent example of an experimental research design is the randomized controlled trial (RCT).

The specific experimental design selected by the researcher depends on several factors. Although these factors include the nature of the exposure (disease or treatment) or the anticipated outcome (poorer or better health), the overriding consideration is the ethical imperative to do no harm.

Because of the dictum to do no harm, it is unethical to expose patients to a condition if there is evidence that the exposure may be harmful. For example, let's say we wished to study the effect of exposure to cigarette smoke (the independent variable) on some aspect of the health of nonsmokers (the dependent variable) who live with people who smoke. Because of the dictum to do no harm, it would be unethical to use an experimental research design in which individuals were exposed to tobacco smoke against their will. However, an observational research design might provide pertinent information. With this design, the investigator might compare the frequency of lung cancer among spouses of smokers to the frequency of lung cancer among spouses of nonsmokers.

Descriptive Research Designs

CASE STUDY AND CASE SERIES

A **case study** is a description of an individual with a novel or unusual condition. A **case series** is a summary of the health status of several individuals who all display a similar novel clinical finding or condition. The main purpose of these communications is to notify the healthcare community of an unusual clinical event. Often, a case study or case series report will stimulate corroborating evidence from other clinical investigators, and the true characteristics of the novel event will emerge.

Case studies and case series are not intended to provide inferential evidence or to provide evidence of a cause-and-effect relationship. Often, they are the early warning signs of emergent diseases such as severe adult respiratory syndrome (SARS). Early reports of SARS included case reports of a cluster of 10 patients in China[2] and its spread to Toronto, Ontario.[3]

Case studies and case series are also used to report emerging adverse effects from drugs. After the introduction of atypical antipsychotic medications in the early 1990s, several case reports appeared in the psychiatric literature suggesting that these medications might be associated with onset of diabetes insipidus and with diabetic ketoacidosis.[4-7] These case reports alerted providers that they must closely monitor glucose levels in patients taking these drugs. These case reports also stimulated research that better defined and quantified the association between atypical antipsychotic drugs and the onset of diabetes mellitus.

Case series protocols are valuable in identifying the sources of *outbreaks*, which are rapid increases in the number of those afflicted in a population. When an outbreak occurs, such as the outbreak of food poisoning in a school, case series methods are quite effective in tracking down the source of the contamination (likely the school cafeteria).

Case series reports do not always involve small numbers of patients. To determine whether higher mortality rates are seen among infants born on weekends than among those born on weekdays in California hospitals, Gould et al.[8] examined 1,615,041 birth certificates of infants born between 1995 and 1997. The authors reported that, after adjusting for several extraneous factors such as birth weight, there was no difference in mortality between infants born on weekdays versus weekends.

Case study and case series reports do not usually include efforts to control extraneous variables. For example, rather than being selected by a random process, the individuals included in the case report are selected purposely by the investigator to dramatize and reinforce the aspects of the condition that the investigator considers to be of major importance. Furthermore, there is no control condition, so the effects of many potentially extraneous variables are not taken into account.

Good sources of case study and case series reports are the journals *Pharmacotherapy, Annals of Pharmacotherapy, New England Journal of Medicine*, and *Morbidity and Mortality Weekly Report* published by the Centers for Disease Control and Prevention (CDC). In fact, an editorial in the *New England Journal of Medicine* illustrates the power of modern electronic communications and the pivotal role of the Internet, in the rapid and worldwide dissemination of information concerning the SARS outbreaks in Hong Kong and Toronto.[9]

Observational Research Designs

Observational research study designs are those in which the investigator assesses the status of the exposure and the outcome. In a study of drug abuse and memory function, for example, the researcher would search out individuals who already abused drugs and then test their memory. Observational research study designs include case-control studies, cohort studies, and cross-sectional or survey research studies.

THE CASE-CONTROL STUDY DESIGN

A **case-control study** uses an **observational study research design** in which the groups are defined in terms of the outcome (e.g., the disease state), and a relationship is sought

TABLE 3-1	Features of the Case-Control Observational Study Design
FEATURE	DESCRIPTION
Goal	Determine exposure variables associated with an outcome
Strategy	Assemble groups that differ only in the exhibiting outcome Determine if groups differ with respect to suspected antecedent exposure factors
Group assignment	Study group selected based on the exhibiting outcome of interest Control group matched on all relevant variables except the outcome of interest
Strengths	Efficient design for rare outcomes, long exposure outcome intervals Comparatively inexpensive and easy to conduct Can be completed quickly
Weaknesses	Susceptible to many different forms of bias Groups cannot be matched on *all* variables except exposure May be difficult to determine time relationship between exposure and outcome At best, evidence indicates an association between exposure and outcome

between the disease state and one or several antecedent exposure variables (Fig. 3-1A; Table 3-1). Note particularly the inclusion of a control or nondisease group in the study design. This group provides baseline data to which information from the case patients can be compared. Furthermore, control group members are matched as closely as possible to study group participants to minimize the effects of extraneous variables. It is not uncommon, in fact, for a case to be matched with more than one control. Differences among case and control groups suggest variables that might be associated with the disease state.

One of the earliest uses of the case-control research design was the classic study by Doll and Hill,[10] suggesting the first clear association between cigarette smoking and carcinoma of the lung (Fig. 3-1B). The study compared the smoking habits of two groups of patients in London hospitals: those with carcinoma of the lung (cases) and those with other cancers (controls). Several aspects of smoking behavior were investigated as potential antecedent events, including the number of cigarettes smoked, history of smoking, and whether the smoker inhaled. Although both groups contained a great proportion of smokers, evidence for an association between cigarette smoking and lung cancer was obtained from observations such as these:

- Only 2 of 646 lung cancer patients (0.3%) were not cigarette smokers, whereas 27 of 622 non-lung-cancer patients (4.2%) were nonsmokers.
- There was a positive relationship between the number of cigarettes smoked and having lung cancer.

PERSPECTIVE 3-1

The paper by Doll and Hill[10] not only was among the first to implicate cigarette smoking as a potential cause of lung cancer but was also among the earliest case-control studies. It bears reading for the careful attention paid to some of the extraneous variables and because of the evidence it provides with respect to the association between tobacco use and lung cancer. In addition, it is a powerful example of scientific writing in plain English, uncluttered by the jargon of many contemporary researchers. Finally, the findings from this case-control study provided the foundation for other studies of the health consequences of smoking tobacco and ultimately to the declaration by the U.S. government that the inhalation of cigarette smoke was harmful to the smoker.[11]

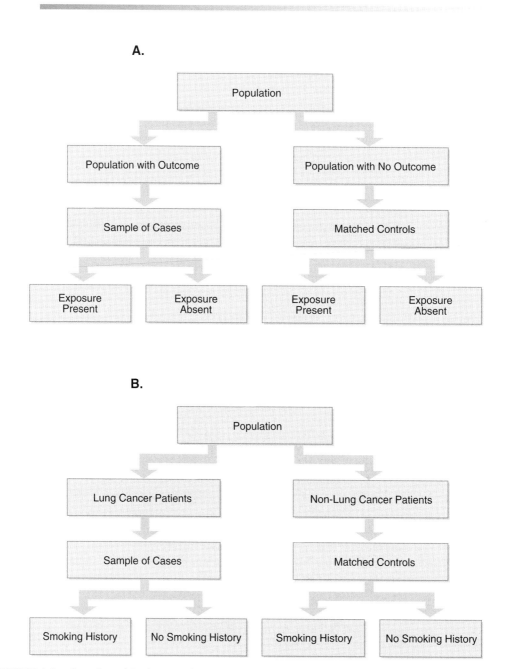

FIGURE 3-1 A. Case-Control Study: General. From the general population with the outcome of interest, a sample of cases is selected and matched to similar, but nonexposed, controls. Differences between the groups in the frequency of the exposure variable suggest an association between the exposure and the outcome. **B.** Case-Control Study: Doll and Hill. Evidence of an association between tobacco smoking and lung cancer was derived from the finding that of patients with lung cancer a greater proportion had smoked than had not smoked.

Case-control studies are usually used as an initial demonstration of an association between an event and an outcome. However, the results of a case-control study, by themselves, cannot demonstrate a cause-and-effect link. Indeed, Doll and Hill were careful to avoid any suggestion that cigarette smoking clearly caused lung cancer.

Case-control studies are relatively quick to conduct. Because participants already have the disease, a case-control research design is particularly well suited to diseases with long incubation periods and to diseases that occur only rarely. However, much thought should be given to the characteristics of the control group because they provide a key to controlling bias in the investigation.

Notice that more than one antecedent condition may be studied in a single case-control study. For example, a population-based case-control study design was used to examine the association between gastroesophageal reflux symptoms, obesity, and estrogen levels.[12] Data were obtained from two surveys administered approximately 10 years apart. More than 47,500 individuals participated in both surveys, representing ~ 73% of the residents of Nordtrandelag, a county in Norway. According to the authors, gastroesophageal reflux symptoms increased with obesity in both men and women but were more pronounced in women than in men. Furthermore, the association was more apparent in premenopausal than in postmenopausal women. However, hormone-replacement therapy in postmenopausal women restored the premenopausal relationship somewhat. The authors concluded that gastroesophageal reflux symptoms were associated in a dose-dependent manner with body mass and estrogen levels.

The case-control design has several potential drawbacks. The most serious is **bias**. Bias is a systematic error introduced into some aspect of the study by the experimental design or methods.[13] There are many different types of bias. Errors caused by **selection bias** are related to the process by which study subjects are chosen and then classified into cases and controls. For example, in the study of cigarette smoking and lung cancer, Doll and Hill examined the possibility that the interviewers had selected a "disproportionate number of light smokers" for the control group. However, there was no statistical evidence that smoking habits of patients comprising the control group differed from the population of control patients available for interviews, arguing against selection bias. However, if the selected control patients had differed from the population in some clinically meaningful way, a selection bias would be evident. Another source of bias is **recall bias**, which refers to the finding that, because of different life experiences, cases and controls may have different recollections of events. For example, a parent of a child who has asthma may be more likely to recall his or her child's gasping or wheezing than a parent of child who does not have asthma.

The consequences of bias are difficult to gauge. Bias may either increase or decrease group differences. Therefore, it is impossible to discover whether the outcome observed is the result of exposure or bias. Because there is no way to remove the bias after the data are collected, biased data are meaningless and have no value for testing a hypothesis.

Another shortcoming of a case-control study is that the data cannot be used to calculate the incidence or prevalence of the condition under study. This is because the participants are selected by the investigator and thus do not constitute a random sample of all those with the disease from the general population. One consequence is that measures of risk, either absolute or relative, have no meaning in a case-control study odds must be used instead.

In summary, a case-control study is an observational study design in which study groups are defined by the outcome and the investigator is interested in identifying an antecedent exposure. Case-control studies are particularly advantageous for studying outbreaks of diseases. Case-control studies also have traditionally provided the first evidence of an association between an event and a disease and have provided the evidence to justify more sophisticated study designs. Case-control study designs are considered in greater detail in Chapter 6. Table 3-1 summarizes the features of the case-control study design.

PERSPECTIVE 3-2

Case-control studies are sometimes dismissed as not very important. However, such a view is short sighted. The specific application of a case-control study is to isolate the antecedent condition that is most closely related to the outcome of interest. In a classic example, case-control studies were used to establish a link between toxic shock syndrome and the use of a particular brand of tampon.[14] In some circumstances, case-control studies represent the only ethical approach to a research problem. In industrial settings, for example, case-control studies have been used to examine cancer rates among those who live near nuclear power plants.[15]

THE COHORT STUDY DESIGN

In a **cohort study research design** groups are defined with respect to their exposure to a particular variable and a relationship is sought between this factor and several outcome variables (Table 3-2). Because the groups are distinguished based on an event not arranged by the investigator, the cohort study is an observational study research design.

One kind of cohort study design is the *prospective cohort design*. With this arrangement, the study begins after the exposure has occurred but before the outcome appears (Fig. 3-2A). This study design was used to examine changes in the incidence of thyroid tumors in children after a nuclear accident in which radioactivity was released into the atmosphere (Fig. 3.2B). After the accident at the Chernobyl nuclear power plant in the Soviet Union in 1986, epidemiologists examined differences in the frequency of thyroid tumors between children living downwind of the reactor (children exposed to the radiation) and those living upwind of the reactor (children of similar socioeconomic status who were not exposed to the radiation).[16] During the 5-year period after the nuclear accident, the frequency of thyroid tumors increased only among children exposed to the radiation.

TABLE 3-2   Features of the Cohort Observational Study Design

FEATURE	DESCRIPTION
Goal	Determine outcomes associated with exposure variables
Strategy	Assemble groups that differ only in exposure Determine if groups differ with respect to suspected outcomes
Group assignment	Study group selected on the basis of exhibiting exposure of interest Control group matched on all relevant variables except exposure of interest
Strengths	Can be used to study harmful exposures Can establish incidence (i.e., frequency of cases) of outcome Exposure effects can be examined retrospectively or prospectively Best with rare exposures
Weaknesses	Susceptible to confounding Groups cannot be matched on *all* variables except exposure Inefficient for long exposure–outcome intervals May be expensive Requires more patients than a case-control study

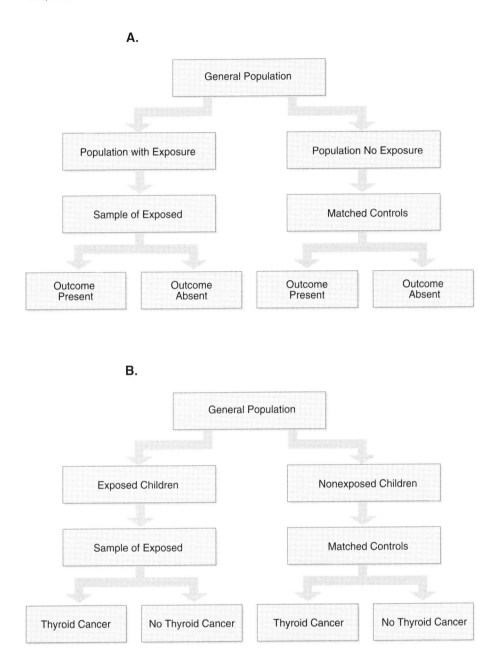

FIGURE 3-2 A. Cohort Study: General. From the general population with the exposure of interest, a sample of cases is selected and matched to similar, but nonexposed, controls. Differences in the frequency of the outcome variable in the two groups suggest an association between the exposure and the outcome. **B.** Cohort Study: Radioactivity Exposure and Thyroid Cancer Children exposed to radioactivity after a nuclear accident were matched with children who were not exposed. Both groups were followed for a 5-year period. Evidence of an association between radioactivity and thyroid cancer was derived from the finding that of children with thyroid cancer a greater proportion had been exposed to the radiation than had not been exposed.

Retrospective cohort designs are those in which both the exposure and the outcome have occurred before the investigation begins. However, because the groups are defined in terms of an antecedent condition, it is still a cohort study design. An everyday example of this design is to ask whether the practice of cramming for tests (the exposure variable) affected final grades in a therapeutics course (the outcome variable) the previous semester. To answer this question, historical records would be searched to sort therapeutics students into those who crammed and those who did not and to examine whether there were differences in the final grades of the two groups.

An example of a historical or retrospective cohort study design is a report of the association between obesity and future healthcare costs (Fig. 3-3).[17] For the data analysis, conducted in 1998, subjects were grouped into normal, overweight, and obese categories based on self-reported data collected in 1990. Subsequent healthcare use and costs for the period between 1990 and 1998 were extracted from electronic records of a health maintenance organization. The results suggested that overweight and obese respondents received a greater number of pharmacy orders than people of normal weight. Furthermore, whereas the normal-weight and overweight participants had mean cumulative prescription drug expenses of $2450 and $3310, respectively, drug-related expenses for the obese subjects were an average of $5000. These discrepancies were particularly pronounced for expenses related to diabetic and cardiovascular disorders.

PERSPECTIVE 3-3

One extremely important cohort study is the Framingham Heart Study. Begun in 1948, it is a continuing investigation of the inhabitants of the town of Framingham, Massachusetts. Findings from this study have been published periodically for more than 50 years and have provided event–outcome associations that are the bedrock of modern medical practice. For example, data from this project were used to identify risk factors for heart disease and to suggest a relationship between elevated blood lipid levels and stroke. A complete summary of the Framingham Heart Study reports is available at www.framingham.com/heart.

The cohort study design is efficient when a disease is relatively common and when the interval between the event and the outcome is short. The cohort study design is also valuable in estimating the incidence of the disease under study. Finally, this design allows several different antecedent conditions to be studied simultaneously.

The major threat to the integrity of a cohort study is **confounding**. Confounding occurs when an uncontrolled variable is correlated with the exposure variable and is an independent risk factor for the outcome. For example, in a study of fiber intake and cardiovascular disease, the level of physical activity, if uncontrolled, could be a confounding variable. That is because both physical exercise and fiber intake are components of a healthy lifestyle and therefore likely to occur together; in addition, physical activity alone has been shown to reduce the risk of cardiovascular disease.

One method of controlling the effects of confounding factors, once they are identified, is to match participants in the groups based on the confounding factor, thereby ensuring that the effect is the same in all groups. Another method is to divide the participants in both groups into subgroups (called strata) based on the confounding factor (for instance, individuals > 65 years of age vs. those < 65 years). Then an analysis can be conducted on each stratum separately. Finally, sophisticated multivariate statistical techniques can be

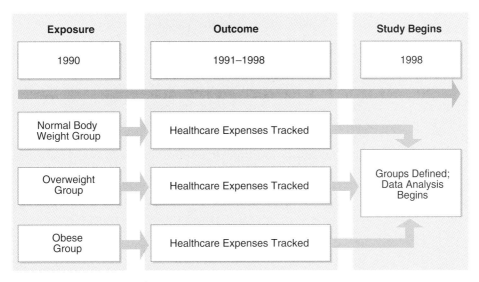

Exposure	Outcome	Study Begins
1990	1991–1998	1998

Normal Body Weight Group	Healthcare Expenses Tracked	
Overweight Group	Healthcare Expenses Tracked	Groups Defined; Data Analysis Begins
Obese Group	Healthcare Expenses Tracked	

FIGURE 3-3 Retrospective Cohort Study. Both the exposure and the outcome occurred before the study began. Body-weight data were collected in 1990, and healthcare costs were accrued for the following 8 years. In 1998, the subjects were sorted into groups based on body weight, and their healthcare expenses were analyzed.

used to remove the effect of the confounding factor. These statistical techniques are discussed in more detail in subsequent chapters.

Another potential difficulty is that an outcome may occur many years after exposure to a variable. Thus prospective cohort designs may require years of data collection before a definitive association is established, meaning these studies may be quite expensive.

In summary, a cohort study design is an observational study in which groups are defined with respect to exposure to an antecedent event; researchers then examine an outcome variable. Cohort studies have traditionally been used to establish associations between events and outcomes. However, although the results of cohort study designs are generally considered to be more persuasive than case-control study results, the findings do not establish a cause-and-effect relationship. Cohort study designs are considered in more detail in Chapter 7. The major features of the cohort study design are presented in Table 3-2.

PERSPECTIVE 3-4

Although the cohort study is an observational study design, it nevertheless can provide information essential to establishing an association between an antecedent event and an outcome. In fact, in circumstances in which it is suspected that the antecedent condition exerts a deleterious effect on health, a cohort study may represent the only ethical research tool.

THE CROSS-SECTIONAL STUDY DESIGN

A third observational study design, the **cross-sectional study research design**, is used to determine the prevalence of an exposure, an outcome, or an exposure–outcome association at a single point in time or during a brief time interval (Table 3-3). It is thus useful in providing a snapshot of the number of individuals who exhibit the variable in question.

TABLE 3-3	Features of the Cross-Sectional Observational Study Design
FEATURE	DESCRIPTION
Goal	Obtain evidence of exposures, outcomes, or their association
Strategy	Gather information on exposure and outcome at a single point in time
Group assignment	Group membership may be determined before or after data are gathered
Strengths	Can be used to study many potential exposure–outcome associations Can be used to examine many subgroup variables Subgroups can be oversampled Can be used to study harmful exposures Data can be obtained easily, rapidly, and cost-effectively
Weaknesses	Susceptible to biases, especially recall bias and volunteer bias Often relies on nonverified, self-reported information Susceptible to cause-and-effect conclusions

For example, a cross-sectional study design was used to assess the prevalence of herbal product use in a major metropolitan area.[18] First, a questionnaire was developed to collect the following data: demographic information about the participant, whether the participant had used an herbal product in the past 12 months, and what specific herbal products had been used. For those who had used herbal products, additional information was collected regarding the reason for using the herb, the perceived efficacy of the herb, and the source of information recommending the herbal product.

Recipients of the survey were selected randomly from the state registry of individuals holding a valid driver's license, who were at least 18 years old, and whose address included a ZIP code in the St. Paul, Minnesota, metropolitan area. Those who returned the survey received $10.00.

Of the 752 surveys mailed, 62% were returned. Compared to the general St. Paul population, the survey sample contained a greater proportion of women and a smaller proportion of those without a high school education. Of the study sample, 61% had used an herbal product in the past 12 months. These individuals were more likely to be women and to have used a multivitamin or a nutritional supplement during the same time frame. Although responses to individual herbal products varied, in general < 60% of the respondents considered the herbal product to be effective. Information about herbal products was obtained most frequently from family or friends and least often from healthcare professionals.

This example typifies the advantages and disadvantages of many cross-sectional study designs. On the plus side, the design permits the simultaneous study of many different variables and thus many possible associations among them. Studies can be completed rapidly, easily, and cost-effectively. Furthermore, groups of participants may be preselected. For example, in a study of attitudes toward physician-assisted suicide, physicians were selected randomly from the rolls of the state medical association.[19] In addition, however, the survey was sent to doctors who, because of their medical specialty, dealt with the problem of euthanasia most frequently. This technique, known as oversampling, ensured that a sufficient number of specialists would be studied to provide accurate population estimates from the subgroup of physicians.

The major difficulty with the cross-sectional study design is bias. Surveys that request information of events that occurred in the past are susceptible to recall bias. Because not all who are invited to participate in the survey do so, the final sample of participants may not be representative of the population of interest. In addition, many responses merely represent unverified self-reports, and respondents may be providing the information they anticipate will find favor with the investigators.

Another problem with the cross-sectional study design is that it is sometimes difficult to determine timing relationships between events. A recent paper, for example, suggested that teenagers were more likely to have tried smoking tobacco if they had viewed motion pictures in which an actor smoked tobacco.[20] Based on these data, the conclusion might be reached that viewing motion pictures with smokers leads to increased tobacco use in teens. However, such a conclusion may be unwarranted. If, for example, no evidence is presented with respect to the timing of the two events, a cause-and-effect relationship cannot be claimed. Notice that the reverse conclusion is also possible: Teenage smokers may be more likely to select films in which the actors smoke. A final, and perhaps most likely alternative, is recall bias: Teenage smokers may be more likely to remember films in which they and the actors shared a common habit—smoking.

Cross-sectional surveys may consist of administering a one-time questionnaire to participants, as in the herbal product study. These studies may also be designed to obtain information from the same population at different points in time. Such longitudinal cross-sectional surveys have been a rich source of information on the health status, changes in health status, healthcare use, and the prevalence of disease and drug use in the United States and elsewhere. The following are U.S. government–sponsored longitudinal cross-sectional surveys: the National Health and Nutrition Examination Survey (NHANES);[21] the National Hospital Discharge Survey (NHDS);[22] and the National Cancer Institute's Surveillance, Epidemiology, and End Results (SEER) database.[23] Cross-sectional research designs are considered in more detail in Chapter 7. The major features of the cross-sectional research design are presented in Table 3-3.

PERSPECTIVE 3-5

Not all cross-sectional surveys attempt to sample a group that is representative of the general population. Two important longitudinal surveys—the Nurses Health Study[24] and the Physician's Health Study[25]—specifically sampled particular healthcare professionals. The subjects were selected as participants because of the conviction that, owing to their commitment to healthcare, these individuals would be more compliant in completing the surveys, be more likely to understand medical terminology, and not be put off by questions regarding intimate personal details. Both surveys have provided important information that is relevant to the general population.

PERSPECTIVE 3-6

Whether observational studies provide convincing proof of a cause-and-effect relationship is a continuing controversy. The basic argument against using case-control and cohort studies to reach cause-and-effect conclusions stems from the lack of a random assignment of subjects to conditions. For example, because subjects are not assigned randomly to exposure conditions in a cohort study, the investigator cannot be sure that the relationship observed is actually the result of a confounding factor. From this viewpoint, the only study designs that can provide proof of causality are those in which participants are assigned randomly to experimental conditions. If this is the case, however, how do we prove cause-and-effect relationships in situations in which it would be unethical to assign participants to particular experimental conditions?

For example, case-control studies have been the traditional research design for identifying and evaluating health risks associated with specific industrial settings, such as nuclear energy and rubber plants, and with particular products, such as tampon use and toxic shock syndrome. They have also been used to study war-related health problems such as mental disturbances resulting from exposure to Agent Orange.

Perhaps the issue is one of prudence rather than scientific proof. That is, human beings often modify their behavior when there is evidence that it is prudent to do so, whether or not the evidence is based on a cause-and-effect relationship. For example, many individuals have stopped using tobacco products even though the precise biologic mechanism by which the tobacco smoke causes cancer had not been identified. Thus, though information derived from observational research study designs may not be sufficient to prove cause-and-effect relationships, the strength of the association (either in terms of intensity or consistency) may be compelling.

Randomized Controlled Trial Study Designs (Experimental Designs)

The **randomized controlled trial (RCT)** is a prospective, experimental study design in which the investigator controls the application of the independent variable among two or more groups of individuals to assess its effect on outcome variables (Table 3-4). One feature of the RCT is that it is always a prospective study design—the treatment is always administered before changes in the outcome variables are sought. Furthermore, participants are assigned to the experimental conditions by a random (i.e., chance) process. This manipulation controls for many forms of bias encountered with observational research designs.

There are two principal types of RCT study designs. One includes a group of individuals who receive a placebo, or surrogate treatment. The purpose of this design is to delineate differences between the experimental treatment and the placebo condition. The other type, the **active controlled trial**, compares a novel treatment to a standard treatment. Active controlled trials are discussed in greater detail in Chapter 8.

TABLE 3-4	Features of the Randomized Controlled Trial Study Design
FEATURE	DESCRIPTION
Goal	Establish cause-and-effect relationships between interventions and outcomes
Strategy	Examine differences in outcomes among groups receiving intervention compared to a placebo or active control group
Group assignment	Assignment to an intervention or a control group is result of a random process
Strengths	Randomization minimizes bias Control group accounts for change in response variables over time Can examine more than one intervention; more than one outcome Can be used to establish cause-and-effect relationships CONSORT guidelines increase study quality
Weaknesses	Cannot be used to study effects of harmful interventions Can be expensive and labor intensive Participants who drop out can compromise advantages of randomization Multicenter patient group may not be similar to an individual clinician's patient group Must consider role of commercial sponsors who have a vested interest in study outcome

The RCT design that includes a placebo group is considered the gold standard for determining the efficacy and safety of a novel drug or other intervention, and the findings provided by RCTs have contributed evidence critical to contemporary healthcare. The significance of RCTs is underscored by the establishment of a panel—the Consolidated Standards of Reporting Trials (CONSORT) group—that periodically publishes guidelines to foster consistency in the design, conduct, analysis, and reporting of RCTs.[26,27]

Several types of RCTs may be distinguished in the healthcare literature. One type of study design is the **parallel-groups RCT study design**. In this schema, a researcher assigns patients at random to one or more treatment groups and to a control group (Fig. 3-4). The design is termed *parallel* because subjects receive only one treatment for the duration of the study. The study is ended after either a specific time period has elapsed or a predetermined number of primary outcomes has occurred.

The Anglo-Scandinavian Cardiac Outcomes Trial—Lipid Lowering Arm (ASCOT—LLA) trial is an example of a placebo-control, parallel-group RCT study design.[28] The purpose of the trial was to study the effects of lipid lowering in hypertensive patients who were at high risk for cardiovascular disease yet displayed normal lipid levels. The experimental plan of the study can be gleaned from the **trial profile**. The trial profile is an important part of the reporting of a RCT because it indicates the fate of each participant who was considered for inclusion in the study. In addition, the trial profile presents a concise depiction of the study design.

As indicated in the trial profile for the ASCOT—LLA trial, of 19,342 individuals who had participated in a previous portion of the ASCOT trial that focused on normalizing blood pressure in hypertensive patients, 10,305 were eligible and randomized to the lipid-lowering arm of the study (Fig. 3-5). From this group, 5,168 patients were assigned randomly to receive atorvastatin, 10 mg daily, and 5,137 patients were assigned to receive a placebo. At the end of the study, complete information was available for 4,928 patients in the atorvastatin group and 4,861 patients in the placebo-control group.

Originally, a 5-year follow-up period was planned to detect group differences in the primary end point: the frequency of nonfatal myocardial infarction or fatal coronary heart disease. After 3.3 years, however, the study was stopped because statistical analyses

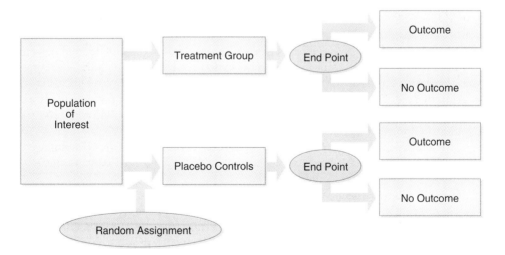

FIGURE 3-4 Randomized Controlled Study: Parallel Groups. From the population of interest, participants are assigned by a random process either to the treatment group or to the placebo control group and are tracked to an end point. Evidence of an association between the outcome and treatment is determined by comparing the difference in the proportion of participants exhibiting the outcome in the two study groups.

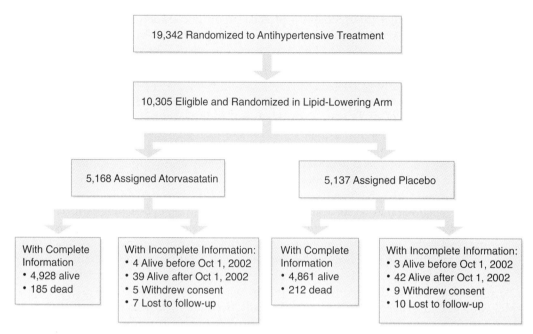

FIGURE 3-5   Randomized Controlled Trial, Parallel Groups: ASCOT-LLA. Note the general study plan and the fate of those considered for inclusion in the Anglo-Scandinavian Cardiac Outcomes Trial—Lipid Lowering Arm (ASCOT—LLA) study are indicated. Adapted with permission from Sever PS, Dahlof B, Poulter NR, et al. Prevention of coronary and stroke events with atorvastatin in hypertensive patients who have average or lower-than-average cholesterol concentrations, in the Anglo-Scandinavian Cardiac Outcomes Trial—Lipid Lowering Arm (ASCOT—LLA): A multicenter randomized controlled trial. Lancet 2003;361:1149–1158.

indicated a dramatic benefit of lipid lowering in the treatment group. For example, whereas 154 primary events had occurred in the placebo group during the 3.3-year interval, only 100 primary events had been reported in the atorvastatin group. Given the efficacy of the statin in affording cardiovascular protection, it was judged unethical to deprive the placebo-control patients of this benefit. The results of this study were among the first to suggest that lipid-lowering agents may be efficacious in reducing cardiovascular events among patients who were not dyslipidemic and thus might not normally receive lipid-lowering treatment.

Another type of RCT is the **crossover RCT study design**, in which individuals initially assigned to one condition or treatment are switched to the other condition at some point in the trial. Thus each subject in the crossover RCT study design is exposed to both the treatment and the placebo condition. The order of treatment and placebo administration, however, should be randomized for each patient to minimize potential confounding of the results by the order of administration.

An example of crossover RCT study design is provided by a report examining the efficacy of an angiotensin II receptor blocker for the treatment of migraine headaches.[29] The crossover scheme is made clear from the trial profile of this study (Fig. 3-6). According to this experimental plan, during the first 12 weeks, 30 participants received candesartan, 16 mg once a day, while 30 other patients received a placebo. During the next 4 weeks, participants received no treatment to clear lingering drug effects. For the final 12 weeks, 28 patients originally assigned to the drug condition were crossed over to the placebo regimen, and 29 patients who had received the placebo crossed over to the drug-treatment group. The results of the study indicated a reduction in the primary end point—the number of days with headache—and several secondary end points. Tolerability was judged to be comparable in both placebo and treatment conditions.

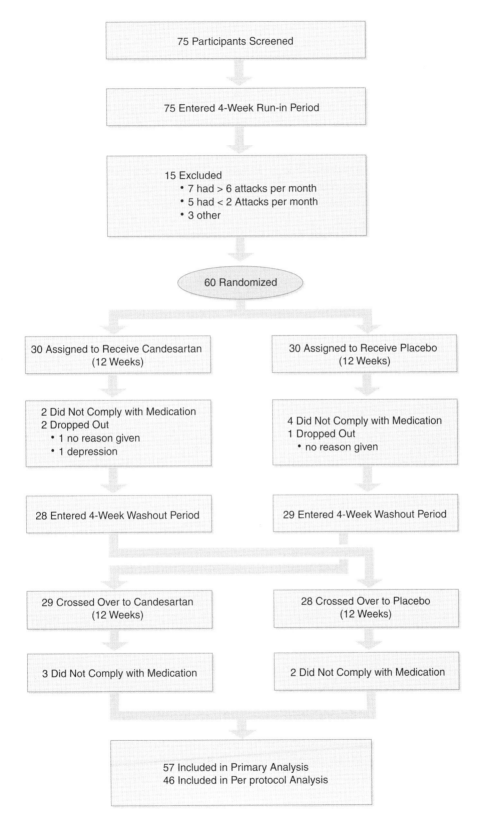

FIGURE 3-6   Crossover Randomized Controlled Trial. Adapted with permission from Tronvik E, Stovner LJ, Helde G, et al. Prophylactic treatment of migraine with an angiotensin II receptor blocker. JAMA 2003;289:65–69.

The crossover RCT design has the advantage that each patient serves as his or her own control, leading to a considerable reduction in experimental error. However, the design assumes that drug effects do not carry over from the first to the second period. A general rule of thumb is to allow at least 5 half-lives of the drug to pass before crossing over to the subsequent treatment. Another assumption is that the disease course remains stable during the course of the study. Thus crossover designs are best used when studying diseases or conditions that are relatively stable and do not involve unpredictable or phasic changes in symptom patterns. For example, studying antibiotic treatment of a bacterial infection would not lend itself well to a crossover design because once the subjects complete the first treatment phase (e.g., have taken an antibiotic for 7 days), the infection is cured and the effects seen during the crossover phase would be distorted.

PERSPECTIVE 3-7

Be alert that data from RCTs may be analyzed in several different ways. One method is called an **intention-to-treat** *(ITT) analysis. In an ITT analysis, the data for each participant who enters the study are included in the final data analysis, even if the person fails to complete the study protocol. To accomplish this, data for patients who do not complete the study are estimated in one of several ways. One common method is to use the last observations from the participant to estimate the missing data, a method termed* **last observation carried forward** *(LOCF). Because such an analysis will include data from individuals who failed to benefit from the entire treatment regimen, the true magnitude of the treatment effect may be underestimated. On the other hand, by including data from all individuals in the final data analysis, researchers obtain a more accurate estimate of the effect of the treatment in the general population, in which some patients will not comply. Such information is of interest to public health officials and epidemiologists.*

Another technique is to analyze data only from those participants who complete the entire study protocol. This is termed a **per-protocol analysis**, *or an on-treatment data analysis. The advantage of the on-treatment method is that it provides an accurate estimate of the treatment effect among those who comply fully with the treatment regimen, and results are not diluted by the data from noncompliant participants. As such, the on-treatment analysis provides a best-outcomes estimate of the safety and efficacy profile of the intervention.*

Since the on-treatment method provides a best-outcome result, the clinician needs to remember that the result obtained in his or her patient pool will be diluted by those who are noncompliant with medications because of adverse effects or lack of efficacy.

In general, the ITT analysis provides a more realistic estimate of efficacy and safety effects in the general population, and the on-treatment analysis provides an idea of the outcomes in compliant patients. Many contemporary studies provide both an ITT and a per-protocol analysis of the data for comparison.

In summary, RCTs provide the best evidence of cause-and-effect relationships for the following reasons. First, they are true experiments, in that the investigator controls changes in an intervention to examine the effect on an outcome variable. Second, the random assignment of participants to study conditions minimizes several kinds of bias, notably selection bias. Randomization also matches participants in the different groups on a number of variables, thereby minimizing the role of confounding variables. Finally, guidelines provide quality assurance that the data being presented have been processed in a standardized manner.

RCTs are not without limitations, however. One of these is that ethical considerations limit treatments to those that will not harm the participants. Furthermore, RCTs that involve many participants are expensive to conduct, often involving massive amounts of money, labor, and time. A current trend is to conduct multicenter RCTs, in which the protocol is carried out in many different clinical settings and even in many different countries. The contribution of individual locations to the final database is not always reported, although the geographical distribution of subjects may affect the results. Finally, the role of sponsors who have a vested interest in the outcome of the RCT needs to be considered. Randomized controlled trial designs are discussed in more detail in Chapter 8.

Pharmacoeconomic Study Designs

The study designs just discussed help clinicians determine associations between diseases and risk factors or efficacy and safety of medications, but another facet that clinicians must consider when deciding on appropriate patient care is economic issues. Thus **pharmacoeconomic studies** provide insight into the costs associated with drug therapy (both benefits and consequences) to individual patients, healthcare systems, and society. Pharmacoeconomic studies help healthcare providers evaluate the total costs of a treatment option (e.g., actual drug costs plus drug-monitoring costs) and the outcomes associated with that treatment (e.g., the money saved by avoiding a myocardial infarction).

The four principal types of pharmacoeconomic studies are cost-minimization analysis, cost-benefit analysis, cost-effectiveness analysis, and cost-utility analysis. Costs examined in these analyses can include:

- Direct medical costs (hospitalizations, doctor's office appointments, drug costs, medical procedures)
- Direct nonmedical costs (travel to and from physician appointments or the hospital, any cost associated with the treatment that are not medical in nature)
- Indirect costs (time missed from work, lack of productivity)
- Intangible costs (pain and suffering)

Often, healthcare decisions are based on a cost-benefit analysis. For example, from an economic perspective, should college students be vaccinated against meningococcal disease? Jackson et al.[30] estimated the rate of vaccine-preventable meningococcal disease among adults 18–22 years of age in the United States to be 0.5 per 100,000 per year. The estimated cost of the vaccine was $30 per person (including actual vaccine cost plus vaccine administration cost), and the cost of treatment for meningococcal disease was on average $8,145 per case (including cost of 7 days of hospitalization plus one doctor's visit per day). Because meningococcal disease is associated with a 15% death rate, the researchers also factored in a cost estimate per death amounting to $1 million. Using a cost-benefit pharmacoeconomic analysis schema, the conclusion was reached that the total cost for the vaccination program ($56.2 million) would not result in a net savings to society, unless the incidence of meningococcal disease among college students increased 13-fold. As this seemed unlikely, the authors concluded that the vaccination program was not feasible. Pharmacoeconomic studies are discussed in greater detail in Chapter 9.

PERSPECTIVE 3-8

One aspect to consider when reading pharmacoeconomic studies is the viewpoint from which the study was designed. Is the analysis looking at costs to society, the patient, healthcare systems, or third-party payers? This is an important distinction to bear in mind because different viewpoints can lead to dissimilar results and recommendations. For instance, if looking from a patient perspective, a higher cost may be estimated for patient pain and suffering compared to the cost estimated for drug therapy to treat that pain. Performing a similar pharmacoeconomic analysis from a managed care organization's viewpoint, the estimated cost of the drug may be higher than cost associated with patient pain and suffering.

Systematic Reviews

The research designs discussed so far involve examining the effect of an exposure on an outcome. However, at some point, the results of individual research studies must be compared to determine the consistency of results among individual studies and the generality of the composite findings to the population. The traditional method of accomplishing this is the narrative review, in which a leader in the field conducts a qualitative review of relevant papers and reaches conclusions on the current status of knowledge in the field. As the general field of evidence-based medicine has evolved, however, a more objective, rigorous approach to data synthesis has emerged: the **systematic review** (Table 3-5).

Systematic reviews may be either qualitative or quantitative. Researchers conducting **qualitative systematic reviews** use rigorous logic and critical thinking to evaluate and synthesize the results of individual investigations. For **quantitative systematic reviews**, researchers use statistical methods to describe the magnitude and consistency of the experimental effect. This latter approach is also termed meta-analysis.

There are two different methods for conducting a meta-analysis (Fig. 3-7). One analytical method is to pool the raw data from individual studies into one large database and

TABLE 3-5	Features of the Systematic Review Study Design
FEATURE	**DESCRIPTION**
Goal	Synthesize findings from individual studies to provide a coherent, integrated answer to a focused research question
Strategy	Use critical thinking approach to gather, evaluate, and synthesize information from individual research studies to address a question of clinical relevance
Group assignment	Study results are weighted with respect to methodologic quality
Strengths	Strict methodologic guidelines, developed a priori, keep review focused, transparent, and objective Can detect intervention–outcome relationships that may be obscured in individual studies Can explore differences among studies (i.e., sources of heterogeneity) Extremely cost-effective Study is quickly completed
Weaknesses	Weaknesses of any observational study, notably selection bias Studies with large samples, or higher quality, count more Studies with methodologic flaws are included The data summary methods obscure fine points of subject, setting, and methods that are the essence of clinical practice Meta-analysis of observational studies is not recommended Results of systematic reviews are sometimes at variance with large, well-conducted RCTs May be labor intensive

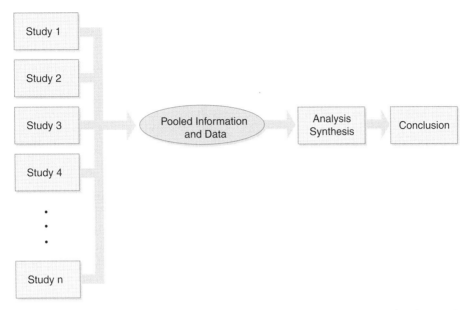

FIGURE 3-7   Systematic Review. Following a protocol for the identification of appropriate articles, the investigator selects individual research papers and evaluates and synthesizes them using critical thinking or statistical techniques.

then conduct statistical analyses as if the data had been part of a single investigation. The other method is to convert the results of each individual study into a common measure. Statistical testing can then be used to compare the findings from different studies to gauge their consistency and provide an integrated, composite estimate of the effect.

Systematic reviews are conducted according to a rigorous, prospectively delineated protocol that consists of a focused clinical question; a comprehensive literature search using an explicit search strategy; a systematic plan for evaluating the utility and quality of the research studies; and a plan for summarizing, synthesizing, and reaching inferences from the data. The question addressed in the systematic review is narrow and clinically focused. It enumerates explicitly a particular patient population exhibiting a condition of interest, a particular exposure or treatment, and a specific set of outcomes.[31]

For example, a combined qualitative systematic review and meta-analysis has been reported examining the adequacy of the currently used level of warfarin-induced anticoagulation in preventing hemorrhages and stroke in patients with nonvalvular atrial fibrillation.[32] To address this question, 714 published and unpublished articles, reports, and abstracts were identified, reviewed, evaluated, rated, and distilled to a final data set of 11 RCTs, 9 observational studies, and 1 uncontrolled case series. Both the qualitative systematic review and the meta-analysis evaluated data from the RCTs and the observational studies separately. Results from both study designs were consistent in suggesting that patients in whom anticoagulation was inadequate were at an increased risk of stroke, whereas patients in whom anticoagulation was above recommended levels were at increased risk of bleeding.

Systematic reviews have significant advantages over narrative reviews. The rigorous nature of the evaluation process reduces subjectivity in the selection and evaluation of individual studies. Furthermore, the synthesis of data from a number of smaller studies may provide a more accurate estimate of safety and efficacy effects than estimates from each individual study alone.

However, a systematic review uses essentially an observational research methodology in which the individual reports are the subjects. As such, bias, while limited by the protocol, may still affect the selection, evaluation, data extraction, analysis, and reporting of the data. Of necessity, the data evaluation ignores the details of patient characteristics, treatments, and outcomes, even though these elements are critical in determining the applicability of the results within a clinician's practice setting. Finally, it is not uncommon for the conclusions reached by systematic reviews to be at variance with the results of large, well-conducted RCTs. Systematic reviews are considered in greater detail in Chapter 10.

Applying the Results from Healthcare Research Designs

The findings from healthcare research designs have several applications. One, of interest to the general healthcare community, is to provide evidence of an association between an exposure and an outcome. Another application is to assist the healthcare professional, including the pharmacist, in making treatment decisions that affect the well-being of the individual patient. Thus the pharmacist must be able to evaluate evidence provided by individual healthcare research studies both for general scientific quality and for relevance to his or her specific therapeutic situation.

The general scientific quality of an individual research paper is called its **internal validity**. Basically, this is a determination that the methods and results of the study are believable and have not been contaminated by other factors, termed **threats to internal validity**. Two threats to internal validity, bias and confounding, have already been discussed. Two others involve error and chance. **Measurement error**, for example, is a systematic lack of precision in assessing the outcome variables, such as a body-weight scale that reads several kilograms less than the person's true body weight. Another threat to the internal validity of a research study is **chance**. Chance is the likelihood that an association occurred as the result a random, unpredictable process. A chance outcome is often referred to as luck, providence, destiny, or accident.

No study is perfect, so it is well to remember that each of the four threats to internal validity occur to some extent in all research. Thus, even though bias was discussed with case-control studies and confounding was described with cohort studies, these factors may affect the veracity of any study design. When evaluating research papers, then, the first task is to determine that the association claimed between the variables is not the result of bias, confounding, measurement error, or chance.

The next step is to review evidence that the association is due to a cause-and-effect relationship. To reach the conclusion of a cause-and-effect relationship, many researchers contend that the data must meet the criteria of causality promulgated by Hill.[33] In the following list, the most important elements are presented first:

- **Temporal relationship**: The cause must *precede* the effect.
- **Strength of association**: For an individual study, the greater the size of the effect, the more confidence is placed in its causal interpretation.
- **Consistency or replicability**: This is an issue of **external validity**. Causal associations that appear consistently and repeatedly in different patient groups, in different clinical settings, and among different investigators are judged to have much merit.
- **Dose-response relationship**: The study should note whether changing the strength of the causal agent (either increasing or decreasing it) leads to proportionate modifications in levels of the outcome.

- **Plausibility**: The report should discuss a likely mechanism to explain the causal association. For example, if a new drug claims to restore glycemic control in diabetic patients, mechanisms by which this might be achieved need to be enumerated.
- **Alternative explanations**: The study should address the four threats to the internal validity: bias, confounding, measurement error, and chance.
- **Experimental evidence**: Experimental studies (RCTs) provide more convincing evidence of causal relationships than do observational studies. In fact, some researchers claim that RCTs provide the best evidence, followed by systematic reviews, cohort studies, case-control studies, and case series and case reports. Remember, however, that some types of associations (harmful exposures) can be addressed by only certain study types (observational studies), and some research questions (cause of an outbreak) can be addressed adequately by only specific research designs (case series).
- **Specificity**: The same outcome should be associated with the same exposure. This refers to the consistency with which the outcome flows from the exposure or intervention.
- **Coherence**: The proposed causal relationship must be consistent with existing knowledge.

Finally, there is an assessment of whether the data are relevant to the pharmacist's patients. This means that the subject characteristics, practice environment, methods of drug delivery, methods for monitoring efficacy and safety, etc., are comparable to those of the pharmacist.

Summary

Researchers who study the effects of variables on the health status of human populations have developed a set of research designs that provide for the systematic collection, analysis, and reporting of data. Each research design has been formulated to address the study of an exposure–outcome relationship in a unique way. These healthcare research study designs are part of a larger scheme used to determine whether an exposure–outcome association is causal. This process includes demonstrating that the association is not likely the result of bias, confounding, measurement error, or chance.

The implications of this information for pharmacists are profound. In today's world, information diffuses through the population at a rapid rate. Many people look to their pharmacist as the expert on drug information. However, this expertise can be acquired only by adopting an evidence-based approach to acquiring, evaluating, and applying healthcare information. A major component of this evaluation process is the ability to understand biostatistics, because biostatistics is the method used to indicate the extent to which the association may be the result of chance. A foundation for biostatistics is presented in Chapter 4.

STUDY PROBLEMS

1. In the middle of the 20th century, diethylstilbestrol was administered to pregnant women to prevent miscarriages. Years later, evidence suggested that daughters of these women displayed an excessive number of reproductive problems.[34] Evaluate the appropriateness of the case-control, cohort, cross-sectional, and randomized controlled trial designs for follow-up studies of this report.

2. Enumerate several variables that might bias healthcare results and several that might confound the results.

3. Select a study summarized in this chapter and evaluate the potential effects of bias and confounding on the results. How might the study be redesigned to avoid the pitfalls of the biasing and confounding variables?

4. A telephone survey was conducted to characterize stress and coping reactions after the terrorists attacks of September 11, 2001.[35] An association was reported between the level of stress and the extent of television viewing. Are there problems (bias, confounding, or measurement error) in considering this association to be causal? If you wanted to research this relationship further, what type of study would you perform next and why?

5. A new drug, X, has been found to increase the CD4 count in a small group of HIV-positive patients. Design a randomized controlled trial to test whether the relationship is causal. Could another study design be used rather than an RCT? What are the advantages and disadvantages of each study design for this application?

REFERENCES

1. Sackett DL. Evidence-Based Medicine. How to Practice and Teach EBM. 2nd ed. New York: Churchill Livingstone, 2000.

2. Tsang KW, Ho PL, Ooi Gc, et al. A cluster of cases of severe acute respiratory syndrome in Hong Kong. N Engl J Med 2003;348:1977–1985.

3. Poutanen SM, Low DE, Henry B, et al. Identification of SARS in Canada. N Engl J Med 2003;348:1995–2005.

4. Ai D, Roper TA, Riley JA. Diabetic ketoacidosis and clozapine. Postgrad Med J 1998;74:493–494.

5. Muench J, Carey M. Diabetes mellitus associated with atypical antipsychotic medications: New case report and review of the literature. J Am Board Fam Pract 2000;14:278–282.

6. Ragucci KR, Wells BJ. Olanzapine-induced diabetic ketoacidosis. Ann Pharacother 2001;35:1556–1558.

7. Takahashi, M., Ohishi S, Katsumi, C, et al. Rapid onset of quetiapine-induced diabetic ketoacidosis in an elderly patient: A case report. Pharmacopsychiatry 2005;38:183–184.

8. Gould, JB, Qin C, Marks AR, et al. Neonatal mortality in weekend vs. weekday births. JAMA 2003;289:2958–2962.

9. Drazen JM, Cazion EW. SARS, the Internet, and the journal. N Engl J Med 2003;348:2009.

10. Doll R, Hill AB. Smoking and carcinoma of the lung. Preliminary report. Br Med J 1950;143:329–336.

11. Lopez AD. Measuring the health hazards of tobacco: Commentary. Bull World Health Organ 1999;77:82–83.

12. Nilsson M., Johnsen R, Ye W, et al. Obesity and estrogen as risk factors for gastroesophageal reflux symptoms. JAMA 2003;290:66–72.

13. Hennekens CH, Buring JE. Epidemiology in Medicine. Boston: Little, Brown, 1987.

14. Latham RH, Kehrberg MW, Jacobson JA, Smith CB. Toxic shock syndrome in Utah: A case-control and surveillance study. Ann Intern Med 1982;96;906–908.

15. Gardner MJ, Snee MP, Hall AJ, et al. Results of case-control study of leukemia and lymphoma among young people near Sellafield nuclear plant in West Cumbria. Br Med J 1990;300:423–428.

16. Kazakov VS. Thyroid cancer after Chernobyl. Nature 1992;??:359.

17. Thompson D, Brown JB, Nichols GA, et al. Body mass index and future healthcare costs: A retrospective cohort study. Obes Res 2001;9:210–218.

18. Harnack LJ, Rydell SA, Stang J. Prevalence of use of herbal products by adults in the Minneapolis/ St. Paul, Minn., metropolitan area. Mayo Clin Proc 2001;76:688–694.

19. Cohen JS, Fihn SD, Boyko EJ, et al. Attitudes toward assisted suicide and euthanasia among physicians in Washington State. N Engl J Med 1994;331:89–94.

20. Sargent JD, Beach ML, Dalton MA, et al. Effect of seeing tobacco use in films on trying smoking among adolescents: A cross sectional study. Br Med J 2001;323:1–6.

21. Centers for Disease Control and Prevention. National Health and Nutrition Examination Survey. Available at: www.cdc.gov/nchs/nhanes.htm. Accessed Feb 2007.

22. Centers for Disease Control and Prevention. National Hospital Discharge Survey. Available at: www.cdc.gov/nchs/about/major/hdasd/nhdsdes.htm. Accessed Feb 2007.

23. National Cancer Institute. Surveillance Epidemiology and End Results. Available at: www.seer.cancer.gov. Accessed Feb 2007.

24. Nurses Health Study. Available at: www.channing.harvard.edu/nhs. Accessed Feb 2007.

25. Physicians Health Study. Available at: phs.bwh.harvard.edu. Accessed Feb 2007.

26. Begg C, Cho M, Eastwood S, et al. Improving the quality of reporting of randomized controlled trials. The CONSORT statement. JAMA 1996;276:637–639.

27. Moher D, Schulz KE, Altman D, et al. The CONSORT statement: Revised recommendations for improving the quality of reports of parallel-group randomized trials. JAMA 2001;285:1987–1991.

28. Sever PS, Dahlof B, Poulter NR, et al. Prevention of coronary and stroke events with atorvastatin in hypertensive patients who have average or lower-than-average cholesterol concentrations, in the Angle-Scandinavian Cardiac Outcomes Trial—Lipid Lowering Arm (ASCOT—LLA): A multicenter randomized controlled trial. Lancet 2003;361:1149–1158.

29. Tronvik E, Stovner LJ, Helde G, et al. Prophylactic treatment of migraine with an angiotensin II receptor blocker. JAMA 2003;289:65–69.

30. Jackson LA, Schuchat A, Gorsky RD, et al. Should college students be vaccinated against meningococcal disease: A cost-benefit analysis. Am J Public Health 1995; 85:843—845.

31. Cook DJ, Mulrow CD, Haynes RB. Systematic reviews: Synthesis of best evidence for clinical decisions. Ann Intern Med 1997;126:376–380.

32. Reynolds MW, Fahrback K, Hauch O, et al. Warfarin anticoagulation and outcomes in patients with atrial fibrillation. A systematic review and meta-analysis. Chest 2004;126:1938–1945.

33. Bradford-Hill A. The environment and disease: Association or causation. President's address. Proc R Soc Med 1965;9:295–300.

34. University of Louisville Birth Defects Center. DES, a generation later. Birth Defects Center Res Newslett 2003;14:3. Available at: louisville.edu/hsc/birthdefectscenter/newsletters/publication72.pdf. Accessed Feb 2007.

35. Schuster MA, Stein BD, Jaycox L, et al. A national survey of stress reactions after the September 11, 2001, terrorist attacks. N Engl J Med 2001;345:1507–1512.

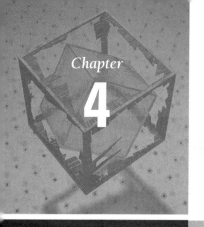

Chapter 4

Biostatistics Concepts—The Building Blocks for Evaluating Biostatistical Methods in Clinical Research

After studying this chapter, the student should be able to:

1. Appreciate the many different ways that numbers are used to convey information.

2. Recognize the different properties of variables.

3. Calculate measures of central tendency, dispersion, and shape.

4. Integrate basic descriptive measures to describe the shape of distributions.

Inevitably, authors of scientific articles use numbers. In a typical research article numbers may be used to suggest the magnitude of the problem under study (e.g., the number of people afflicted by a disease or the economic costs of a disease), to describe the methods used to address the problem (e.g., the number of patients studied, the drug regimen used), and to communicate the findings and implications of the study results (e.g., the outcomes of the statistical tests). In the clinical realm, pharmacists and other healthcare providers use numbers in various ways to describe patient attributes, as in the following case example.

Case Example 4-1

CHIEF PATIENT COMPLAINT

I'd like to cut down on my blood pressure (BP) medications if that's okay because, lately, I've felt off balance. Yesterday I was dizzy when I stood up after watching a movie.

HISTORY OF PRESENT ILLNESS

LT is a 65-year-old white female who presents to the pharmacy clinic for follow-up. Patient was first diagnosed with hypertension (HTN) approximately 1 year ago (BP 154/98 and 160/96 on two separate occasions). Lisinopril 5 mg/day was started after 3 months of lifestyle changes did not decrease BP to goal. Nisoldipine 10 mg/day was then added 2 months ago as BP remained above goal while on lisinopril 5 mg/day (BP was 136/90).

PAST MEDICAL HISTORY

Diabetes mellitus type 2
Hypertension
Hyperlipidemia

MEDICATIONS

Nisoldipine 10 mg daily (started 2 months ago)
Lisinopril 5 mg daily (started 9 months ago)
Aspirin (ASA) 81 mg daily (started 5 years ago)
Metformin 1000 mg b.i.d. (started 4 years ago)
Glyburide 5 mg b.i.d. (started 2 years ago)
Lipitor 20 mg h.s. (started 3 years ago)

SOCIAL HISTORY

Lives with husband. Denies alcohol or illegal substances. States that she quit smoking 10 years ago. Tries to follow an American Diabetes Association–recommended diet but sometimes has a weakness for cookies and chocolate. Goes to a gym 3 times weekly for 30-min intervals.

FAMILY HISTORY

Parents died of natural causes in their 80s. Has 1 sister with diabetes.

ALLERGIES

Sulfa (rash)

VITALS

Respiratory rate: 20 breaths/min
Weight: 145 lb
Height: 64 in.
Temperature: 36.2 °C
Sitting blood pressure = 98/62; pulse = 72
Standing blood pressure = 86/60; pulse = 78

REVIEW OF SYMPTOMS

Dizziness upon standing in clinic, no other current complaints

PHYSICAL EXAMINATION

General: overweight female in no apparent distress   [AU1]
Head, ears, eyes, nose, throat (HEENT): unremarkable
Neck: no jugular venous distention (JVD), bruits, or masses
Lungs: clear to auscultation
Neuro: alert and oriented $\times$ 3; cranial nerves intact
Cardiovascular: normal S_1 and S_2; no m/r/g
Extermities: no edema, redness

LABORATORY

Aspartate aminotransferase (AST): 11 U/L
Alanine aminotransferase (ALT): 19 U/L
Hemoglobin A_{1c}: 7.2%

Low-density lipoprotein (LDL): 95 mg/dL
Total cholesterol (TC): 175 mg/dL
Triglycerides (TG): 100 mg/dL
High-density lipoprotein (HDL): 60 mg/dL
Chem-7
Glucose: 130 mg/dL
  Serum chloride: 101 mmol/L
  Blood urea nitrogen (BUN): 10 mg/dL
  Serum sodium: 154 mEq/L
  Serum potassium: 3.7 mEq/L
  Carbon dioxide (CO_2): 24 mmol/L
  Creatinine: 1.1 mg/dL
Urinalysis (UA): 1+ protein
Ejection fraction (EF): 60%

HOME BLOOD SUGAR READINGS

A.M. (fasting): average of 120; range of 72 to 140 mg/dL
P.M. (preprandial): average of 130; range of 88 to 155 mg/dL
h.s.: high of 200; low of 132 mg/dL

To make the clinical decision concerning the dosage of this patient's blood pressure medication, the pharmacist needs to evaluate the correspondence between the evidence provided by the medical literature and the particular circumstances of the patient. For example, the pharmacist must consult the medical literature to determine morbidity and mortality risks associated with the discontinuation of nisoldipine in patients similar to this one. Only with such evidence can the pharmacist make a rational, effective, and defensible recommendation regarding patient therapy.

Evaluating medical literature and understanding a patient's situation require an appreciation of numbers. Indeed, the language of contemporary healthcare practice is numbers. The goal of this chapter is to describe the different ways that numbers are used to convey information. Methods used to summarize and group numbers are discussed. The chapter begins by providing a context for understanding basic concepts.

Numbers are critical to effective evidence-based health care decision making, and inherent in the use of numbers is *variability*. Differences arise in the diagnosis of patients; laboratory values not only differ among similar patients but change with repeated assessments of the same sample; treatment regimens differ in the time of administration. Statistics is the science of classifying, measuring, analyzing, and interpreting information in the face of variability and uncertainty. **Biostatistics** is the application of the principles and methods of statistics to healthcare data.

Biostatistics can be used in two different ways. One application is to describe the major features of a set of data. For example, a pharmacist might use **descriptive statistics** to explore the demographic composition of patients with diabetes who visit the clinic. Such descriptive statistics include the average age of the patients, the proportion of women, and the severity of the disease. Notice that descriptive statistics are used only to summarize and characterize information from the group at hand.

In contrast, a research pharmacist might be studying the efficacy of a novel drug for diabetic patients. In this case, the pharmacist is primarily interested in generalizing the results of an experiment to all patients with diabetes. Generalizing the findings from a small subset of patients to all similar patients is an example of **inferential statistics**. In this process, a statistical test is used to determine the extent to which differences between the treatment and the control groups may have been the result of chance. This statistical test uses numbers derived from the data, such as averages and frequencies.

The chapter provides basic information about numbers, including the ways numbers are used to convey information and the ways in which numbers can be clustered into distributions. A major portion of the chapter deals with descriptive statistics—that is, with techniques that can be used to convey the salient features of data sets. Chapter 5 continues this discussion by building on the principles described here to explain how data from a subset of a population can be used to characterize the entire population.

Properties of Variables

Numbers are used in a bewildering variety of ways. In Case Example 4-1, numbers were used to indicate the age of the patient, pretreatment and post-treatment blood pressure levels, doses of the drugs, duration of treatment, and indices of a healthy lifestyle. However, numbers have only one function: to specify that the objects being measured are different in a qualitative or a quantitative way. That is, numbers are used to designate different values that a variable might take on.

A **variable** is a characteristic of an entity that can assume different values. For example, take the variable *gender*: a person is assigned either to the category *male* or to the category *female*. When determining compliance with a drug regimen, the pharmacist may count the number pills returned by a patient. The severity of postoperative pain may be determined by having the patient rank pain intensity on a 10-point scale. Finally, some aspect of the entity, say bone mineral density, may be assessed as part of an examination of osteoarthritis.

Thus variables are used to *categorize, count, rank*, or *measure* some aspect of a person or thing. Variables differ in other ways. Categorical variables, like hair color, differentiate objects by *type* and are termed **qualitative variables.** Counting, ranking, and measurement variables, in contrast, represent differences in *amount* and are termed **quantitative variables.** Another difference is that the values or levels of some variables can be expressed only in whole numbers, such as counts and ranks. These are termed **discrete variables.** Other variables, called **continuous variables,** involve measurements, such as lipid levels, that may assume many different values.

When used to designate persons by type, variables are categorical, qualitative, and discrete. The distinction between male and female is used only to differentiate one type of patient from another. Often, different levels of the gender variable may be coded by assigning males a value of 0 and females a value of 1. Note that the quantitative value of the number is meaningless: 1 is not better or worse than zero, it simply shows that a person is of a specific type. This is an example of a **nominal scale of measurement.**

Numbers may also be used to indicate differences in quality and quantity, but still be discrete. Suppose a person is asked to rank his or her 10 favorite movies, with 1 indicating the most preferred film. There is little doubt that the film receiving the rank of 1 is most preferred, and that with a rank of 2 is less preferred. However, the difference in preference between films 1 and 2 may not be the same as the difference in preference between films 9 and 10. The **ordinal scale of measurement** is used to indicate such differences in rank. Ordinal scale variables have wide application in healthcare research. For example, a visual-analog scale (VAS) may be used to assess differences in postoperative pain intensity by having the patient indicate the pain level on a scale of 1 to 10.

Another type of ordinal measurement is a **Likert scale.** While Likert scales are used frequently to obtain self-reports from patients, they are also used by clinicians to rate signs

TABLE 4-1	Brief Psychiatric Rating Scale	
MEASURE	**POINTS**	
Not present	1	
Very mild	2	
Mild	3	
Moderate	4	
Moderate to severe	5	
Severe	6	
Extremely severe	7	

Adapted with permission from Overall JE, Gorham DR. The Brief Psychiatric Rating Scale. Psychol Rep. 1962;10:799–812.

and symptoms. Table 4-1 is an example of a Likert rating scale, the Brief Psychiatric Rating Scale (BPRS), which is used to quantify 16 signs and symptoms such as level of anxiety, hostility, depressive mood, and hallucinatory behavior on a 7-point scale. The scores for each area are then summed and interpreted. In the BPRS, the lowest possible score is 16, the highest possible score is 112. Higher scores indicate a more severe psychiatric disorder.

Variables may also indicate differences in quantity. One major use of quantitative variables is to express differences in the frequency of an event, such as the incidence of acute myocardial infarction. The use of variables to count events is an example of a quantitative, discrete variable.

Quantitative variables may also be expressed along a **continuous scale of measurement**. Variables measured on continuous scales can exhibit a wide range of values that depend only on the resolving power of the measuring device. It is possible, for example, given a sensitive enough measuring instrument, body weight can be determined to many decimal places.

One characteristic of continuous measurement scales is that the intervals between adjacent levels represent equal quantities across the entire measurement range. For example, the same amount of heat is required to increase the temperature of distilled water by 1 °C whether the change is from 10° to 11° or from 100° to 101°. The Celsius temperature scale is an example of an **interval scale of measurement**.

The fourth scale of measurement, the **ratio scale of measurement**, also displays equal intervals between adjacent levels of the variable. However, it possesses two characteristics that differentiate it from the interval scale. First, its 0 value indicates a true null quantity for the variable. Thus a drug level of 0 indicates an absence of drug activity, but 0 °C does not indicate an absence of heat. Second, the ratio of two values in a ratio scale is meaningful: 100 mg of a substance is twice as much as 50 mg, but 100 °C is not twice as hot as 50 °C.

In addition to the scale of measurement, variables may differ by being fixed or random. A **fixed variable** is one whose levels are deliberately selected by the investigator. These are commonly independent variables. In studies of drug efficacy, for example, only two or three doses of the drug are studied, not all possible doses. A **random variable**, in contrast, is one whose value cannot be determined with certainty before its actual measurement. These are commonly dependent variables. For example, a person's blood pressure cannot be known with certainty until it is measured. Remember, however, that random does not mean that the variables were chosen haphazardly and without care or are the result of chaos.

Distributions of Numbers

Grouping numbers is an efficient way to convey information about a variable. **Distributions** of numbers are arrangements of data in a manner that makes it easy for an observer to grasp its meaning. Two ways of arranging data are the ordered array and frequency distributions.

An **ordered array** is an arrangement of individual values of a dependent variable in ascending order. Table 4-2 presents an ordered array of t_{max} values from 14 patients who received a dose of a drug. Note that the value for each participant is presented, even if values are duplicated. Examination of the array suggests that it is easy to find the lowest and highest values of t_{max}, but discerning other characteristics of the data set is more difficult.

Ordered arrays are informative when there are few patients and the values of the variable under study show little duplication. Ordered arrays, however, are cumbersome if large numbers of patients are studied or if many patients display the same value of the dependent variable. In these cases, a frequency distribution is preferred.

A **frequency distribution** is a way of organizing data by combining adjacent numbers into class intervals and indicating the number of cases included in each interval. Table 4-3 presents a frequency distribution of the ordered array given in Table 4-2 using 0.5-hr class intervals. Notice that presenting data in a frequency distribution makes it easier to visualize that the most frequent t_{max} was between 1.5 and 1.9 hr, but the exact value might be a little as 1.0 hr or as many as 2.9 hr.

Notice these other characteristics of the frequency distribution:

- Intervals are arranged in ascending order, with no overlapping values.
- The lower limit of the first interval is equal to or less than the smallest value.
- The upper limit of the last interval is equal to or greater than the largest value.
- Class intervals are all the same size; intervals in the extremes of the distribution are not combined.

TABLE 4-2	Ordered Array of t_{max} Values from 14 Patients Who Received a Hypothetical Drug
PATIENT CODE	t_{max} (HR)
1	1.2
2	1.3
3	1.4
4	1.5
5	1.6
6	1.6
7	1.7
8	1.8
9	1.9
10	2.3
11	2.4
12	2.6
13	2.8
14	3.2

TABLE 4-3	A Frequency Distribution of the Data Presented in Table 4-2
t_{max} (HR)	FREQUENCY
1.0–1.4	3
1.5–1.9	6
2.0–2.4	2
2.5–2.9	2
3.0–3.4	1

Two other ways of presenting frequency data are the **relative frequency distribution** and the **cumulative frequency distribution.** A relative frequency distribution displays the proportion (rather than the number) of the total values falling within each class interval. A cumulative frequency distribution displays the sum of the relative frequencies of the present and all previous intervals. Table 4-4 presents the relative and cumulative frequency distributions of the ordered array given in Table 4-2.

The relative frequency distribution reveals the proportion of patients falling into each of the categories. It is easy to see, for example, that 0.429 (~43%) of the patients displayed a t_{max} between 1.5 and 1.9 hr. The information provided by the cumulative frequency distribution shows that about 0.79 (79%) of the patients reached t_{max} within 2.4 hr of drug administration.

In addition to presenting data in tables, it is often effective to display data graphically. **Frequency charts** depict the dependent variable on the ordinate (or y axis) and the independent variable on the abscissa (or x axis). A frequency chart of the t_{max} data from Table 4-3 is presented in Figure 4-1. In addition to the number of individuals appearing in each class interval, frequency charts provide an idea of the shape of the distribution of scores. In Figure 4-1, for example, it seems that most t_{max} values occur within first 1.9 hr of drug administration, and then decline slowly.

Charts may also be used to display relative and cumulative frequency data (Figs. 4-2 and 4-3). Notice that the shapes of the frequency and the relative frequency charts are the same, yet each chart emphasizes a different aspect of the data. It is easy to determine the contribution of each class interval to the total result with a relative frequency chart.

TABLE 4-4	Frequency, Relative Frequency, and Cumulative Frequency Distributions of the Data Presented in Table 4-2		
t_{max} (HR)	FREQUENCY	RELATIVE FREQUENCY[a]	CUMULATIVE FREQUENCY[b]
1.0–1.4	3	0.214	0.214
1.5–1.9	6	0.429	0.643
2.0–2.4	2	0.143	0.786
2.5–2.9	2	0.143	0.929
3.0–3.4	1	0.071	1.000
Total	14	1.000	

[a]Relative frequencies are calculated as the number of patients in each class interval divided by the total number of patients.

[b]Cumulative frequencies are the sums of all frequencies up to and including the designated class interval. Thus the cumulative frequency of scores for the class interval 2.0–2.4 is the sum of relative frequencies from lower class intervals, including the current class interval.

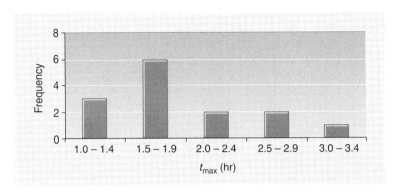

FIGURE 4-1 Frequency Chart. Data from Table 4-4; $n = 14$.

This is because a distinctive feature of the relative frequency distribution is that the sum of the relative frequencies is equal to 1.0. Thus the area under the curve (AUC) of a relative frequency distribution is equal to 1.0. As a consequence, the relative frequency of any class interval (or combination of class intervals) is a proportion of the total AUC. In Figure 4-2, scores in the interval 1.5–1.9 represent about 43% (0.43) of the total number of t_{max} values.

 EXTRA CREDIT 4-1

One additional chart used often in healthcare is the **Pareto diagram.** *This diagram combines a relative frequency chart with a cumulative frequency chart. It is used to express the comparative contribution of individual components to the total.*

For example, suppose a pharmacist, wishing to identify the major factors contributing to the loyalty of her customers, obtained the data in Table 4-5. The table suggests that pharmacist counseling services and the friendly staff are major contributors to customer loyalty but does not suggest the relative contributions of each of the factors to the total effect. Such an expression, however, can be achieved with a Pareto diagram (Fig. 4-4).

To construct a Pareto diagram, both the relative and the cumulative frequencies of each factor are plotted on the same graph. On the left, or y, coordinate are plotted the relative frequencies of each factor. Note that the factors are arranged on the abscissa in descending order

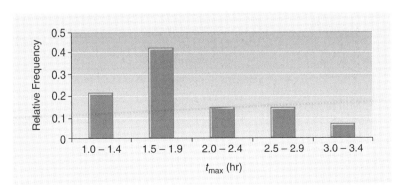

FIGURE 4-2 Relative Frequency Chart. Data from Table 4-4; $n = 14$.

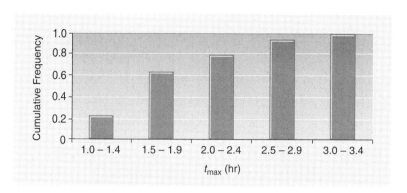

FIGURE 4-3 Cumulative Frequency Chart. Data from Table 4-4; $n = 14$.

of relative frequency: The factor with the greatest relative frequency is first, and the factor with the least relative frequency is last. The cumulative frequency is then plotted on the right, or z, coordinate.

A Pareto diagram depicts not only the portion of the total effect attributable to each factor but also indicates the sum of relative frequencies for the factors that make the greatest contribution. In this application, it suggests that 80% of customer satisfaction is the result of three factors: pharmacist counseling, friendly staff, and speed of prescription fulfillment.

Armed with this information, the pharmacist can either build loyalty by strengthening the first three factors or increase loyalty by addressing the remaining issues: pricing of over-the-counter (OTC) and prescription drugs and the availability of herbal products.

Describing Data

As the amount of information becomes large, listing and arranging the numbers in intervals may not provide a summary of the data set that is easy to comprehend. Because of this, large data sets are described by three factors:

- An index of the center of the distribution of scores, called a **measure of central tendency**
- An index of the variability of the scores in the distribution, called a **measure of dispersion**
- An idea of the shape of the distribution of scores, called **indices of shape**

TABLE 4-5	Relative Frequency Distribution of Factors Affecting Customer Loyalty
CUSTOMER LOYALTY FACTORS	**RELATIVE FREQUENCY**
Friendly staff	0.27
Herbal Products	0.08
Pharmacist consulting	0.31
Prescription drug pricing	0.04
Price of OTC products	0.12
Speed of order fulfillment	0.19

OTC, over the counter.

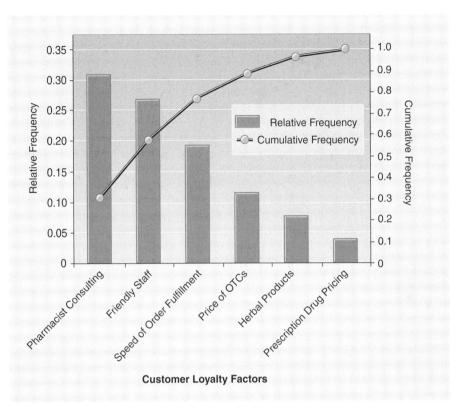

FIGURE 4-4 Pareto Diagram of Factors Affecting Customer Loyalty. By plotting the relative frequency, in descending order, and the cumulative frequency an analyst can determine not only the contribution of the major factors but their relative contribution to the total outcome. *OTCs*, over-the-counter products.

MEASURES OF CENTRAL TENDENCY

Measures of the center of a distribution are termed measures of central tendency and include the arithmetic mean, the median, and the mode. The **arithmetic mean**, or the average, is the sum of all scores divided by the number of scores. The formula for the mean is

$$\bar{y} = \frac{\sum y_i}{n}$$

The equation indicates that the mean ($\bar{y}$) is equal to the sum ($\sum$) of each individual score (y_i) divided by the total number of scores, n. For example, the mean t_{max} for the set of scores in Table 4-2 is calculated as follows.

$$\frac{(1.2 + 1.3 + 1.4...2.6 + 2.8 + 3.2)}{14} = \frac{27.3}{14} = 1.95 \text{ hr}$$

That is, the sum of the t_{max} values for all patients equals 27.3 hr. Because there are 14 patients, n equals 14. Dividing 27.3 hr by 14 patients yields a mean of 1.95 hr.

The arithmetic mean (or simply the mean) is used quite often as a measure of central tendency for interval and ratio data because it is *unique*, there is only one mean per data set, it is *simple* to compute and to understand, and it uses all the numbers in the data set.

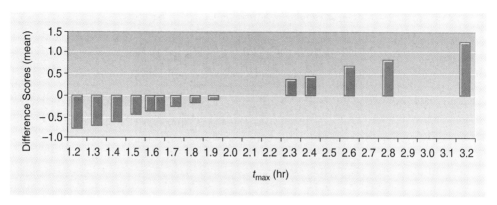

FIGURE 4-5 Group mean vs. individual t_{max} values. Notice that the mean of a set of scores (here, 1.95 hr) is the balance point of that set of scores. Data from Table 4-2.

The mean is often considered to be the "balance point" of a data set, in the sense that the sum of the deviation scores about the mean is zero. Mathematically,

$$\sum (y_i - \bar{y}) = \o$$

This equation indicates that the differences between each patient's score (y_i) and the group mean ($\bar{y}$), when summed over all the patients' scores, will equal zero. The difference scores for the data in Table 4-2 are presented in Figure 4-5.

One difficulty with the mean is that it may be affected disproportionately by extreme values. For example, in the data set 1, 3, 5, 7, 9 the mean is calculated to be 5. If the data set were 1, 3, 5, 7, 29, the mean value would be 9. When such extreme scores are encountered, the **median** is used to indicate the middle value of the data set. The median is the middle score of the data set. It is often applied to ordinal data. To find the median, the scores in the data set are first ranked or ordered. Then the number of scores plus 1 is divided by 2. This dividend indicates the rank of the score that is the median. If n is an even number, the dividend will not be an integer, and the median is calculated as the average of the two adjacent middle scores.

Returning again to Table 4-2, we find that $n = 14$, so the median score is the average of the values of the 7th and 8th scores. These scores equal 1.7 and 1.8 hr, respectively. So the median of the data set is 1.75 hr.

Like the mean, there is only one median per data set, its calculation is simple and uses all numbers in the data set. Unlike the mean, however, the median is not affected by extreme scores. Referring to our example, the average t_{max} was 1.95 hr, and the median is 1.75 hr. This difference arises because the value of the mean is affected by the few long intervals to attain t_{max}, but the median is not.

The **mode** is the most frequent score in a data set. It is often used to characterize nominal data. Although the mode is simple to compute, it is not unique because a data set may have more than one mode. The presence of such a bimodal or multimodal distribution usually indicates that an underlying variable, not accounted for at present, is affecting the data. For example, a frequency distribution of the combined heights of adult men and women is characterized typically by two modes.

MEASURES OF DISPERSION

Indices of the spread of scores around the measure of central tendency include the range, the variance, the standard deviation, and the coefficient of variation.

The **range** is the *difference* between the largest and smallest scores in the data set. Therefore, the range, although it is unique and simple to compute, uses only two numbers in the data set. In Table 4-2, the range is 3.2 − 1.2, or 2.0. It should be evident that the range is affected by extreme values.

The **variance** and the **standard deviation** are related in that the standard deviation is the square root of the variance. The variance may be defined as the average of the squared difference scores in a data set. This is the formula:

$$\text{variance } s^2 = \frac{[\Sigma(y_i - \bar{y})^2]}{(n - 1)}$$

$$\text{standard deviation} = s = \sqrt{s^2}$$

To calculate a variance (s^2), the difference score (equal to $y_i - \bar{y}$) is first detemined for each individual score (y_i). These difference scores are then squared, and the sum of these squared difference scores is obtained. (The difference scores must be squared because the sum of a set of difference scores about its mean is always zero.) This sum of the squared difference scores is divided by the number of scores (n) minus 1. The computation of the s^2 of the t_{max} scores in Table 4-2 is presented in Table 4-6. The standard deviation is abbreviated s, and is calculated as the square root of the variance.

Notice that the sum of the deviation scores is divided by one less than the total number of scores in the sample. This number of scores, $n − 1$, is called the degrees of freedom, and abbreviated *df*. More formally, **degrees of freedom** refers to the number of scores in a sample that may assume more than one value in the calculation of a statistic. For example, a pharmacist is given a list of 5 patients who have volunteered to be screened for hypertension and is asked to assign each patient to 1 of 5 examination rooms. The first patient

TABLE 4-6	Calculation of Variance for Data in Table 4-2		
PATIENT NUMBER	t_{max} **(HR)**	$(Y_I - \bar{Y})$	$(Y_I - \bar{Y})^2$
1	1.2	−0.75	0.5625
2	1.3	−0.65	0.4225
3	1.4	−0.55	0.3025
4	1.5	−0.45	0.2025
5	1.6	−0.35	0.1225
6	1.6	−0.35	0.1225
7	1.7	−0.25	0.0625
8	1.8	−0.15	0.0225
9	1.9	−0.05	0.0025
10	2.3	0.35	0.1225
11	2.4	0.45	0.2025
12	2.6	0.65	0.4225
13	2.8	0.85	0.7225
14	3.2	1.25	1.5625
Sum	$\Sigma y_i = 27.3$	$\Sigma(y_i - \bar{y}) = 0$	$\Sigma(y_i - \bar{y})^2 = 4.855$
Variance = 4.855 ÷ (14 − 1) = 0.373			

may be assigned to any of the 5 rooms, but the second patient can be assigned to only one of the 4 remaining unoccupied rooms. As the process continues, the pharmacist discovers he has no choice: the 5th patient must be assigned to the last unoccupied examination room. Therefore, the pharmacist is able to assign only 4 of the 5 patients to more than one examination room, so the degrees of freedom in this example are equal to $n - 1$; in this case, $5 - 1 = 4$.

In the calculation of s^2 for the t_{max} values, all the scores in the data set but one are free to vary. The value of the last number is determined by the constraint that the sum of the deviation scores equals 0. Hence there are $14 - 1 = 13$ degrees of freedom.

A unique index of variability is the **coefficient of variation** (*CV*), which is a measure of *relative* variability in a data set. The *CV* is calculated by dividing the standard deviation by the absolute value of the mean and multiplying this value by 100. The coefficient of variation is thus the variability of the data set expressed as a percent of the mean.

$$CV = \left(\frac{s}{\bar{y}}\right) \times 100$$

Although the coefficient of variation is not often encountered in published literature, it is a handy statistic for those versed in evidence-based medicine. This is because the *CV* can be used as an index of the consistency of an effect or the precision of a result. Here is an example, albeit a theoretical one. Consider two studies of the effects of statins on low-density lipoprotein (LDL). Results from both studies indicate a decrease in average LDL levels of 20 mg/dL. Was the drug effect comparable in both studies? To find out, compute the *CV*. From the published tables we can estimate that the standard deviation of the data in the first study was 5 mg/dL and that in the second study was 10 mg/dL. The *CV* for the change in LDL levels in the first study is thus $(5/20 \times 100) = 25\%$ and that for the second study is $(10/20 \times 100) = 50\%$. This finding suggests that although the average response to the statin was similar in both groups, the variability in the second group was twice that in the first group.

In addition to comparing the results of two studies using the same variable, the *CV* can be used to examine differences in the same variable studied under two measurement scales and to examine the comparability of several estimates of theoretical values.

Indices of Shape

The third feature of interest in characterizing a data set is its *shape*. It is not surprising that measures of central tendency and dispersion can be used to convey indices of shape. Two common ways of conveying the shape of a data set are the box plot and the normal distribution.

BOX PLOTS

A **box plot** is a graphical display that divides a data set into four parts so that each part contains 25% of the total sample in the data set. These divisions are achieved using the median and two other values termed **quartiles.** The *first quartile* delimits the bottom 25% of the data set, and the *fourth quartile* delimits the top 25% of the data set.

The first and fourth quartiles are calculated in a manner similar to the median, which is the *second quartile.* As with the median, the first step in finding a quartile is to arrange the numbers in an ordered array. Then

- The first quartile (Q_1) is determined to be the number associated with a rank equal to the number of scores $n + 1$ multiplied by 0.25. The interval between the smallest value in the data set and this number contains the lowest 25% of the data set values. For the data in Table 4-2, the first quartile is the $(14 + 1) \times 0.25$ or 3.75th score. So the 3rd and 4th scores are averaged, making the value of the first quartile 1.45.

- The second quartile (Q_2) is calculated as the number of scores $n + 1$ multiplied by 0.50. This is the median: half of the scores lie below this value, and half of the scores lie above this value. The median for the data in Table 4-2 was determined earlier to be 1.75.
- The third quartile (Q_3) is calculated as the number of scores $n + 1$ multiplied by 0.75, which for our example is the average of the 11th and 12th scores. It is equal to 2.50.
- The fourth quartile (Q_4) is the interval between the value of the third quartile and the highest value in the ordered array.

Figure 4-6 presents the box plot of the data from Table 4-2. The central area of the diagram, delineated by the box, contains the middle 50% of the scores, and is termed the **interquartile range (IQR)**. The lower bound of the IQR is the first quartile, and the upper bound is the third quartile. The median bisects the IQR. Lines extending below the first quartile and above the third quartile indicate the extent of these segments, respectively.

Fences are limits that define acceptable values from **outliers**. Outliers are values that are so different from the remaining numbers in the data set that they raise doubt as to whether they belong to the data set. The lower fence is set to exclude values that are less than a specified criterion, which equals the value of the first quartile minus 1.5 times the IQR. Similarly, the upper fence is set to exclude values that exceed the value of the third quartile plus 1.5 times the IQR. The lower and upper fences for the data in Table 4-2 are 0 and 4.10, respectively.

The shape of the box plot conveys much information about a data set. An examination of the box plot in Figure 4-6 suggests the following:

- Because the median is not located in the middle of the IQR, the distribution of scores is not symmetric about the median.

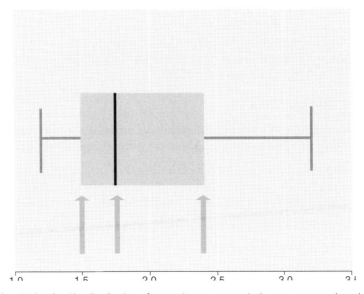

FIGURE 4-6 Box Plot. Notice that the distribution of scores is not symmetrical; scores greater than the median are more spread out than scores less than the median. T_{max} values are on the abscissa. Q_1 through Q_4 indicate the four quartiles. Interquartile range (IQR) is delineated by the box. Median is heavy line bisecting IQR. Lines extending from sides of box indicate the first and fourth quartiles. Data from Table 4-2.

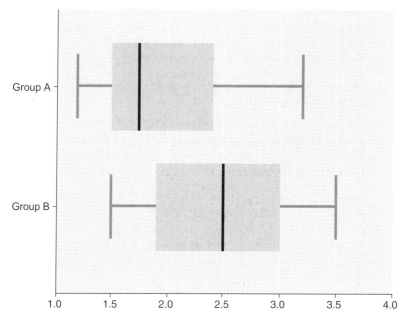

FIGURE 4-7 Box Plots: Comparing Two Data Sets. Although the range of scores is rather similar, the group B scores are distributed more symmetrically about the median. In addition, although the distribution of scores overlap, more than half of the group B scores fall in the uppermost quadrant of the group A scores. Group A data from Table 4-2.

- More evidence of the asymmetry of the data set scores is derived from the observation that the line depicting the extent of Q_1 is shorter than the line depicting the length of Q_4.
- The scores in Q_2 are closer together than the scores in any other quadrant.

Box plots can also be used to identify differences between data sets. Figure 4-7 presents the t_{max} values for two groups, A and B. Group A contains the data from Table 4-2, and Group B is made up of data from another patient group. Both sets of scores display a similar range and show many overlapping values. Further examination suggests, however, that three-quarters of group B scores exceed the median of group A scores. Furthermore, group B scores are distributed more symmetrically.

NORMAL DISTRIBUTION

For many continuous variables, a **normal distribution** is used to convey the shape of the data set. This is the familiar bell-shaped curve, which displays two characteristics:

- The mean of the variables designates the center of the distribution, bisecting the distribution into two parts, each containing 50% of the scores in the data set.
- The standard deviation is used to indicate the variability of scores about the mean.

Because of these two properties, the following relationships hold:

- About 68% of the scores in the data set lie in an interval from $\bar{y} - (1 \times s)$ to $\bar{y} + (1 \times s)$.
- About 95% of the scores in the data set lie in an interval from $\bar{y} - (2 \times s)$ to $\bar{y} + (2 \times s)$.
- About 99.7% of the scores in the data set lie in an interval from $\bar{y} - (3 \times s)$ to $\bar{y} + (3 \times s)$.

The normal distribution shown in Figure 4-8 demonstrates these relationships. In this characterization, Greek letters are used to designate the mean (μ) and the standard deviation (σ). This is a convention to indicate that the distribution represents the relative

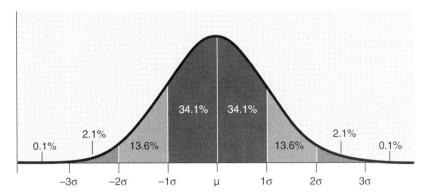

FIGURE 4-8 Normal Distribution. In a normal distribution, the areas under the curve are symmetric about the mean (μ). For example, 68.2% of the total area is within 1 standard deviation (σ) of the mean, and 95.4% of the total area is within 2 σ of the mean.

frequencies of all possible members of a group and thus constitutes a **population**. In reality, assessing a characteristic of all members of a population is impossible. As a result, data are obtained from a subset or **sample** drawn from the population, and the **parameters** of the population (e.g., μ and σ) are estimated by the statistics calculated from the samples (e.g., $\bar{y}$ and s).

It is important to emphasize that the relationships between the percentage of numbers in the data set and the interval described by the mean and standard deviation are valid for *any* variable that is normally distributed. As such, they provide the foundation for many applications of statistics encountered in the healthcare literature.

Summary

Numbers are the foundation of evidence-based medicine. Understanding the nature and application of numbers is of paramount importance for the practicing pharmacist. Individual values of a variable are important because they provide information unique to an individual patient. However, diagnosis and treatment of the individual patient are often facilitated by knowledge of similar cases. The role of statistics is to provide this information. This chapter presents an overview of descriptive statistics. Chapter 5 builds on this to explain inferential statistics.

STUDY PROBLEMS

1. Select 10 of your classmates and collect demographic information from them (height, body weight, hair color, age, etc.). Determine the scale of measurement for each variable. Draw frequency distributions of several of the variables and compute the measures of central tendency, dispersion, and shape.

2. The following table contains information about the sales of herbal products for one week at an independent pharmacy. Construct Pareto diagrams to determine which herbal products accounted for 80% of the total sales and which herbal products accounted for the top 20% of total units sold that week.

HERBAL PRODUCT	SALES	UNITS
Aristolochia	$1,410.00	300
Cynarol	$3,565.10	333
Echinacea	$3,130.20	666
Ephedra	$2,707.20	576
Kava kava	$4,215.90	897
St. John's wort	$4,694.20	786

3. In a recent paper, Jacobson et al.[1] reported on the association of body mass and symptoms of gastroesophageal reflux in women. Women claiming frequent bouts of gastroesophageal reflux exhibited an average body mass index of 27.8 kg/m^2 with a standard deviation of 5.3. Women without gastroesophageal reflux exhibited an average body mass index of 25.6 $kg.m^2$ with a standard deviation of 5.0. Assuming that these distributions are normal, use your knowledge of the relationship of the mean and standard deviation to the shape of the distribution to generate normal curves. How much overlap is there between the values in the two groups?

REFERENCE

1.   Jacobson BC, Somers SC, Fuchs CS, et al. Body-mass index and symptoms of gastroesophageal reflux in women. N Engl J Med 2006;354:2340–2348.

Foundations of Statistical Inference

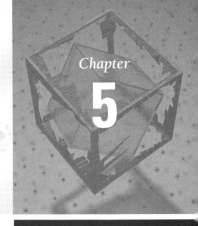

After studying this chapter, the student should be able to:

1. Describe the fundamentals of probability.

2. Comprehend the rationale for screening tests and the use of measures derived from them.

3. Describe the important properties of probability distributions.

4. Understand the significance of the central limit theorem for statistical inference.

5. Describe the role and significance of confidence intervals in published literature.

6. Understand the rationale and principles of hypothesis testing and be able to compute and interpret a *t* test.

In Chapter 4, numbers were used to characterize the major features of data sets using measures of central tendency, dispersion, and shape. A pharmacist, for example, might use such **descriptive statistics** to characterize factors affecting polypharmacy among his or her patients or clients. Another application of statistics is to extend the findings from a small group of individuals to all similar individuals. In this circumstance, the pharmacist may wish to generalize the factors affecting polypharmacy among his or her patients or clients to all patients and clients in similar healthcare settings. This use of statistics—to generalize to a population the characteristics of a subset drawn from that population—is termed inferential statistics, or statistical inference, and is the topic of this chapter.

A **population** is the set of all observations of interest. For example, a population may consist of bone mineral density determinations of all women diagnosed with osteoarthritis. A population is considered to be a very large or infinite set of observations. Characteristics of a population, such as measures of central tendency and dispersion, are termed **parameters**. Population parameters are assumed to be constants and are symbolized using Greek letters, such as μ (mu) for the mean of the population, σ (sigma) for its standard deviation, and N (nu) for the number of values in the population.

A **sample** is a subset of a population. So, for example, a researcher may obtain bone mineral density observations from a subset of patients who have osteoarthritis. Characteristics of a sample, such as measures of central tendency and dispersion, are termed statistics and are symbolized using English letters, such as $\bar{y}$, s, and n. The size of the sample is envisioned to be very small compared to the size of the population. Consequently, membership of various samples drawn from the population will differ, as will the statistics computed from them. Thus statistics provide only approximations of population parameters. The discrepancy between the value of the statistic and that of the population parameter is termed **sampling error.** Sampling error is the result of chance.

Statistical inference may be used in three different ways. **Statistical estimation** is the use of a sample statistic to characterize a population parameter. Thus an epidemiologist may use statistics from a sample of patients to estimate the prevalence of adverse drug reactions among children who have asthma. Another application of statistical inference is **hypothesis testing**, in which statistics from two or more samples are compared to ascertain whether the corresponding population parameters differ. This application has wide application in healthcare as part of the decision-making process regarding the safety and efficacy of a drug. The third use of statistical inference is **statistical modeling**. This technique uses mathematical formulas to describe relationships among variables or to control for the effects of potentially confounding variables. For example, in a study of the relationship between physical activity and the risk of breast cancer, a statistical model was used to control for the confounding effects of variables such as age, body weight, and the use of hormones.[1]

These applications of statistical inference depend on a statistical theory. This theory provides both the rationale and the rules governing the appropriate use of these methods. The goal of this chapter is to describe the basis and applications of this theory because it is a major component of the foundation of evidence-based medicine.

The chapter begins by exploring the properties of sampling error, the variability in statistics computed from different samples as a result of chance. First, the basic principles of probability are described as a prelude to introducing the topic of probability distributions. Probability distributions provide a way to use mathematics to associate a probability of occurrence with every possible outcome of an event. Next, these principles are extended to probability distributions of statistics, termed *sampling distributions*. Sampling distributions possess several unique attributes that are fundamental to the theory of statistical inference. Finally, the principles developed in this chapter are used to estimate population parameters from sample statistics and to test statistical hypotheses.

Probability

Measurement invariably involves variability. Patients participating in a study of the efficacy of a novel pain-relief medication will report different levels of analgesia and different combinations of side effects. The assumption in statistics is that these errors are random— that is, they are caused by chance variation. By *chance* is meant that the different values are unpredictable and are not the result of a systematic bias. The principles of probability can be used to provide an idea of the role of chance in the results of an experiment.

One approach to the principles of probability builds on knowledge of the relative frequency distribution. Recall that a relative frequency distribution indicates the proportional contribution of each outcome to the total of all possible outcomes. Refer again to the t_{max} data originally presented Chapter 4 and reprinted here in Table 5-1. The relative frequency of the interval 1.5–1.9 hr is 0.429, indicating that t_{max} values within this interval occurred among almost 43% of the patients sampled. In the sample so constituted, the relative frequencies of all possible outcomes have been tabulated so that the sum of all the relative frequencies is 1. Because of this, the relative frequency of any single interval also describes its probability of occurrence. For example, if a patient is selected at random from this sample, the probability that the patient displays a t_{max} value between 1.5 and 1.9 hr is 0.429.

TABLE 5-1	Frequency, Relative Frequency and Cumulative Frequency Distributions of t_{max} Data from 14 Patients[a]		
t_{max} (HR)	FREQUENCY	RELATIVE FREQUENCY[a]	CUMULATIVE FREQUENCY[b]
1.0–1.4	3	0.214	0.214
1.5–1.9	6	0.429	0.643
2.0–2.4	2	0.143	0.786
2.5–2.9	2	0.143	0.929
3.0–3.4	1	0.071	1.000
Total	14	1.000	

[a]Data Presented in Table 4-2.
[b]See Table 4-4 for details.

Relative frequency distributions thus provide a way to describe the probability of an event. That is, the **probability** of an event is equal to the ratio of the number of times a specific outcome occurs to the total number of events for all possible outcomes.

The basic principles of probability may be illustrated using examples that involve flipping a fair coin (the chances of obtaining heads or tails is 0.5). For example, if a coin is flipped 10 times, what are the probabilities associated with each possible outcome? In this demonstration, there are 11 possible outcomes, ranging from 10 tails and 0 heads to 10 heads and 0 tails. The probability of obtaining specific combinations of heads and tails can be obtained by flipping the coin many times, tracking the numbers of heads and tails obtained, and then determining the relative frequencies of the different possible outcomes.

In this demonstration, note the following:

- On any one coin flip (called an *event*) only two outcomes are possible, a head or a tail. Such an event is termed a **binomial event**. Furthermore, the outcomes are **mutually exclusive**, only one of the two outcomes can occur on any one coin flip. Finally, the outcomes are **exhaustive**, in that only a head or a tail and no other outcome may occur one any coin flip.
- A series of events is called a *trial*. Thus flipping a coin 10 times is a trial of 10 coin-flipping events. The events constituting a trial are **independent**. That is, the outcome of one event does not affect the outcome of any other event.

The actual procedure of flipping a coin is a chance or **random event**. That means that the outcome of the event cannot be determined until the operation is carried out. In other words, for any one coin flip, the outcome cannot be determined with certainty until the coin has been flipped and the result observed. Random does not mean chaos. There are precise mathematical methods that characterize these outcomes.

If a coin is flipped once, either a head or a tail will be obtained, and, assuming the coin is fair, each of the two outcomes has a probability (i.e., a relative frequency) of 0.50. If the coin is flipped twice, there are 4 possible outcomes: 0 heads and 2 tails, 1 head and 1 tail, 1 tail and 1 head, and 2 heads and 0 tails. The probability of the occurrence of two events is the product of their individual probabilities. So, the probability of obtaining two heads with two coin flips is $0.5 \times 0.5 = 0.25$. Furthermore, if there is no interest in the order in which heads and tails are obtained, the outcomes in which one head and one tail were obtained can be combined, so that the probability of obtaining "1 head and 1 tail" with two coin flips is $0.25 + 0.25 = 0.50$.

The result of a series of two coin flip events is shown as a probability tree in Figure 5-1. Each branching of the tree represents an event, each of which has two outcomes: a head or

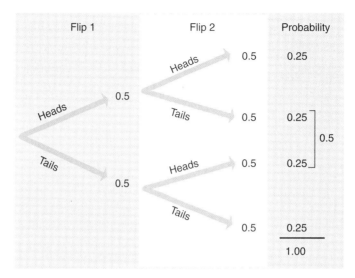

FIGURE 5-1 Probability Tree: Coin Flipping. For each coin flip, the probability of heads equals the probability of tails, which is 0.5. The probability of each outcome for two coin flips is shown in the rightmost column.

a tail. Because there are two events, the tree branches twice. The column on the far right contains the probabilities of the occurrence of the possible joint outcomes. Notice that the sum of the probabilities is equal to 1.00, indicating that all the possible outcomes have been included.

Probability trees are very useful in understanding more complex probability outcomes. For example, Figure 5-2 presents a probability tree depicting the possible outcomes associated with selecting two people at random from a population in which 20% are diagnosed with macular degeneration. Notice that since the probability of selecting a person with

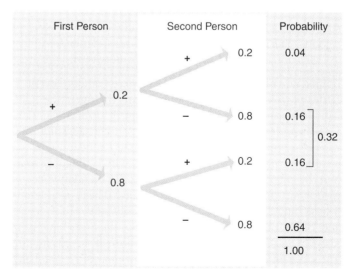

FIGURE 5-2 Probability Tree: Selecting Two Patients with Macular Degeneration. The proportion of the population with macular degeneration is 0.20. The first branching of the tree indicates the probability that the first person selected will have (+) or will be free of (−) macular degeneration. The second branching indicates the same for the second person selected. The probability of each possible joint outcome is shown in the rightmost column.

macular degeneration is 0.20, the probability of selecting a person without macular degeneration is its *complement*, calculated as $1 - 0.20$, or 0.80. The first branch of the tree displays the results of the first random event, the probability of selecting a person with macular degeneration versus a person without macular degeneration. The second branch of the tree indicates the outcomes of the second random event—selecting the second person. Probabilities associated with the outcomes of both events (the joint probabilities) are presented in the rightmost column.

The first person selected has a 0.20 chance of being diagnosed with macular degeneration, as does the second person. Thus the probability of both people exhibiting macular degeneration is 0.20×0.20, or 0.04. Alternately, the probability of obtaining two people who are not diagnosed with macular degeneration is 0.80×0.80, or 0.64. The probability of selecting one person with macular degeneration and one without macular degeneration is equal to 0.20×0.80, or 0.16. If the sequence of selection is not important, the probability of obtaining one person with macular degeneration and another without macular degeneration is 2×0.16, or 0.32.

Probability trees can also provide valuable information in understanding the results of diagnostic screening tests. Assume that a screening test has been developed for osteoarthritis, which is known to afflict 25% of the population being studied. Preliminary work indicates that 95% of those with osteoarthritis exhibit a positive test result. This is the **sensitivity of a screening test.** Alternately, 88% of those who do not have osteoarthritis test negative, a concept termed the **specificity of a screening test.**

The probability tree of the screening test for osteoarthritis applied to this population is presented in Figure 5-3. The first branch indicates the proportion of the population with osteoarthritis, and the second branch reflects the **sensitivity** and specificity characteristics of the screening test. The results indicate that a person chosen at random from this population has

- A probability of 0.2375 of being afflicted with osteoarthritis and testing positive (a *true positive* result)

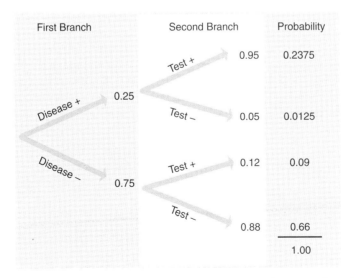

FIGURE 5-3 Probability Tree: Screening Test for Osteoarthritis. The first branch of the tree reflects the proportion of the population with the disease (0.25). The second branch of the tree indicates the effects of sensitivity (0.95) and specificity (0.88) of the test on this population. The final probabilities are presented in the rightmost column.

- A probability of 0.0125 of being afflicted with osteoarthritis and testing negative (a *false negative* result)
- A probability of 0.09 of not being afflicted with osteoarthritis and testing positive (a *false positive* result)
- A probability of 0.66 of not being afflicted with osteoarthritis and testing negative (a *true negative* result)

Other aspects of a screening test may be illustrated by arranging the probabilities of various outcomes in a table, such as Table 5-2. The table presents disease status and screening test results. Cell entries were determined by assigning 1000 patients to the different cells according the probabilities given in Figure 5-3.

Some of the information in Table 5-2 confirms information already available. For example, the sum of the "disease present" column, divided by the total number of individuals, is the prevalence of the disease, 0.25. Furthermore, the sensitivity of the test is equal to the proportion of subjects who have the disease and who test positive, which in this example is 238/250, or 0.95. Specificity is the proportion of subjects who do not have the disease and who test negative, which is 660/750, or 0.88.

In general, when a diagnostic test exhibits high sensitivity, a negative test result will rule out the disease. A good mnemonic is SnOUT, for sensitivity negative rules the diagnosis out. Similarly, for a diagnostic test with a high specificity, a positive result rules the diagnosis in. The mnemonic for this is SpIN, for specificity positive rules the diagnosis in.[2]

Unfortunately, to be useful, sensitivity and specificity values must attain levels that are rare for most diagnostic indicators. Furthermore, this application is limited to cases in which there are only two test outcomes.

An alternative method of using the information in Table 5-2 is to compute predictive values. The **positive predictive value (PPV)** is the proportion of subjects who test positive and who have the disease. Using the data in from example, PPV = 238/328 = 0.73. The **negative predictive value (NPV)** is the proportion of subjects who test negative and who do not have the disease; in the example, NPV = 660/672 = 0.98. Thus the clinician might expect that only about 73% of the patients with a positive test result really have the disease. However, a person who tests negative will almost always be disease free (at least 98% of the time).

Although these numbers may seem useful, one difficulty is that PPV and NPV are affected by the prevalence of the disease in the population. As a consequence, applying a screening test developed in a research hospital in which the condition is common to a general hospital setting in which the condition is rare will provide different PPV and NPV values. To illustrate, assume that the data in Table 5-2 are from a specialty clinic in which the disease prevalence is 25%. Data in Table 5-3, in contrast, are obtained from a population in which the disease prevalence is 15%. Notice that each table contains the same

TABLE 5-2	Results for Osteoarthritis Screening Test: Example 1		
	DISEASE STATUS		
TEST RESULTS	PRESENT	ABSENT	TOTAL
Positive	238	90	328
Negative	12	660	672
Total	250	750	1000

[a]Sample (*n*) = 1000 people. Proportion of population with osteoarthritis = 0.25. Sensitivity = 238 ÷ 250 = 0.95. Specificity = 660 ÷ 750 = 0.88. Positive predictive value = 238 ÷ 328 = 0.73. Negative predictive value = 660 ÷ 672 = 0.98. Likelihood ratio positive = (238 ÷ 250) ÷ (90 ÷ 750) = 7.93. Likelihood ratio negative = (12 ÷ 250) ÷ (660 ÷ 750) = 0.05. See text for definition of terms.

TABLE 5-3	Results for Osteoarthritis Screening Test: Example 2		
	DISEASE STATUS		
TEST RESULTS	PRESENT	ABSENT	*TOTAL*
Positive	142	102	244
Negative	8	748	756
Total	150	850	1000

[a]Sample (*n*) = 1000 people. Proportion of population with osteoarthritis = 0.15. Sensitivity = 142 ÷ 150 = 0.95. Specificity = 748 ÷ 850 = 0.88. Positive predictive value = 142 ÷ 244 = 0.58. Negative predictive value = 748 ÷ 756 = 0.99. Likelihood ratio positive = (142 ÷ 150) / (102 ÷ 850) = 7.93. Likelihood ratio negative = (8 ÷ 150) / (748 ÷ 850) = 0.06. See text for definition of terms.

values for the sensitivity and specificity of the screening test. However, the PPV now equals 142/244 = 58% rather than 73%, and the NPV has increased from 98% to 99%. These measures appear to be on shaky ground if the prevalence of the disease is not known, which is a common occurrence in a specific healthcare setting.

A third method of assessing the outcomes of a screening test is to use likelihood ratios (LRs). In general, a likelihood ratio expresses the chance of observing a test result in a person who has the disease versus a person who does not have the disease. A **likelihood ratio positive (LR+)** indicates how much more likely a person with the disease is to test positive compared to a person who does not have the disease. The LR+ is calculated as the ratio of the true positive rate (the sensitivity) to the false positive rate (1 − specificity). For Tables 5-2 and 5-3, the LR+ is 7.9. Thus a positive test result is almost 8 times more likely to be found in a person who has the disease than in a person who does not have the disease.

The **likelihood ratio negative (LR−)** indicates how much more likely a negative test result will be obtained from a person who has the disease compared to a person who does not have the disease. The LR− is the ratio of the false negative rate (1 − sensitivity) to the true negative rate (specificity). In this example, LR− is about 0.06. Because the LR− is a fraction, it is often difficult to interpret for patients. A simple calculation makes this number an integer and thus understandable to most patients. The calculation is to take the reciprocal of the LR−, which in this example is 1/0.06 = 16.7. Interpret this to mean that a person who does not really have the disease is 16.7 times more likely to score negative on the screening test than a person who has the disease.

Here is an example of a clinical application of the likelihood ratio from the Oxford Centre for Evidence Based Medicine.[3] While reading a clinical report, a pharmacist finds that 90% of patients with iron-deficiency anemia exhibit serum ferritin values of 60 mmol/L but that only 15% of patients with other maladies have a ferritin value close to this. If the pharmacist has a patient with a ferritin value about 60 mmol/L, the likelihood that the person is iron deficient is 0.90/0.15 = 6. Thus the patient is 6 times more likely to be iron deficient than to be normal.

Guidelines for the interpretation of likelihood ratios are presented in Table 5-4. As might be expected, an LR+ > 10 is strong evidence of the disease, and LR− < 0.1 is strong evidence against the presence of disease. The closer an LR value is to 1, the less convincing the evidence.

Probability Distributions

The techniques just reviewed are quite useful in addressing problems involving specific probabilities or combinations of probabilities. In many situations, however, interest is in the relative frequency of all possible values that might be assumed by a variable. Such a

TABLE 5-4	Common Interpretations of Likelihood Ratios
LIKELIHOOD RATIO	**INTERPRETATION**
> 10	Persuasive evidence of the likelihood of disease
5–10	Moderate evidence of the likelihood of disease
2–5	Minimal evidence of the likelihood of disease
1	No evidence of the likelihood of disease
0.2–1.0	Minimal evidence against the likelihood of disease
0.1–0.2	Moderate evidence against the likelihood of disease
< 0.1	Persuasive evidence against the likelihood of disease

distribution is termed a probability distribution. A **probability distribution** associates a probability of occurrence with each possible value of a variable. Probability distributions form the foundation of statistical theory and underlie the rationale for many statistical tests. Two probability distributions, one for discrete variables and one for continuous variables, are explored in this section.

THE BINOMIAL DISTRIBUTION

Although probability trees are convenient for visualizing the outcomes of binomial events, they become cumbersome rapidly as the number of branches of the probability tree increases. For example, determining the probability of all possible outcomes of flipping a coin twice was determined easily using a probability tree. Determining all possible outcomes of a trial of 10 coin flips requires another approach.

The approach uses (simple) mathematics instead of tree branches to achieve the same end. The product is a **binomial distribution**, a relative frequency distribution that associates a probability with every possible outcome of a series of discrete, binomial events. Understanding this material is enhanced if the student is clear that each coin flip is an *event*, and the series of events is called a *trial*.

To begin, consider determining the probability of obtaining 6 heads and 4 tails when a fair coin is flipped 10 times. As with the probability tree, determining this requires consideration of three factors:

- The probability of obtaining one of the two outcomes (e.g., a head, with each coin flip)
- The probability of obtaining the alternative outcome (e.g., a tail, with each coin flip)
- The number of sequences in which heads and tails can occur

Applied to our example, the probability of obtaining one outcome, say a head, on any one coin flip is p. Thus the probability of obtaining a tail on any one coin flip is $(1 - p)$. Over series of n coin flips, the probability of obtaining several heads will equal

$$p^j$$

where j is the number of successful event outcomes. The probability of obtaining $j = 3$ heads in a row is 0.5^3 or 0.125. Similarly, the probability of obtaining a tail is $(1 - p)$ for any one coin flip so the probability of obtaining a series of $(n - j)$ tails is

$$(1 - p)^{(n-j)}$$

In our example involving 6 heads and 4 tails in 10 coin flips, then, these two factors are multiplied together like so:

$$p^j \times (1 - p)^{(n-j)}$$
$$0.5^6 \times 0.5^4$$

The final component is the number of ways that j heads and $(n - j)$ tails might occur. This term is called the binomial coefficient, and is abbreviated $_nC_j$. Table B-1 (Appendix B) contains binomial coefficients for various values of n (read down the leftmost column) and j (read across the first row). Reference to the table indicates that there are 210 different ways to obtain 6 heads and 4 tails when a coin is flipped 10 times.

In the present example, the binomial equation can be used to calculate the probability of obtaining 6 heads and 4 tails with 10 coin flips:

$$\Pr\{j = 6 \text{ and } (n - j) = 4\} = 210 \times 0.5^6 \times 0.5^{(10-6)}$$

Figure 5-4 presents the probability distribution for all possible outcomes of heads and tails when $n = 10$ coin flips. Notice that every possible outcome, from 0 heads to 10 heads, appears with an associated probability of occurrence. All outcomes are not equally probable, however. It appears that obtaining 4, 5, or 6 heads would occur quite frequently, almost two-thirds of the time, in fact. In contrast, obtaining 0 heads or 0 tails is a rare event.

Notice how the results of the coin-flipping experiment substitute specific quantities for expectations based on experience and expressed in general terms. That is, one expectation is that outcomes close to 5 heads in 10 coin flips will occur frequently, whereas more extreme outcomes will occur rarely. However, instead of describing outcomes of an experiment as frequent or rare, the binomial distribution assigns specific probabilities to each individual outcome.

In addition, inspection of the binomial distribution in Figure 5-4 confirms some expectations and provides some surprises. The expectation that 5 heads is somehow the center of the distribution is confirmed by the calculation of the mean as:

$$n \times p = 10 \times 0.5 = 5$$

Furthermore, the expectation that the results of most coin-flipping trials will cluster around this value is reinforced by the computation of the standard deviation of this distribution:

$$\sqrt{[n \times p \times (1 - p)]} = \sqrt{10 \times 0.5 \times 0.5} = 1.58$$

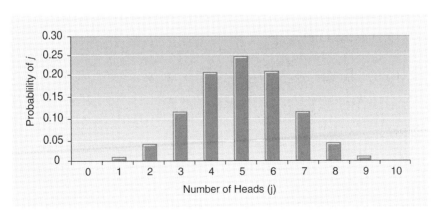

FIGURE 5-4 Binomial Distribution. The bars indicate the probability of obtaining the indicated number of heads (j) in 10 coin flips. $n = 10$; $p = 0.5$.

As mentioned, Figure 5-4 also reveals several surprising outcomes. The first is that, although the mean of this binomial distribution is 5, obtaining exactly 5 heads in 10 coin flips occurs only about 25% of the time, despite its also being the modal value. Note, however, the occurrence of 4, 5, or 6 heads has a combined probability of around 65%. So, obtaining a number of heads within 1 unit of the mean would occur rather frequently, as suggested by the standard deviation.

The general formula for the binomial equation is:

$$\Pr\{j\} = {}_nC_j \times p^j \times (1 - p)^{(n - j)}$$

For any binomial event, then, knowledge of only two parameters, n and p, make it possible to associate a probability of occurrence with each possible outcome of a series of binomial events.

In addition to the examples described in this section, binomial events play an important role in healthcare research. Binomial distributions provide a means for quantifying and analyzing many different types of nominal and ordinal data and are explored in more detail in chapter 6.

THE NORMAL DISTRIBUTION

Another relative frequency distribution with wide application in biostatistics is the normal distribution, the familiar bell-shaped curve. The normal distribution is used to describe quantitative, continuous variables that characterize a very large, if not infinite, number of elements, μ.

Actually, a family of normal distributions exists, each of which is defined in terms of its two parameters: a mean (μ) and a standard deviation (σ). As demonstrated in Figure 5-5A, changing μ alters the distribution's position on the abscissa but does not change its shape. Changing σ, in contrast, alters the dispersion of the distribution's values, and thus its shape, but does not change the distribution's position on the abscissa (Fig. 5-5B).

Because continuous variables have an unlimited number of values, probability distributions of continuous variables have a smooth, continuous surface. Theoretically, at least, this means that the area under the curve (AUC) associated with any specific value, and therefore its relative frequency, is quite small. It makes more sense, then to refer to intervals of the continuous variable.

The AUC of the normal distribution can be described using its two parameters, μ and σ. Recall that about 68% of the AUC lies within 1 σ of μ, about 95% of the AUC lies within 2 σ of μ, and more than 99.7% of the AUC lies within 3 σ of μ.

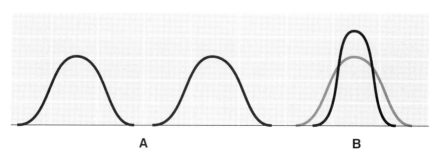

A   **B**

FIGURE 5-5 Normal Distributions. **A**. Altering the mean of the distribution changes its position along the measurement scale but does not affect its shape. **B**. Altering the standard deviation of the normal distribution changes the shape of the curve but not its position along the measurement scale.

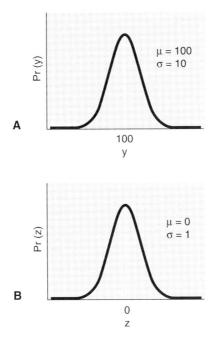

FIGURE 5-6 Normally Distributed Variable and the Standard Normal Distribution. Independent of the parameters of the original distribution (**A**), the mean of the standard normal distribution (**B**) equals 0 and the standard deviation equals 1. The shapes of the two distributions are the same.

However, obtaining AUCs that differ from these benchmarks using the equation for the normal distribution is cumbersome and inconvenient. Fortunately, there is a relatively simple solution that consists of transforming the data of the parent distribution into values of another population for which AUC quantities have been calculated.

This process is demonstrated in Figure 5-6. Values of a continuous variable are presented in the upper trace, with $\mu = 100$ and $\sigma = 10$. Beneath this distribution is the **standard normal distribution**, with $\mu = 0$ and $\sigma = 1$. Mathematically, this is a linear transformation of the data, so the shape of the two distributions is the same.

Individual values of the standard normal distribution are called *z scores*, and the standard normal distribution is often called a *z* score distribution. Any variable (y) that is normally distributed may be converted into a z score by subtracting its value from μ and dividing the difference by σ:

$$z = \frac{(y - \mu)}{\sigma}$$

For example, from a population with normally distributed mean blood pressure levels with $\mu = 100$ mmHg and $\sigma = 10$, a mean blood pressure value of 97 mmHg is obtained from a patient. The corresponding standard score value is obtained as follows:

$$z = \frac{(97 - 100)}{10} = \frac{-3}{10} = -0.30$$

To find the AUC corresponding to this value of z, a table of standard score values is consulted, such as Table B-2, as found in Appendix B. Notice that the z scores are expressed to two decimal places. The first two digits of the z score make up the rows (under heading "z") and the second decimal place is indicated by the column headings. The entries in the body of the table indicate the area under the standard normal distribution from minus infinity to the value of z indicated. For example, for a z score of -0.30, find the row labeled "-0.3" and the column labeled "00." The table gives a value of 0.3821, which means that 0.3821 of the AUC is located between minus infinity and the z score -0.30. Because -0.30 corresponds to the mean diastolic blood pressure value of 97 mmHg, we may also conclude that 38.21% of the population displays a mean blood diastolic pressure value ≤ 97 mmHg.

The z score distribution is important for several reasons. First, the distribution provides a simple way to analyze the many biological variables that display a normal distribution. Instead of creating tables for each variable, the variables are first converted to z scores, for which the probabilities have already been calculated. Second, the distribution reduces variables quantified in several measurement scales to a common metric. That is, a change in a variable—whether body temperature or blood pressure or mental status—of 1σ reflects the same amount of change no matter the nature of that variable. Third, the z score distribution provides indices of the probabilities of events, if the mean and the standard deviation of the population are known. These features are illustrated by the following examples.

1. In a population, the mean total cholesterol level of the men is 225 mg/dL and the standard deviation is 5. What is the probability that a man selected at random from this population would have a total cholesterol level of 220 mg/dL or less?
   - To solve this problem, first convert the individual value to a z score:

$$z = \frac{(220 - 225)}{5} = \frac{-5}{5} = -1.00$$

   - By referring to a table of z scores, you find that the area under the standard normal curve between minus infinity and a z score of -1.00 is 0.1587. Thus 15.87% of the men would be expected to display a total cholesterol level ≤ 225 mg/dL.
2. Using the parameters from the first example, what is the probability that a man selected at random from this population would have a total cholesterol level between 220 and 227 mg/dL?
   - Again, the first step is to convert each of the total cholesterol levels to z scores. The first value, already calculated, is equal to -1.00. The second z value is equal to $(227 - 225) \div 5 = 0.4$.
   - From the first example, 15.87% of the AUC is located between minus infinity and the z score of -1.00; and from the table of z scores, 65.54% of the AUC is located between minus infinity and the z score of 0.4. Therefore, the area between these two values is $(65.54\% - 15.87\%) = 49.67\%$. This result indicates that almost half of men selected from this population will have a total cholesterol level between 220 and 227 mg/dL.
3. Finally, what are the highest 20% of total cholesterol levels in this population?
   - Here the procedure is reversed: the z score table is first consulted to find the z score value that most closely indicates the highest 20% of the population of standard scores. This value is found to be 0.84, which is actually the z value indicating z scores of the lower 80% of the distribution.
   - The formula for determining the value of z is then used to calculate the value of y for a z score of $= 0.84$:

$$0.84 = \frac{(y - 225)}{5}$$

$$y = (5 \times 0.84) + 225$$

$$y = 229.2 \text{ mg/dL}$$

Therefore, the highest 20% of the scores in the distribution are ≥ 229.2 mg/dL.

The number of variables that can be described using a normal distribution is almost limit-less. Even moderate departures from normality do not radically affect its application to real data. In addition to describing data, normal distributions are essential for using statistics to generalize from samples to populations. This is because they characterize the shape of probability distributions of statistics, termed *sampling distributions.*

Sampling Distributions

In the previous section, properties of relative frequency distributions as probability distributions of measured values were described. In this section, those same principles are extended to probability distributions of statistics.

Recall that statistics are computed from samples, which are subsets of populations. Because populations are considered to be very large or infinite, many different samples may be obtained from them. Although population parameters such as μ and σ remain constant, statistics such as $\bar{y}$ and s change as the membership composition of the samples from which they are computed change. A sampling distribution is simply a frequency distribution of all possible values a statistic might attain when computed from all possible samples. More formally, the **sampling distribution of a statistic** is defined as a probability distribution of all possible values of a statistic obtained from random samples of the same size.

To illustrate the construction of a sampling distribution, imagine that a clinic is attended by 25 patients who have diabetes and interest is in the proportion of these patients who exhibit good glycemic control, defined as a glycosylated hemoglobin (Hba1c) level < 7%. The procedure would consist of drawing all possible samples of, say, 5 from the population of 25 patients, determining the proportion of each sample with good Hba1c control, and then summarizing the findings by expressing each possible outcome as a proportion of all possible outcomes. Unfortunately, this process would be very time- and energy-consuming because data from 53,130 different possible samples would need to be processed.

Fortunately, sampling distributions do not have to be constructed empirically. Like other distributions, probabilities for these variables can be calculated mathematically if the parameters of the distribution are known. If the distribution of the variable conforms to a normal distribution, the parameters required are μ and σ. This is often the case.

Sampling distributions can be constructed for a wide variety of statistics, including the sample mean, the sample proportion, the difference between two sample means, and the difference between two sample proportions. In the next section, the sampling distribution of the sample mean is used to exemplify the rationale, applications, and implications of all sampling distributions.

SAMPLING DISTRIBUTION OF A SAMPLE MEAN

The sampling distribution of the sample mean consists of a relative frequency distribution of all possible values of the sample mean, calculated from random samples of size n drawn from a population of size N. The number of elements available to be sampled from the parent population is considered to be very large, if not infinite, compared to n.

An important attribute of the sampling distribution is the correspondence of its parameters to the parameters of the parent population. These are, specifically:

1. The mean of the sampling distribution of sample means, $\mu_{\bar{y}}$, equals the mean of the population, μ. In symbols:

$$\mu_{\bar{y}} = \mu$$

2. The standard deviation of the sampling distribution (termed the standard error), $\sigma_{\bar{y}}$, is equal to the standard deviation of the parent population, σ, divided by the square root of the sample size:

$$\sigma_{\bar{y}} = \frac{\sigma}{\sqrt{n}}$$

3. The distribution of sample means is a normal distribution if:
   - The parent population is known to be a normal distribution and the sample size is small, <30
   - The shape of the parent population is either unknown or known not to be normal and the sample size is large, >30

The **central limit theorem** summarizes the salient items succinctly: Given a population with a mean (μ) and a finite standard deviation (σ), the probability distribution of the means of samples of size n drawn from this population will have a mean of μ, will have a standard deviation of $\sigma/\sqrt{n}$, and will exhibit a normal shape as long as n is large.

Almost all decisions made using statistics rely on the central limit theorem. Whether estimating the prevalence of patients with diabetes under good glycemic control or testing a hypothesis about differences in the safety of drugs, the shape of the population of these values is unknown. The critical importance of the central limit theorem is that, if a sufficiently large sample size is obtained, the shape of the sampling distribution of the statistic will be normal. Consequently, statistics such as a sample mean can be referred to the sampling distribution of the sample mean to determine its probability of occurrence.

For the use of the central limit theorem to be valid, the following requirements must be met.

1. *The manner in which the sample data are obtained is critical.* Commonly, data are obtained using a **simple random sample.** This is a method of obtaining samples in which the selection of each participant is a chance event, and each potential participant has a constant probability of being selected from the population. In large populations, the change in the probability of the second person being selected owing to the reduction in population size when the first person is selected can be neglected. Other sampling techniques may be permitted, but the ultimate requirement is that the sample must be a microcosm of the population.
2. *The statistic used to estimate the population parameter must be an unbiased estimator.* Using the sample mean as an example, the notion is that the deviation of individual sample means from the mean of the sampling distribution is the result of sampling error. When the mean of the sampling distribution is calculated, these sampling errors average out, and $\mu_{\bar{y}}$ will equal μ. Thus with an **unbiased estimator,** the mean of the sampling distribution of the statistic equals the mean of the population.
3. *The population studied must be representative of the population of interest, the target population.* This is not always the case. In a study of the effect of a drug in patients with severe Alzheimer disease, for example, the most profoundly afflicted may not be able to participate fully in the experiment. Often the problem is that the composition of the study sample is not under the investigator's control. Many studies nowadays use only volunteer patients, who necessarily are different from patients who refuse to participate.

Because sampling distributions are normal distributions, the principles of the normal distribution can be applied to sampling distributions if the parameters are known. But how are the parameters of the sampling distribution obtained? They are not derived from the parent population. If the parent population parameters were known, then sampling distributions would not be necessary to characterize them. The only information at hand is the data from the patients who make up the sample.

So sample data, or more precisely statistics calculated from sample data, are used to estimate parameters of the parent population. The rationale for this procedure is that, owing to the sampling techniques used, the sample is a mini-representation of the parent population. Therefore, the value of the sample mean, $\bar{y}$, should be similar to the parent population mean, μ, and the sample standard deviation, s, should be similar to the parent population standard deviation, σ. Variations in the sample statistics are attributed to sampling error. In short, because of the sampling technique used, sample statistics can be used instead of the parameters of the parent population to estimate the parameters of the sampling distribution.

For example, consider the population of total cholesterol levels for all males over the age of 50 in North America. The mean, standard deviation, and shape of the parent population are unknown. However, suppose blood samples are obtained from 100 men using a simple random sampling method. The following sample statistics are calculated: $\bar{y} = 180$ mg/dL and $s = 20$.

First, sample data are used to estimate the parameters of the sampling distribution: $\bar{y}$ is assumed to be equal to $\mu_{\bar{y}}$, so $\mu_{\bar{y}} = 180$; and because $\sigma_{\bar{y}} = \sigma/\sqrt{n}$, the value of $\sigma_{\bar{y}}$ can be calculated from the sample data s, and n as $20/\sqrt{100}$ or 2.0. Second, because the sample size and sampling technique met the criteria of the central limit theorem, the shape of the sampling distribution is normal.

The objection might be raised that, if a second sample were drawn, different values of $\bar{y}$ and s, would be obtained, resulting in a different set of parameters for the sampling distribution. This is true: The probability that $\bar{y} = \mu_{\bar{y}}$ exactly is extremely small, and the value of $\bar{y}$ will vary with different samples.

However, because the distribution of $\bar{y}$ values is normal, $\bar{y}$ and s can be used to calculate an interval of values that should include $\mu_{\bar{y}}$. These are similar to the benchmark intervals calculated previously to contain 68%, 95%, and 99.7% of all the scores in the population. The general formula to calculate an interval that would be expected to include a specific percentage of the sample means has the following form:

$$\text{Estimate} \pm \text{reliability coefficient} \times \text{standard error}$$

The estimate, or more properly the point estimate, of $\mu_{\bar{y}}$ is $\bar{y}$. The standard error is $\sigma_{\bar{y}}$. The reliability coefficient reflects the number of standard deviation units to be included in the interval. For example, we know that 95% of the sample means will lie within ± 1.96 standard deviation units of the mean of a normal distribution.

In this example, then, the interval equals:

$$\text{Sample mean} \pm z \times \text{standard error}$$

$$180 \pm 1.96 \times 2.0$$

$$(176.1, 183.9)$$

From these data, it is estimated that 95% of the sample means in the sampling distribution lie between 176.1 and 183.9 mg/dL. This interval is termed the 95% **confidence interval** (95% CI). In addition to a 95% CI, other CIs, such as 90% CI or 99% CI, can be calculated by changing the reliability coefficient, z.

Several properties of the CI merit emphasis. The first is that the CI describes the probability of an event. In the above example, the results indicate that 95% of sample means obtained from samples of size 100 will lie in the interval between 176.1 and 183.9 mg/dL. This can also be a probability statement: A random sample of $n = 100$ drawn from this population has a 95% probability of exhibiting an average total cholesterol level between 176.1 and 183.9 mg/dL. The complement can also be stated: There is only a 5% probability that the mean total cholesterol concentrations obtained from a sample of 100 men will fall outside the interval between 176.1 and 183.9 mg/dL.

Second, the shape of the sampling distribution of a statistic changes with sample size. This is because the dispersion of scores in a normal distribution is the result of $\sigma_{\bar{y}}$. The values of $\bar{y}$ and s do not change with sample size; however, $\sigma_{\bar{y}}$, because it is calculated as $s/\sqrt{n}$, is sensitive to changes in n. In fact, the larger the n, the smaller the σ. For example, if 10,000 men were included in the sample for cholesterol levels, $\sigma_{\bar{y}}$ would have equaled 0.20, and the 95% CI would have extended from 179.6 to 180.4 mg/dL.

This is why the standard deviation of a sampling distribution is called a *standard error*: It is a measure of the extent to which the sample means will vary about the true mean, $\mu_{\bar{y}}$. In this sense, $\sigma_{\bar{y}}$ is an estimate of the *precision* with which $\mu_{\bar{y}}$ estimates μ.

The third property of sampling distributions requires special comment. As pointed out earlier, the sample mean, $\bar{y}$, will rarely equal the mean of the sampling distribution, $\mu_{\bar{y}}$, because of sampling error. However, CIs can be used to suggest the location of the true value of $\mu_{\bar{y}}$. Figure 5-7 presents a sampling distribution of the sample mean. To simplify the example, assume that $\mu_{\bar{y}}$ is the mean of the sampling distribution in which $\mu_{\bar{y}} = \mu$ and thus is the true $\mu_{\bar{y}}$. Below the sampling distribution are three 95% CIs based on three different samples of the same size (so all three CIs are the same width). Each sample provides an independent estimate of $\mu_{\bar{y}}$. CI a is a case in which the estimated mean of the sampling distribution equals the true $\mu_{\bar{y}}$. Its 95% CI is thus the "true" CI in that every sample mean it encompasses is within 1.96 σ of the mean of the population of y values. For CI b, the estimated mean of the sampling distribution is not equal to the true $\mu_{\bar{y}}$. However, the 95% CI includes the true value of $\mu_{\bar{y}}$. Notice how much the 95% CI can vary and still include $\mu_{\bar{y}}$. CI c indicates that the estimated mean of the sampling distribution would need to attain very extreme values before its 95% CI would not include the true $\mu_{\bar{y}}$. In fact, such extreme values of $\mu_{\bar{y}}$ should occur fewer than 5% of the time.

Thus although the sample mean will rarely be identical to $\mu_{\bar{y}}$, the 95% CI computed from the sample mean will almost always contain $\mu_{\bar{y}}$. The implications are profound: Because of the central limit theorem, estimation of population parameters using the 95% CI of statistics will include the true population parameter 95% of the time. Only 5% of the

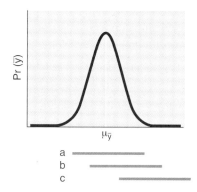

FIGURE 5-7 The Effect of Sampling Error on the Relationship of Confidence Intervals to the Sampling Distribution. The normal curve represents a sampling distribution in which $\mu_{\bar{y}}$ 5 m. The 95% CI for this distribution is shown by line *a*. For CI *b* the estimate of $\mu_{\bar{y}}$ does not equal the true $\mu_{\bar{y}}$, but the CI contains the true $\mu_{\bar{y}}$. This situation seems to occur quite frequently. For CI *c*, the estimate of $\mu_{\bar{y}}$ does not equal the true $\mu_{\bar{y}}$, and the CI does not contain the true $\mu_{\bar{y}}$. Such an outcome is expected to occur < 5% of the time.

time will the estimate be erroneous. These relationships are true as long as the sample statistic is an unbiased estimate of the population parameter, the sample is obtained using a random sampling method, and the data in the sample mimic the characteristics of the target population.

It bears repeating that this information about populations can be derived from sample statistics alone—it is not necessary to have knowledge of the parameters of the parent population. Indeed, the true value of many of these parameters cannot be ascertained by direct measurement.

One modification of the formula for calculating CIs is necessary, however. Recall that the population standard deviation, σ, is required to calculate the appropriate values of the reliability coefficient, z. However, it is usually the case that neither the μ nor σ is known. Estimating σ from s is biased unless $(n - 1)$ rather than n is used as the divisor, particularly when sample size is small. To compensate for this error, the CI is calculated using the statistic t as the reliability coefficient. Like the z distribution, the mean of the t distribution is zero. The shape of the t distribution is symmetric. In contrast to the one z distribution, however, there are many different distributions of t, which vary with the degrees of freedom (df) used to estimate $\sigma_{\bar{y}}$.

Values of the t distributions are presented in Table B-3 found in Appendix B. The leftmost column identifies the df associated with various distributions of t. The columns identify the AUC for values of t equal to or greater than the critical values appearing in the body of the table. For the distribution associated with any df, separate critical values are used to define specific regions of the t distribution. For example, with a sample size of 25, for which $df = 24$, only 5% of the t values in the distribution equal or exceed $t = 1.711$, and only 1% of the t values in this distribution are ≥ 2.492.

The method of computing a CI using the t statistic is similar to that using the z score. Here's an example. From a sample of $n = 16$, with $\bar{y} = 45$ and $s = 10$, compute the 95% CI for $\mu_{\bar{y}}$: $\sigma_{\bar{y}} = 10/\sqrt{16} = 2.50$. The value of t is selected so that the total area excluded by the interval is $1 - 0.95$, or 0.05. Because the t distribution is symmetric, the critical value of t is selected to demarcate the most extreme 0.025 or 2.5% of the values in both the lower and the upper tails of the distribution. With 15 df, the critical value of t is 2.131. Thus the 95% CI for this sample is

$$45 \pm 2.131 \times 2.5$$
$$45 \pm 5.3$$
$$(39.7, 50.3)$$

Confidence intervals appear quite commonly in healthcare literature. Many clinicians consider them to be valuable because they provide an interval in which the true value lies. Furthermore, narrow intervals are preferred to wide intervals because they provide more precise and accurate estimates of the population parameter values. In addition, CIs can be used to quantify the probability that two statistics are different. That is, CIs, as explained in the next section, can be used to test statistical hypotheses.

Hypothesis Testing

Hypothesis testing is a method of using statistics to make decisions. The process involves quantifying the probability that an experimental outcome occurred by chance and then deciding whether to attribute the experimental outcome to chance.

The general method of hypothesis testing begins with a statement of the way nature works, called a **research hypothesis.** For example, a research hypothesis might be that a novel drug improves the breathing ability of children who have asthma. This notion is tested by prescribing one group of children a drug and another group a placebo. Evidence regarding the efficacy of the drug is provided by group differences in an index of breathing ability, for example the volume of air a child can forcibly expel in 1 second (forced expiratory volume at 1 sec; FEV_1).

If there is no effect of the drug, then there should be no difference in the average FEV_1 values between the drug group and the placebo group. If, however, the drug is effective, then the FEV_1 values of the drug group should be greater than the FEV_1 values of the placebo group. These alternatives are formalized as **statistical hypotheses.** One hypothesis, the **null hypothesis (H_0),** is a statement that there is no difference between the two group means. Thus the H_0 is that the difference between the average FEV_1 values of the two groups is 0. The other hypothesis, the **alternative hypothesis (H_A),** is that there is a difference between the FEV_1 values of the two groups. The H_A is accepted if the H_0 is rejected.

Owing to sampling variability, however, it is unlikely that the difference between the means will exactly equal 0. This adds uncertainty to the decision-making process. A critical question arises: if the difference between the group means does not equal 0 because of sampling variability, how far does the group difference have to be from 0 before the investigator can reject the notion that the mean difference is the result of chance?

The solution adopted by healthcare researchers is to suggest that values of the group means that are so extreme that they occur $\leq 5\%$ of the time if the H_0 is true provide sufficient evidence to reject H_0 and accept H_A. If the difference between the groups is not that extreme, the investigator fails to reject H_0.

In the following sections, hypothesis testing methods are illustrated using both the CI and a test statistic. In the process, these principles are elaborated.

HYPOTHESIS TESTING USING CONFIDENCE INTERVALS

Table 5-5 presents data for two groups of children who have asthma. Children in the placebo group received a placebo treatment, and children in the drug group received a novel agent. The table contains the mean for FEV_1, the standard deviation, and the number of children in each group.

The research hypothesis is that the novel agent affects the respiratory function of the drug group compared to the placebo group. The H_0 is that the difference between the mean FEV_1 of the two groups is 0. The H_A is that the difference between the mean FEV_1 of the two groups is some nonzero value.

The H_0 is tested by constructing a 95% CI of the difference between the group means from the sample data. This interval provides an index of the variability in the group mean differences that would be expected by chance. The decision rule is as follows: If H_0 is true, then a 0 difference between the means is a quite likely outcome. In fact, the value 0 would be expected to be included in the 95% CI. If, however, the value 0 is not included in

TABLE 5-5	FEV$_1$ Data: Hypothesis Testing Example	
	FEV$_1$ (L)	
STATISTIC	PLACEBO GROUP	DRUG GROUP
$\bar{y}$	2.20	2.50
s	0.71	0.81
n	140	138

the 95% CI, then H_0 would only rarely be true under these experimental conditions. This is evidence in favor of rejecting H_0.

Thus the process begins by calculating the 95% CI for the difference between the two group means. The general formula follows the familiar format:

$$\text{Estimate} \pm \text{reliability coefficient} \times \text{standard error}$$

$$(\bar{y}_1 - \bar{y}_2) \pm t \times \sigma_{(\bar{y}_1 - \bar{y}_2)}$$

The estimate is the difference between the two means, $(\bar{y}_1 - \bar{y}_2)$, and is equal to $2.50 - 2.20 = 0.30$.

The term $\sigma_{(\bar{y}1 - \bar{y}2)}$ is the pooled standard error of the difference between the two group means and is equal to 0.09. (The formula for the pooled standard error of the estimate is beyond the scope of this text, but is available in many statistical textbooks.)

The reliability coefficient, t, is selected from Table B-3 (Appendix B). The df are determined as follows:

$$df = (n_1 + n_2 - 2) = (138 + 140 - 2) = 276$$

The critical value of t for $df = 276$ is not present in the table. Instead the value of t for 140 df, 1.977, is substituted.

The calculation of the 95% CI for the difference between the two means is thus:

$$(0.30) \pm 1.977 \times (0.09)$$

$$(0.12, 0.38)$$

The results of this calculation are given in Figure 5-8. The 95% CI suggests that the true difference between the means lies in an interval from 0.12 to 0.38 L. Under the conditions of this experiment, a mean difference of 0 would occur < 5% of the time. The decision rule is thus to reject H_0 and to conclude that the drug improved the respiratory function of children who have asthma.

It is important to note that the decision rule is not foolproof. Although the 95% CI makes it *likely* that an investigator will fail to reject H_0 when it is true, there is a 5% chance that this decision will be erroneous. The probability of rejecting the H_0 when it is indeed true is called alpha (α), and this type of error is termed an **α error**, or type I error. Alternately, H_0 may not be rejected even though it is false. This is a **β error**, or type II error. The complementary probability, that a false H_0 is rejected, is equal to $1 - \beta$, and is called the **power** of the statistical test.

These various correspondences between the statistical decision based on the experimental outcome and the veracity of the H_0 in nature are presented in Table 5-6.

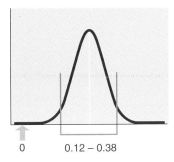

0   0.12 – 0.38

FIGURE 5-8 Confidence Interval Analysis: Novel Agent in Children Who Have Asthma. The 95% CI for the difference between the sample means does not include the value specified by H_0, (i.e., 0); therefore, conclude that H_0 is false.

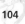

TABLE 5-6	Correspondence of the State of Nature and Probabilities Associated with Hypothesis Testing Decisions: 1	
	STATE OF NATURE	
STATISTICAL DECISION	**H_0 TRUE**	**H_0 FALSE**
Reject H_0	α (type I error)	$1 - \beta$
Fail to reject H_0	$1 - \alpha$	β (type II error)

The columns represent whether the difference between the groups is real or not real (the truth of the H_0). The rows indicate the statistical decision concerning the H_0: whether it is rejected or not. The cells contain probabilities associated with various decisions.

Some healthcare workers find a table such as Table 5-7 informative. Here, the difference in nature is either true or false, and the statistical decision either confirms the state of nature or it does not. The correspondence between the state of nature and the experimental evidence determines the correctness of the decision. For example, the statistical decision to fail to reject the H_0 is a negative decision. If in nature there really is no difference between the groups, then the decision is true. If, however, there really is a difference in the groups, then the decision to fail to reject H_0 is false.

The probability of a type I error, α, is set by the experimenter before the beginning of the study and is traditionally set at 0.05. Thus the researcher is accepting the possibility of making an α error by rejecting H_0 when it is indeed true 5% of the time.

The other major factor under the investigator's control is the power of the statistical test. The power of a statistical test is the probability that the H_0 will be rejected when it is really false. Commonly, power is set no lower than 80%, and frequently higher, around 90%. Control of power is through a variety of factors that determine its complement: β.

The factors that determine β include the true difference between the group means, the standard deviations of the groups, the level of α, and the sample size, n. The first two factors are obtained from the literature or from preliminary research. As noted, the α level is traditionally set at 5%. Thus the level of β, and therefore power, is determined by sample size.

Calculations of sample size appear frequently in the reporting of randomized controlled trials. Here is an example from the Incremental Decrease in End Points through Aggressive Lipid Lowering (IDEAL) Study, which examined the efficacy of four different diets on weight loss:[4]

> The primary end point was mean absolute change from baseline weight at 1 year. Using t tests and a 2-sided type I error of 5%, we estimated that 40 participants in each group would be necessary to achieve 80% power to detect a weight change of 2% from baseline or 3% between diets.

TABLE 5-7	Correspondence of State of Nature and Probabilities Associated with Hypothesis Testing Decisions: 2	
	STATE OF NATURE	
STATISTICAL DECISION	**H_0 TRUE**	**H_0 FALSE**
Reject H_0	False positive	True positive
Fail to reject H_0	True negative	False negative

The statistical decision is positive if it rejects H_0, and negative if it fails to reject H_0.

In summary, CIs provide useful information to healthcare workers because they not only afford a method of testing statistical hypotheses but also specify an interval that contains the true magnitude of the treatment. Another, more traditional, way to test statistical hypotheses is by calculating a test statistic. This is the topic of the next section.

HYPOTHESIS TESTING WITH A TEST STATISTIC

Confidence intervals are used commonly to display the range of expected values of statistics and have wide application in healthcare research. However, their use in hypothesis testing is somewhat limited, particularly when the effect of more than one independent variable is being tested.

Furthermore, contemporary healthcare researchers use a variety of independent variables and study a complex matrix of dependent variables. Consequently, different analytical tools are needed. In this section, a general method of using a test statistic to make decisions concerning hypotheses is described. In subsequent chapters, a variety of statistical tests will be examined in greater detail.

The general process of using a test statistic to make a decision regarding the veracity of an H_0 is similar to that used with CIs. Assuming H_0 is true, a test statistic (for this example, t) is computed. The obtained value of t is then referred to its sampling distribution, the table of critical values of t, and the probability of obtaining that particular test statistic by chance is determined. If the probability is $\leq 5\%$, the statistical decision is to reject the H_0.

The calculation of the test statistic is illustrated using the data in Table 5-5, the same data that were used to calculate the CI for the difference between the two means. Indeed, the same variables are used in the calculation, but they are rearranged as follows:

$$t = \frac{(\bar{y}_1 - \bar{y}_2)}{\sigma_{(\bar{y}_1 - \bar{y}_2)}}$$

$$t = \frac{0.30}{0.09} = 3.33$$

Thus, the t statistic is calculated from the difference between the two sample means, divided by the pooled standard error. This is the formula for the t-test for independent means. The df associated with this t statistic is $(n_1 + n_2 - 2) = (138 + 140 - 2) = 276$, as before.

This t statistic value of 3.33 is referred to the table of critical t values (Table B-3 found in Appendix B). Because there is no listing for $df = 276$, the distribution of the t statistics for $df = 140$ is again substituted. Examination of different values of the t statistic in the t distribution with $df = 140$ indicates that, for a 2-sided test, observed values of $t \leq -1.977$ or ≥ 1.977 would be expected to occurs 5% of the time by chance. Because the obtained value of t, 3.33, exceeds the critical value 1.977, the H_0 is rejected.

This result is given in Figure 5-9, which displays the t distribution for $df = 140$ assuming the difference between the group means is 0. Notice first that the α region has been distributed so that half the total α region is located in each tail of the distribution. Thus values of t that fall into either region will lead to rejection of H_0. This is referred to as a 2-sided test. In contrast, the total α region may be placed in one tail of the distribution, so that only a t value in a specific direction leads to rejection of H_0. This is called a 1-sided test.

Figure 5-9 presents the 2-sided test results. Values of $t < -1.977$ or > 1.977 fall into the α region, and justify rejection of H_0. In the present case, the value of t is 3.33, which is clearly in the α region. Thus H_0 is rejected.

But more information is available. By continuing to examine the critical values of this

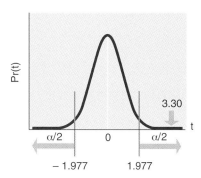

FIGURE 5-9 Statistical Significance. The distribution of the t statistic ($df = 140$) is used to determine statistical significance.

t distribution, it is noted that a t value of 3.33 is > 2.611, the critical value associated with 1% (2-sided test), but < 3.361, the critical value associated with 0.1% (2-sided test). Thus the result obtained would be expected to occur < 1% but > 0.1% of the time by chance.

In sum, calculating values of test statistics is another way of testing hypotheses. Notice that, whereas the CI provides information about the interval that likely contains the true value of the treatment effect, the test statistic indicates the rarity of the obtained effect by chance. Be aware that a rare event provides no information about the size of the effect. To obtain an index of the size of the effect, another statistic must be computed.

Putting It All Together—Understanding the Rationale for Statistical Inference

For many students, understanding the rationale for statistical inference is difficult. The source of this confusion is the failure to distinguish among the different sources of numbers and the formulas used to calculate the same statistics from the different sets of data. Perhaps the following explanation will help.

Begin with a *population*. A population is an aggregation of *all possible values* of a variable. For example, the distribution of all high-density lipoprotein (HDL) values in 44-year-old men living in North America is a population. The parameters of this distribution (μ and σ), as well as its shape, are unknown. It is assumed that σ is finite. It is the characteristics of the population that are of interest.

A *sample* is a subset of the population. Because it is obtained using random sampling techniques, statistics calculated from the sample ($\bar{y}$ and s) will be similar to the population parameters (μ and σ), within the limits of sampling error. That is, $\bar{y}$ is an unbiased estimate of μ, and s is an unbiased estimate of σ. The shape of the two sets of data will be similar. In short, because of the method used to draw the sample from the population, the sample is a miniature population.

So, sample statistics can be used to estimate the population parameters. But the specification of probabilities associated with specific values of the variable requires knowledge of the shape of the distribution, which is unknown. The solution to this problem lies in another population, the *sampling distribution of the statistic*. The sampling distribution of a statistic is a population. It is, more precisely, a frequency distribution of all possible values of a statistic, obtained using a specific sample size. Most important, because of the central

TABLE 5-8	Comparison of Formulas for the Mean and Standard Deviation and Knowledge of the Shape of the Population, Sample, and Sampling Distribution			
SOURCE OF DATA	**MEAN**		**STANDARD DEVIATION**	**SHAPE**
Population	$\mu = \dfrac{\Sigma y}{N}$		$\sigma = \sqrt{\dfrac{\Sigma(y - \mu)^2}{N}}$	Unknown
Sample	$\bar{y} = \dfrac{\Sigma y}{n}$		$s = \sqrt{\dfrac{\Sigma(y - \bar{y})^2}{(n - 1)}}$	Unknown
Sampling distribution	$\mu_{\bar{y}} = \bar{y}$		$\sigma_{\bar{y}} = \dfrac{s}{\sqrt{n}}$	Normal

limit theorem, the *shape* of the sampling distribution of the statistic is known to be a normal distribution. Thus probabilities associated with different values of the statistic can be determined and decisions regarding H_0 can be made.

The parameters of the sampling distribution of a statistic ($\mu_{\bar{y}}$ and $\sigma_{\bar{y}}$) are estimated using sample data ($\bar{y}$ and s). Because $\bar{y}$ is an unbiased estimate of μ, and $\bar{y} = \mu_{\bar{y}}$, $\mu_{\bar{y}}$ is also an unbiased estimate of μ. Because we know that s is an estimate of σ, then $\sigma_{\bar{y}}$ can be calculated using s as a substitute for σ. Thus the central limit theorem and the sampling distribution of a statistic provide the theoretical rationale for using unbiased statistics to make inferences about population parameters. Table 5-8 may help in clarifying these relationships.

Effect Size of Statistically Significant Differences

One difficulty with hypothesis testing using a test statistic is that the standard error depends on the sample size. Although it makes sense that a larger sample would provide a more accurate estimate of the population parameter, it is also possible to pad (use an excessively large) the sample size and thus to obtain statistical significance for clinically meaningless effects. As a result, there is a growing interest in the development of statistical indicants of the size of statistically significant effects.

Several measures of **effect size** (ES) have been suggested. One useful version is that provided by Cohen,[5] and termed Cohen's *d*.[*] The formula for Cohen's *d* is as follows

$$(\bar{y}_1 - \bar{y}_2) \div \text{the larger standard deviation of the two groups}$$

To compute Cohen's *d* from the data used to calculate the *t* statistic in Table 5-5, the following value is obtained:

$$0.30/0.81 = 0.37$$

Published guidelines suggest the following interpretation of Cohen's *d* values:[5]

- *d* of 0.2 is small
- *d* of 0.5 is medium
- *d* of 0.8 is large

---

[*]There are several different equations for calculating effect size; this is the one in Cohen.[5] It is conservative, which means that, compared to other formulas, it will result in a lower effect size estimate.

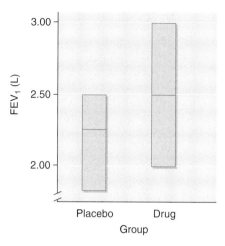

FIGURE 5-10 Calculating Interquartile Ranges (IQRs) from Published Data to Detect Effect Size. FEV_1, forced expiratory volume at 1 sec.

It would seem that, although the difference between the means is statistically significant, the size of the effect is less than medium. Examination of Figure 5-10 suggests the reason for the small ES. In this figure, the interquartile ranges (IQRs) for the two groups are compared. It seems that, although there are differences in the measure of central tendency, the range of the IQR is rather wide in both groups (i.e., more than 1 L in the drug group), and there is quite a bit of overlap in the scores of the two groups. Finding such a low ES might induce the clinician to reassess the enthusiasm developed for the drug based on only knowledge of statistical significance.

PERSPECTIVE 5-1

As just illustrated, box plots comparing the distributions of scores can be a valuable adjunct to the interpretation of grouped data. An IQR for published data, whether or not an ES is presented, can be approximated using the following method.

Beginning with the mean and standard deviation, the lower and upper limits for the IQR for each group can be approximated by values for the 25th and 75th percentiles using the z score distribution. Instead of the median, the mean value is substituted as an approximation. Assuming that the shape of the distributions is normal, this substitution entails little error.

For the drug group in Table 5-5, the 25th percentile is delimited by 1.96 L (2.50 − 0.67 × 0.81) and the 75th percentile is delimited by 3.04 L (2.50 + 0.67 × 0.81). Values for the placebo group are determined in a similar manner.

While the effect size index is rather crude, it is applicable in many different situations and is easy to calculate. Most important, because it is a dimensionless number it can be used to compare the effects of studies that use different dependent variables. For example, ES is used commonly to compare results from different studies in meta-analyses. Finally, there are other indices of ES that appear commonly in the healthcare literature. One of these, the odds ratio, is discussed in detail in Chapter 6.

Summary

This has been a long journey through statistical thinking. It began with a consideration of probability and probability distributions as ways to quantify the role of sampling variability in the outcome variable. These principles were then extended to probability distributions of statistics, sampling distributions. The essential role of the central limit theorem in providing the theoretical framework for the continuance of the journey cannot be overemphasized because the theorem provides the rationale for the estimation of population parameters from sample data even though the shape of the parent population is unknown. The central limit theorem also provides the foundation for the development of hypothesis testing using both CIs and test statistics. Although the components of the two calculations are similar, the results of the calculations provide fundamentally different types of information. In fact, there is a growing practice of providing both the CI and the test statistic results in many published articles.

STUDY PROBLEMS

1. Using the parameters $n = 10$ and $p = 0.7$, generate the binomial distribution to describe the results of a coin-flipping demonstration. Compute the mean and standard deviation of this distribution. Compare these parameters (including shape) to those of the binomial distribution in Figure 5-4.

2. You are examining the results of a screening test to detect patients at risk of osteoarthritis owing to a previous sports stress injury. About 35% of your population is at risk for osteoarthritis. Of those who are at risk, 90% test positive on the screening test, and 85% of those not at risk test negative. Assuming that you test 1000 people, construct a 2×2 table for the results and calculate the predictive values and the likelihood ratios. Discuss the diagnostic value of SpIN and SnOUT, the predictive values, and the likelihood ratios in this example.

3. Describe the properties of a confidence interval and its significance for estimating population parameters.

4. In one group of 35 patients receiving antihypertensive treatment, the mean blood pressure is 105 mmHg, with a standard deviation of 15 mmHg. In a control group of 35 patients receiving a placebo, the average blood pressure is 115 mmHg, with a standard deviation of 10 mmHg. The pooled standard deviation for the difference between the means is 3.05. Calculate a 95% CI for the difference between the two sample means. Compute a t-test of the difference between the two sample means. Compare the two hypothesis testing methods.

5. What is the significance of the central limit theorem in statistics?

6. In a long-term randomized controlled trial, analyses are conducted periodically. The purpose is not to deprive the control patients of any benefit of the treatment being tested. In these analyses, α is typically set to be very low, for example around 0.001. Why?

REFERENCES

1. McTiernan A, Kooperberg C, White E, et al. Recreational physical activity and the risk of breast cancer in postmenopausal women. The women's health study. JAMA 2003;290:1331–1336.
2. Sackett DL, Haynes RB, Richardson WS, et al. Evidence-based medicine. How to practice and teach EBM. Edinburgh, UK: Churchill Livingston; 2000.
3. Center for Evidence-Based Medicine. Likelihood ratios. Available at www.cebm.net/likelihood_ratios.asp. Accessed February 2007.
4. Dansinge, ML, Gleason JA, Griffith JL, et al. Comparison of the Atkins, Ornish, Weight Watchers, and Zone diets for weight loss and heart disease risk reduction. A randomized trial. JAMA 2005;293:43–53.
5. Cohen, J. Statistical Power Analyses for the Behavioral Sciences. 2nd ed. Hillsdale, NJ: Erlbaum, 1988.

Critical Appraisal of Evidence Derived from Studying Cases

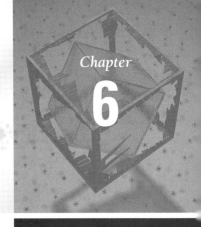

Chapter

6

CHAPTER GOALS

After studying this chapter, the student should be able to:

1. Describe case study, case series and case-control study designs and how they are used clinically.

2. Explain the rationale for these designs.

3. Enumerate the advantages and disadvantages of each study design.

4. Explain and use epidemiologic measures of occurrence.

5. Define and use epidemiologic measures of risk.

6. Interpret statistical tests used to analyze frequency data.

Epidemiology is the study of factors that affect health and disease, particularly from a population or public health perspective. Both the principles and methods of epidemiology are used frequently in evaluating evidence pertinent to healthcare decisions. Indeed, the research designs examined in this chapter and in Chapter 7 were developed originally by epidemiologists and are sometimes termed epidemiologic study designs or **observational study research designs**.

This chapter examines research strategies that involve studying cases, patients who already exhibit a disease or condition, in an attempt to identify potential exposure factors. Several observational study designs focus on cases: the **case study**, **case series**, and the **case-control study** designs.

Examples of investigations focusing on cases follow:

- An elderly woman complains of blood in her urine (hematuria), and the pharmacist suspects that a drug interaction is the culprit. How does he or she gather evidence?
- Several individuals in a clinic display a sudden decrease in international normalized ratio (INR). Why?
- An investigator wishes to provide evidence for the roles of several factors, including acetaminophen, in altering the anticoagulation response to warfarin. How might he or she proceed?

The goal of this chapter is to increase awareness of the value of the case study and case series study designs and to provide a framework for the evaluation of evidence from case-control designs. To accomplish this, statistical methods used in observational study designs, both case-control and cohort paradigms, are examined in some detail.

111

Case Study and Case Series Designs

The case study is a retrospective description of a condition in an individual, whereas a case series is a retrospective description of a condition in several individuals. These reports may appear in bulletins promulgated by government agencies, such as the Centers for Disease Control and Prevention (CDC). Their intent is to inform the healthcare community of novel or unusual clinical findings or conditions or to track the spread of a disease. For example, CDC bulletins were among the first to report the presence of Avian influenza H7N3 in British Columbia and the appearance of West Nile Virus in New York City.[1,2] Case reports of specific interest to pharmacists include descriptions of adverse drug reactions, novel drug uses, and other pharmacist-related matters.[3–5]

The elements of a case study may be illustrated by considering the report of a woman who complained of a 3-day history of hematuria and gingival bleeding.[6] Because she had suffered a stroke 6 years earlier, she had been prescribed a dose of warfarin sufficient to maintain a prothrombin time between 15 and 19 sec, within the normal range. In contrast, her prothrombin time at hospital admission was 96 sec, abnormally high. Her husband indicated that the patient had begun a regimen of acetaminophen plus codeine for backache pain approximately 5 weeks earlier. Administering 3 units of fresh frozen plasma and discontinuing the acetaminophen restored the prothrombin time to its predrug value.

This study exemplifies the typical elements of a case study:

- The case history of the patient is described, including disease history and past and concurrent treatments. Anomalous conditions are also noted. This may be preceded by a more general review of the topic area.
- The exacerbating circumstance, the event that prompted the patient to seek treatment, is then noted in detail and related to potential antecedent factors.
- Finally, changes in treatment based on the patient's history are described, emphasizing those that resolved the problem successfully.

This presentation sequence is also used in case series reports: Several elderly patients who were maintained on an efficacious dose of warfarin for several years suddenly displayed a decrease in INR.[7] A detailed medical history, emphasizing recent changes in medication, revealed that each patient had begun ingesting a dose of ubidecarenone (coenzyme Q10) several weeks earlier. Discontinuing the ubidecarenone regimen restored INR to a normal value in all patients.

Case study and case series reports increase the awareness of healthcare providers regarding conditions or consequences that may be novel, occur rarely, or be currently underappreciated. Case study and case series study designs provide valuable information to pharmacists regarding adverse drug reactions, drug interactions, novel uses of a drug, or unanticipated benefits of treatment.

The results of case study and case series reports, however, provide only *suggestive* evidence of an exposure–outcome association. The evidence is not convincing for several reasons. First, patients are deliberately selected by the investigator. Thus the remarkable consistency of patient histories and outcomes may be the result of that selection process: choosing patients who exhibited exemplary results and excluding patients who did not show results supporting the point the author wished to make.

Second, the possibility of confounding cannot be dismissed. Here is an example. In studying the potential relationship between tobacco use and lung cancer, demonstrating that lung cancer patients have a positive history of tobacco use is not conclusive. The cancer may be the result of a variety of other factors, such as air quality. Often, the control of confounding factors is beyond the scope of the case series report.

Finally, case study and case series study designs lack control groups to gauge the effects of **nuisance variables**. As a result, effects of treatments may be obscured. Changes in variable values over time, for example, are measurable only if a placebo control group is included in the study design. For these reasons, the case-control study design is preferred to the case study and case series designs.

In summary, the case study and case series study designs can provide valuable indications of possible associations between exposures and outcomes. Some applications of the case series report, like a case series investigation of a food poisoning outbreak, provide evidence sufficient to act on. More often, evidence derived by these study designs prompts further research, as in the case of the acetaminophen–warfarin interaction.[8]

The Case-Control Study Design

The case-control study is a sophisticated case series design that incorporates a group of control patients. Theoretically, one or more control participants are matched to each case with respect to all variables except the suspected exposure. The critical comparison is the difference in cases versus controls with respect to the variable under consideration.

Case-control study designs were introduced in Chapter 3. Their features, summarized in Table 3-1, are as follows:

- The goal is to identify exposure variables that are associated with an outcome.
- The strategy is to assemble groups that differ only in exhibiting an outcome, and to then search for differences in antecedent exposure variables.
- The design is particularly prone to bias, although factors such as confounding and measurement error may also affect the exposure–outcome association.

In evaluating a case-control study, it is important to examine two specific aspects of the study design. One is the similarity of case and control participants on variables other than the exposure variable of interest. Another is the extent to which bias may have affected the study results.

A critical component of the integrity of the case-control study design is the extent to which cases and controls differ on variables other than the exposure variable. One aspect of this comparison involves demographic variables such as age, gender, socioeconomic status, and so on. Another facet is health history. Both cases and controls should exhibit similar health histories so that it is unlikely that differences in general health status could affect the results. Finally, cases and controls should be matched on known confounding and other nuisance variables. Ideally, effects of confounding and nuisance variables on the exposure–outcome association should be assessed.

Selecting cases and controls with common characteristics is called **matching**. Matching cases and controls can be accomplished in several ways. In studies in which an entire population of patients is available for study, controls can be selected randomly from the population and compared to case patients. Another method of matching is to select control participants who share important characteristics with case participants. For example, in a case-control study examining the link between toxic shock syndrome and the use of different tampons, investigators interviewed neighbors of cases in the belief that people in the same neighborhood would exhibit similar socioeconomic characteristics and hygienic practices.[9]

In sum, the point of matching cases and controls is to make sure that the two groups differ only with respect to the suspected exposure variable, thus excluding the roles of confounding and nuisance variables in the outcome.

The other aspect of concern with case-control studies is the presence of bias. Bias refers to a systematic difference in the manner in which the cases and controls are treated. Bias makes an appearance in many different forms. It may occur in the process of selecting cases or controls for the study; when interviewing patients or participants; or in data analysis, data interpretation, or data reporting. Three common sources of bias are selection bias, interviewer bias and recall bias.

The method of selecting patients for the case-control study is important. Because patients are not selected randomly, **selection bias** may be a real problem. There may be a tendency to include only the worst cases or the best cases to make a point or to maximize or minimize an association. This can be achieved, for example, by altering the criteria that determine the classification of a patient as a case or a control.

Either standard diagnostic criteria should be used to designate cases or criteria that normally prompt medical intervention should be applied. Otherwise, the composition of the study group is not certain, which diminishes the external validity of the study. For example, the current standard diagnostic criteria for diabetes mellitus include fasting blood glucose measurements > 126 mg/dL obtained on two separate occasions. Adding patients who almost meet this standard, perhaps by including those with impaired glucose tolerance, makes it difficult for the reader to determine precisely which patients are affected by the exposure. Furthermore, mixing patients with different disease severities adds to measurement error, thereby obfuscating the results. In short, criteria for defining cases should be meaningful clinically.

Interview bias occurs when the interviewer treats case patients differently from controls. For example, an interviewer might treat breast cancer patients with more sympathy than controls. As a result, the cancer patient may be more likely to share details of her methods of coping with the disease. Interview bias can be minimized by training personnel to conduct the interview, conducting the interview according to a prepared script, asking closed-end questions, and perhaps even using an electronic device to deliver verbal content.

Recall bias is the tendency of cases to have better retention of circumstances associated with a precipitating event than controls. A common example (as noted earlier) is that parents of children who have asthma are more likely to recall their children's coughing or wheezing episodes than are parents of children who do not have asthma because the former parents are more attuned to such events. Likewise, a woman who has experienced deep vein thrombosis (DVT) secondary to hormonal contraceptives may be more attuned to her past use of birth control pills than a woman who has not experienced DVT.

Finally, investigators may be tempted to focus on aspects of the data that are of interest to them, even though they are not statistically significant. For example, findings that are not statistically significant may be termed *clinically significant* and be discussed as though they had achieved statistical significance. Alternately, results that are not statistically significant may be described as *small*, suggesting perhaps that they were meaningful even though they had not achieved acceptable levels for statistical significance.[10] Finally, a common practice is to describe effects that are not statistically significant as providing evidence of a *trend* in the data.

In summary, studying cases provides much valuable information about the relationship of one or more exposures and an outcome. These studies can be conducted relatively quickly and are inexpensive compared to costs associated with other study designs. Furthermore, the epidemiologic designs are well suited for studying diseases with long incubation periods or diseases that are rare. However, care must be taken in evaluating these reports to make sure that standard definitions of the variables are provided and that all reasonable steps have been taken to limit bias in the design, subject selection, data management, and reporting of the study results.

Expressing Associations Using Case-Control Study Designs

Like the observational research paradigms, the use of numbers to provide estimates of population parameters and to suggest changes in levels of variables as a function of exposure are developments pioneered by epidemiologists. The general interest of epidemiologists is to understand the determinants of health and disease and to identify factors that differentiate those who succumb to the disease from those who do not.

A signal feature of the use of numbers in these situations is that numbers are used to count rather than to measure. That is, epidemiologists are interested in differences in the *frequency* of an event or a condition among different groups of people. The generalization of observational (e.g., case-control and cohort) research paradigms to the study of other areas of healthcare (e.g., disease prevention and health promotion) carries over these uses of numbers and statistics.

WAYS TO EXPRESS DIFFERENCES IN FREQUENCY OF EVENTS

To understand patterns of health and disease, epidemiologists focus on two phenomena: the number of individuals exhibiting an outcome during a specific time period and the number displaying the outcome at any point in time.

The number of new cases of a disease in a specific time period is the incidence of the disease. More specifically, the **incidence** of a disease is the ratio of the number of *new* cases of a disease occurring during a specific time interval divided by the number of *susceptible* individuals. Thus the incidence of benign prostatic hyperplasia is referred to the population of men. In healthcare circles, another term for the incidence of a disease is *risk*.

One apparent difficulty with this definition of incidence is that it does not count every occurrence of the disease. For example, a person who experiences two bouts of the common cold is counted only once under this definition of incidence. To compensate, a different measure of time is used instead of chronological time. This measure of time is **person-time**, expressed in person-years, person-months, and so on.

Person-time is calculated by dividing a person's total participation time into segments and expressing the event rate per segment. For example, assume a study of the incidence of the common cold used three patients: one patient participated 3 months, another patient participated 5 months, and a third patient participated 2 months. To use all the data, the investigator divides the different time intervals into person-months and expresses the incidence of the common cold in terms of this denominator, which is 10 person-months. If 2 cases of the common cold were identified, the rate of the cold would be 1 per 5 person-months, which can be extrapolated to 6 per 2.4 person-year.

This expression of incidence is termed **incidence density.** For this measure to be accurate, the threat of the risk—the probability of a person contracting the common cold as well as the susceptibility of the patient—must remain constant during the measurement period.

Another measure of interest to epidemiologists is the proportion of individuals in a population who exhibit the disease at any point in time. More formally, the **prevalence** of an event is the relative frequency of that event at a specific time. Thus the prevalence of the common cold in a group of students in a pharmacy program is the proportion of those with the condition on, say, January 30, 2007. Although the prevalence is sometimes referred to as a rate, it is really a proportion.

Actually, there are two uses of prevalence. Point prevalence, just defined, is an accurate measure when the disease is characterized by an abrupt onset and is easily diagnosed, as for diseases like the common cold and Asian flu. The onset of other maladies, like Alzheimer disease and osteoarthritis, are not as readily apparent. In these cases, a **period**

prevalence measure is used. The period prevalence is the sum of the number of cases present at the beginning of the measurement interval (i.e., the point prevalence) plus the number of new cases that occur during a specified time period.[11] To obtain the period prevalence of rheumatoid arthritis, participants might be asked whether they had experienced any arthritic symptoms in the previous year.

The prevalence of a disease is the result of several factors. One factor, incidence, is the rate at which new cases are added to the prevalence pool. Two other factors, mortality and recovery, express the rates at which cases are removed from the disease pool. When considering changes in prevalence, each of these factors must be assessed. For example, the prevalence of cystic fibrosis in the United States increased progressively during the 20th century. This change, however, was the result of improvements in treatment, which extended the life span of such patients. The incidence of the disease remained virtually unchanged.[12]

The incidence and prevalence data derived from a research study are *crude* numbers, meaning that they are characteristic of the sample used in the study. Often, however, the characteristics of a study sample do not mirror those of the population of interest to the investigator. In these circumstances, the data may be adjusted to increase the similarity between the characteristics of the sample and those of the population.

As an example, refer to the data in Table 6-1, which shows the prevalence of Alzheimer disease in two communities. The table indicates that there are almost 46% more cases of Alzheimer's disease in community B than in community A. Because the populations of the two communities are different sizes, a more accurate estimate of Alzheimer's disease would be based on a common population index, such as the *rate* of the disease per 100,000 people. When the prevalence of Alzheimer's disease is adjusted for the size difference between the populations, the prevalence of the disease is seen to be similar in the two communities.

Another adjustment of the data may be illustrated with measures of mortality. The overall measure of mortality is **all-cause mortality.** This measure reflects the total mortality in a group from all causes during the study period. Thus it provides an index of the general burden of mortality in the group. In addition to reflecting group differences in overall mortality, discrepancies in all-cause mortality may provide the rationale for examining specific causes of mortality. These are termed **case-fatality rates** and refer to the number of deaths attributable to specific causes during a specific time interval, such as the number of deaths owing to pneumonia during a recent flu season. An **attack rate** refers to the incidence of mortality during an unusually short time interval, such as would occur after the ingestion of tainted food.

In addition to measures of death and disease, there are a number of ways of expressing the likelihood of dying, contracting a disease, or benefiting from a treatment. These are *risk, odds,* and **hazard.** Note that these terms can be used to describe both undesirable events (death and disease) and desirable events (avoidance of death and disease, the increment in a healthy lifestyle). An increase in the risk of an untoward event is tantamount to a decrease in benefit and vice versa.

TABLE 6-1	**Crude and Adjusted Prevalence of Alzheimer's Disease in Two Communities**	
	COMMUNITY	
MEASURE	A	B
Crude prevalence	24,000	35,000
Total population	600,000	875,000
Adjusted prevalence	4,000	4,000

TABLE 6-2   Calculation of Indices of Risk[a]

| LUNG ABNORMALITIES | EXPOSURE STATUS | | TOTAL |
	MINIMAL	MAXIMAL	
Yes	80	467	547
No	1120	883	2003
Total	1200	1350	2550

Risk calculations assuming data from a cohort study

MEASURE	CALCULATION
Risk in maximally exposed group	467/1350 = 0.346
Risk in minimally exposed group	80/1200 = 0.067
Attributable risk	0.346 − 0.067 = 0.279
Relative risk	0.346/0.067 = 5.16

Odds approximations assuming data from a case-control study

MEASURE	CALCULATION
Odds in maximally exposed group	467/883 = 0.529
Odds in minimally exposed group	80/1120 = 0.071
Odds ratio	0.529/0.071 = 7.45

[a]Data indicate the frequency of residents who developed asbestos-related lung abnormalities as a function of the extent of exposure to asbestos.

Data from Miller AK. Libby, MT: Overview of asbestos exposures and health effects. Paper presented at the 101st meeting of the Cordilleran Section, Geological Society of America, San Jose, CA, April 29–May 1, 2005. Abstract available at: gsa.confex.com/gsa/2005CD/finalprogram/abstract_85952.htm. Accessed June 2006.

The calculation of variables to express risk is illustrated by using the data given in Table 6-2. The data are adapted from a case-control study of asbestos-related lung abnormalities among workers and their families in Libby, Montana.[13] The table indicates the number of people with and without such abnormalities who were maximally and minimally exposed to the asbestos mine. Risk, or absolute risk, is the probability of an individual acquiring a condition in a specific time interval. It is calculated as the number of those afflicted divided by the total number of susceptible individuals in the population and is an example of incidence.

In cohort study designs, the calculation of risk is straightforward, because the study design provides an estimate of the incidence of the disease. In case-control studies, participants are selected deliberately because they display the malady of interest and therefore do not provide an accurate index of incidence. However, the determination of risk may still be obtained indirectly, using odds.

To illustrate, first assume that the data in Table 6-2 are derived from a cohort study. During the study period, 80 new cases of asbestos-related lung abnormalities were detected among 1200 citizens who were minimally exposed to the asbestos mine, and 467 of 1350 mine workers displayed asbestos-related lung abnormalities. Thus the risk of asbestos-related lung abnormalities in minimally exposed citizens was 80/1200 or 0.067 and the risk of asbestos-related lung abnormalities among maximally exposed citizens was 467/1350 or 0.346.

Although the absolute risk of asbestos-related lung abnormalities among those maximally exposed to asbestos was 34.6%, this calculation does not suggest that 34.6% of the asbestos-related lung abnormalities were the result of maximal asbestos exposure. Such a conclusion is erroneous because it does not consider the baseline or background rate of asbestos-related lung abnormalities. That is, 6.7% of the residents displayed asbestos-related lung abnormalities even though their exposure to asbestos was minimal. So the risk attributable to maximal asbestos exposure is 0.346 − 0.067 = 0.279. This is the attributable risk or the risk difference and is the risk of asbestos-related lung abnormalities specifically associated with maximal exposure to asbestos.

An expression of the *strength of association* between the exposure and the outcome is the **relative risk** (RR). This is the risk of the exposed group divided by the risk of the unexposed group. In the present example, the RR would equal 0.346/0.067 or about 5.2. This number suggests that those who are maximally exposed to asbestos are 5.2 times more likely to develop asbestos-related lung abnormalities than those minimally exposed.

Another expression of the strength of association between exposure and outcome is the **number needed to harm (NNH).** This is the reciprocal of the risk difference or attributable risk. From the asbestos exposure example, the NNH = 1/0.279 or 3.58. The NNH of 3.58 suggests that 1 person will develop asbestos-related lung abnormalities for every 3.58 persons maximally exposed to asbestos for the time period delineated in the study. A companion measure, the **number needed to treat (NNT)**, is computed in the same manner to convey the beneficial effects of a treatment, and has a similar interpretation.

To illustrate these calculations using odds, assume that the data in Table 6-2 were gathered using a case-control study design. To reiterate, because cases are selected deliberately with this study design, the incidence of the malady cannot be estimated directly. Indirect methods must be used that involve odds. **Odds** is the ratio of the number of ways an event may occur divided by the number of ways it may not occur. In this example, the odds of asbestos-related lung abnormalities with minimal exposure are 80/1120 = 0.071, and with maximal exposure are 467/883 = 0.529.

Like relative risk, an **odds ratio** (OR) can be used to express the *strength of association* between an exposure and an outcome. In this example, 0.529/0.071 = 7.45, meaning that the odds of exhibiting asbestos related lung abnormalities are 7.45 times greater for those maximally exposed to asbestos compared to those minimally exposed.

Note that the RR and OR equal 1 if the risk or odds in the two groups is the same, are > 1 if the risk or odds in the exposed groups exceeds the risk or odds in the unexposed group, and are < 1 if the risk or odds in the exposed group is less than the risk or odds in the unexposed group. In the present example involving asbestos-related lung abnormalities, the RR was calculated to be 5.16, and the OR was determined to equal 7.45. Thus both provide similar estimates of the strength of association between the exposure and the outcome.

 EXTRA CREDIT 6-1

Risk and odds are almost always presented in terms of diseases and other exposures that increase chances of mortality or morbidity. Here's an example of risk calculations from a study in which a drug reduces an untoward symptom.

The data in Table 6-3 are adapted from a study of the effects of ibuprofen, 200 mg and 400 mg, versus placebo in reducing migraine headache pain.[14] Because both doses of ibuprofen were associated with a similar benefit, only data from the 200 mg dose and the placebo are presented. Of 437 patients complaining of headache, 216 received ibuprofen 200 mg and 221 received a placebo. It was found that 90 of those receiving the drug

TABLE 6-3	Efficacy of Ibuprofen 200 mg versus Placebo in Relieving Migraine Headache Pain[a]		
	DRUG TREATMENT		
PAIN RELIEF	IBUPROFEN	PLACEBO	*TOTAL*
Yes	90	62	152
No	126	159	285
Total	216	221	437

[a]Data are frequencies of patients reporting whether they experienced pain relief after treatment with a placebo or ibuprofen 200 mg.

Data from Codispoti JR, Prior MJ, Fu M, et al. Effect of nonprescription doses of ibuprofen for treating migraine headache. A randomized controlled trial. Headache 2001;41:665–679.

and 62 of those receiving placebo reported pain relief. Thus the risk of headache in the treatment group after the intervention was $(216 - 90)/216$ or 0.58, whereas that in the control group was $(221 - 62)/221$ or 0.72.

The **risk difference**, also called the absolute risk reduction, is $(0.58 - 0.72)$ or -0.14. Thus about 14% of the reduction in pain relief can be attributed to ibuprofen 200 mg.

The relative risk reduction is the difference between the two event rates, divided by the control event rate, which is $(0.58 - 0.72)/0.72 = -0.194$. This suggests that the rate of headache was 19.4% less in the group administered ibuprofen 200 mg.

A final measure of risk reduction, the NNT, is equal to the reciprocal of the absolute risk difference, or $1/0.140 = 7.14$. This suggests that 1 patient will obtain pain relief with ibuprofen 200 mg for every 7 patients treated. ■

Analyzing Nominal and Ordinal Data

In chapter 5 a statistical theory was presented for analyzing *quantitative* data based on variables involving interval and ratio scales of measurement. These might include demographic variables or indices of drug activity. That method of statistical analysis depended on estimating population parameters and assumed that the variable could be characterized by a normal probability distribution. These kinds of tests are generally termed *parametric statistics*.

Epidemiologic studies discussed in this chapter and in Chapter 7 however, use frequencies and ranks to characterize *qualitative* differences among observational units. Statistical analyses of these nominal and ordinal data differ fundamentally from analyses of interval and ratio data. First, variable levels reflect differences in count or rank rather than quantity. Second, they rely neither on estimates of population parameters nor on assumptions about the distribution of the variable in the parent population. Instead, these elements are developed from expectations derived from the null hypothesis (H_0). The kinds of statistical tests to be described are therefore termed *nonparametric* or *distribution-free statistics*.

Nonparametric statistical tests are reported frequently in healthcare studies of interest to pharmacists. Statistical tests of frequency data, include the *chi-square test* (χ^2) (which is really a family of tests), *Fisher's exact test*, *McNemar's test*, and the *sign test*. In addition, two tests that allow control for confounding factors, the *Mantel-Haenszel test* and *logistic regression analysis*, are described. This is followed by a brief description of two tests of ordinal data: the *Wilcoxon rank-sum test* and the *Wilcoxon signed-rank test*.

TABLE 6-4	Raw Data for a χ^2 test of the Efficacy of a Novel Pain Reliever[a]			
DRUG RESPONSE	LESS EFFECTIVE	AS EFFECTIVE	MORE EFFECTIVE	*TOTAL*
Count	75	240	35	350

[a]Data are frequencies of patients reporting whether they experienced pain relief after treatment with a placebo or ibuprofen.

CHI-SQUARE (χ^2) Test

The signal feature of data appropriate for the χ^2 test is that they are frequencies. For example, counting the number of people in a sample that display high, medium, and low sensitivity to a drug provides appropriate data for a χ^2 test. A χ^2 test can also be used to analyze the pattern of change in one variable as a function of another variable. Thus a χ^2 test can also be used to examine whether the effects of a drug are the same in men and women or in different age groups. Finally, this test can be applied to continuous data, if the data are first converted to frequency data. This is the procedure followed, for example, when a person is diagnosed with hypertension (a dichotomous categorical variable) based on a diastolic blood pressure reading (a continuous variable).

The simplest application of the χ^2 test is to assess the distribution of scores across different levels of a single variable. For example, the efficacy of a novel pain reliever is to be assessed by having migraine headache sufferers rate it as less efficacious, as efficacious, or more efficacious than their current pain reliever. The data might appear as in Table 6-4. Of 350 patient ratings, 75 judged the drug less effective than their current medication, 240 rated the new drug as equally effective, and 35 rated the new drug as better than the current drug.

The next step is to generate the distribution of the 350 ratings according to a H_0. This is accomplished as follows: If there were no differences in drug effect, the distribution of patient ratings should be random, with 116 in each category. These, then, become the *expected cell frequencies*—they are the outcome expected if the H_0 is true. Table 6-5 displays the both the *observed* and the *expected* cell frequencies for this example.

The rationale for the statistical test is as follows: if the H_0 is true, then differences between observed and expected cell frequencies should be small. If the H_0 is false, these differences should be large. This is the role of the χ^2 test statistic—it compares the extent of the discrepancy between each cell's observed (O) cell frequency and its expected (E) frequency if the H_0 is true. Specifically, the χ^2 statistic is calculated according to this formula:

$$\chi^2 = \Sigma \frac{(O - E)^2}{E}$$

In words, the χ^2 statistic is obtained by determining the difference between the observed and the expected cell frequencies for each cell, squaring the difference, and dividing the

TABLE 6-5	Observed and Expected Frequencies for a χ^2 Test of the Efficacy of a Novel Pain Reliever[a]			
DRUG RESPONSE	LESS EFFECTIVE	AS EFFECTIVE	MORE EFFECTIVE	*TOTAL*
Observed count	75	240	35	350
Expected count	116.7	116.6	116.7	350

[a]Data are observed and expected frequencies of patients reporting whether the pain relief they experienced with a novel agent was less, as, or more effective than their usual pain reliever.

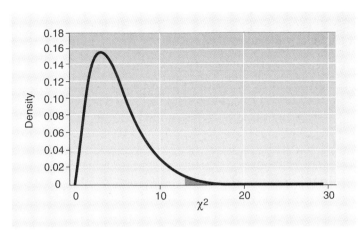

FIGURE 6-1   Probability distributions of the χ^2 statistic with 5 *df*. (Created with aid of the x^2 calculator available at www.stat.tamu.edu/~west/applets/chisqdemo.html.)

product by the expected cell frequency. These values are then summed over all the cells. For this example:

$$\chi^2 = \frac{(75-116.7)^2}{116.7} + \frac{(240-116.6)^2}{116.6} + \frac{(35-116.7)^2}{116.7} = 202.7$$

The statistical significance of the χ^2 statistic is determined by referring to a distribution of all possible values of χ^2 assuming that H_0 is true. Such distributions are based on the degrees of freedom (*df*). The *df* for the χ^2 test statistic are based on the number of *cells* in the analysis, not the number of participants contributing to the frequency count of each cell. In this example, with 3 cells, the *df* equal 2 because once the cell count for the first two cells is determined, the third cell must contain a frequency that guarantees the total is equal to the total frequency count, 350.

The distribution of the χ^2 statistic for five *df*, assuming the H_0 is true, is displayed in Figure 6-1. Note that the χ^2 statistic is not distributed normally. This suggests that values of χ^2 are not distributed symmetrically about the center of the distribution. Thus, for a two-sided test, separate critical values of the χ^2 statistic must be obtained for each tail of the distribution.

Critical values of the χ^2 are found in Table B-4 (Appendix B). For the χ^2 distribution with 2 *df*, the calculated value of χ^2 must exceed 5.991, the χ^2 value delimiting the upper 5% of the probability distribution. The calculated value of χ^2, 202.7, clearly exceeds this critical value, and the conclusion is reached that the rating of drug efficacy was not the result of chance.

A second application of the χ^2 statistic is to compare the frequencies of scores for one variable as a function of changes in a second variable—a cross tabulation. Table 6-6 shows

TABLE 6-6	A 2 × 2 Contingency Table: Hypercholesterolemia and Stroke[a]		
	HYPERCHOLESTEROLEMIA		
STROKE	YES	NO	*TOTAL*
Yes	150	100	250
No	135	130	265
Total	285	230	515

[a]Data are patients characterized with respect to the presence of hypercholesterolemia and stroke.

TABLE 6-7	A 2 × 2 Contingency Table (with Expected Cell Frequencies): Hypercholesterolemia and Stroke[a]		

| | HYPERCHOLESTEROLEMIA | | |
STROKE	YES	NO	*TOTAL*
Yes	150 (138)	100 (112)	250
No	135 (147)	130 (118)	265
Total	285	230	515

[a]Data are patients characterized with respect to the presence of hypercholesterolemia and stroke. Expected frequencies are in parentheses.

a hypothetical relationship between hypercholesterolemia and stroke in a group of patients. This type of table is called a **2 × 2 contingency table**, because each variable has two levels (in this example, yes and no.). Of 285 patients with elevated cholesterol levels, 150 experienced a stroke in the past year, whereas only 100 of 230 patients with normal cholesterol levels suffered a stroke. What is the probability that this difference occurred by chance?

The answer to this question depends on whether the two variables are related. If the two variables are independent, then the proportion of stroke patients should be roughly similar in both cholesterol conditions. This is the H_0. Furthermore, the proportion of stroke patients in both cholesterol groups should be similar to the proportion of stroke patients in the total study (which is equal to 250/515 or 48.5%). In each group, therefore, the expected cell frequency of stroke patients is equal to 0.485 of the total group membership. These expected values are 138 stroke patients in the elevated cholesterol group and 112 stroke patients in the normal cholesterol group. Similar methods generated the expected cell frequencies for the other two cells. Table 6-7 includes the expected cell frequencies in parentheses.

The χ^2 statistic is calculated according to the typical formula:

$$\chi^2 = \Sigma \frac{(O - E)^2}{E}$$

$$\chi^2 = \frac{(150-138)^2}{138} + \frac{(100-112)^2}{112} + \frac{(135-147)^2}{147} + \frac{(130-118)^2}{118} = 4.53$$

The *df* for a 2 × 2 contingency table are equal to 1. This is because the assignment of a frequency to the first cell determines all other cell frequency values if the row and column sums are to equal the total count.

From Table B-4 (Appendix B), the critical value of χ^2 with df = 1 and α = 0.05, for a one-sided test is 3.84. The calculated value of χ^2, 4.53, exceeds this critical value. Thus the H_0 that the two variables are independent is rejected and the conclusion reached is that the frequency of stroke is greater in the hypercholesterolemic group.

These applications of the basic χ^2 test are used commonly in healthcare studies. The χ^2 test is flexible and has wide application. As with other tests, validity of the test results depends on several assumptions being met. The major ones for the χ^2 test are these:

- It is assumed that the data are obtained using random sampling methods.
- It is assumed that the scores are independent. That is, selecting one person does not affect the chances of selecting any other person. As such, the χ^2 test cannot be used to test correlated data.
- It is assumed that there are a minimum number of counts per category. There is general agreement that the expected cell frequency for each cell in a 2 × 2 table should be at least 5. And, even with larger tables, there should be no cells with 0 scores.

- The test must be based on frequencies. χ^2 tests based on percentages are not valid because this implies that the sample size is 100.

Finally, the H_0 is that two variables are related only by chance. Therefore, rejecting the null hypothesis does not provide evidence of a cause-and-effect relationship between the two variables.

The next section examines statistical tests that can be used when these assumptions are not met. For example, Fisher's exact test is used when the number of cell frequencies is small and McNemar's test is applied when data are related rather than independent.

FISHER'S EXACT TEST

Fisher's exact test is used when the numbers in a 2×2 contingency table are too small to compute a χ^2 statistic. It is an exact test because it computes the probability of the H_0 directly rather by than calculating a statistic using the χ^2 formula.

For example, assume the data presented in Table 6-8 are being examined to discern whether a new treatment is superior to a standard treatment in extending the life of terminal cancer patients. There are a total of 44 records. A total of 11 patients were given the standard treatment and 4 died. A total of 33 patients were given the new treatment and 1 died. What is the probability that this result was obtained by chance?

Fisher's probability is computed using the binomial coefficient, $_nC_j$, which was presented in Chapter 5. The test determines the probability of the observed pattern in the data given all possible patterns the data might assume. In essence, we are asking about the number of ways different combinations of events can occur. Specifically:

1. In how many ways can 4 of the 5 people who are fated to die be assigned to the standard treatment group?
2. In how many ways can the 7 of the 39 patients who are fated to survive be assigned to the standard treatment group?
3. In how many ways can 11 of the 44 patients be assigned to the standard treatment group?

The answer to question 1 is $_5C_4$, the answer to question 2 is $_{39}C_7$, and the answer to questions 3 is $_{44}C_{11}$. Fisher's exact probability is computed by multiplying the first factor by the second, and dividing the product by the third factor:

$$\frac{_5C_4 \times _{39}C_7}{_{44}C_{11}}$$

$$\frac{5 \times 15,380,937}{7,669,339,132} = 0.010028$$

TABLE 6-8	**Data for Fisher's Exact Test: Efficacy of a Novel Treatment vs. a Control in Extending the Lives of Terminal Patients[a]**

| | TREATMENT | | |
OUTCOME	STANDARD	NEW	TOTAL
Died	4	1	5
Survived	7	32	39
Total	11	33	44

[a]Data are number of patients receiving either the standard or the novel treatment who survived or died during the study period.

TABLE 6-9	Cross-Tabulation of Drug Compliance and Efficacy of Hypertensive Responsiveness		
	DRUG COMPLIANCE		
HYPERTENSION RESPONSIVE	YES	NO	*TOTAL*
Yes	46	8	54
No	40	9	49
Total	86	17	103

Adapted with permission from Nuesch R. Relation between insufficient response to antihypertensive treatment and poor compliance with treatment: A prospective case-control study. Br Med J 2001;323:142–146.

The computed probability (*p* value) is 0.01. Thus the pattern of the data would occur 1 time in 100 by chance. If the decision rule was to reject H_0 if the calculated probability was < 0.05, the H_A that the new drug was more effective than the standard drug in preventing death would be accepted.

The calculation of Fisher's exact test is typically more complex than was illustrated here, because interest is usually in the cumulative probability of obtaining the current data set as well as all data sets containing more extreme values. One solution is to find and use an interactive calculator on the Internet. A particularly useful one was provided by Preacher and Briggs.[15] The self-learning student may wish to access this site and compare its results with those reported here.

In one study, Fisher's exact test was used to analyze the data from an examination of the research hypothesis that patients whose hypertension was not responsive to therapy would be more likely to be noncompliant with a drug regimen than would patients in whom drug therapy was effective.[16] To test this notion, data from a total of 103 hypertensive patients was aggregated for a case-control study (Table 6-9).

Of 54 patients who responded to antihypertensive medication, 46 were compliant with the drug regimen. Similarly, of 49 patients who were not responding to treatment, 40 were compliant with the drug regimen. Calculation of Fisher's exact test for these data indicated an exact probability (*p* value) of 0.79. Because this probability is larger than the criterion set by the decision rule ($\alpha = 0.05$), H_0 is not rejected, and the conclusion is reached that the evidence was insufficient to suggest that differences in compliance with the drug regimen explained the discrepancy in responsiveness to the medication.

The application of Fisher's exact test is not restricted to observational studies. The data in Table 6-10 were extracted from a randomized controlled trial of the effects of efalizumab

TABLE 6-10	Cross-Tabulation of the Efficacy of Efalizumab 1 mg/kg/week versus Placebo in Reducing Symptoms of Psoriasis		
	DRUG REGIMEN		
SENSITIVITY INDEX	EFALIZUMAB	PLACEBO	*TOTAL*
≥ 75%	52	6	58
< 75%	232	122	354
Total	284	128	412

Source: Lebwohl, M. A novel-targeted T-cell modulator, Efalizumab, for plaque psoriasis. New England Journal of Medicine. 2003; 349: 2004–2013.

1 mg/kg/week versus placebo on the severity of psoriasis symptoms in 412 patients.[17] This example is restricted to patients whose severity score improved at least 75%. Among the 284 patients receiving efalizumab, 52 exhibited an improvement in symptom score of at least 75%. Similar levels of improvement were observed in only 6 of 128 patients receiving placebo. Calculation of Fisher's exact test from these data indicated that the probability of obtaining these results by chance was < 0.001, which exceeds the α level of 0.05 set before the study. Therefore, the H_0 is rejected, and the conclusion is reached that efalizumab was more efficacious than placebo.

In sum, Fisher's exact test can be substituted for the χ^2 test if the assumption regarding the expected cell frequencies cannot be met. However, keep in mind that the number of observations entered into the calculation is small and that the results may vary widely as more observations are made. In other words, conclusions drawn only on the basis of this test are tentative and suggestive only when accompanied by corroborative evidence.

McNEMAR'S TEST

McNemar's test is used to examine frequency data when cases are *not* independent. This may occur if several data points are obtained from the same patient (e.g., repeated measures for a pretest vs. posttest), or data are obtained from related patients (e.g., case-control pairs, twins). McNemar's test is a measure of how well *pairs* of patients are matched with respect to exposure and outcome variables.

Here is an example. A group of investigators wish to study the link between smoking and heart failure (HF). To control for several potential confounding variables, they match individuals on these variables. They thus obtain 53 pairs of individuals in which one member of the pair is a case (has HF) and the other member of the pair is a control (does not have HF). They then sort the pairs with respect to whether pair members were concordant (both smoked or both did not smoke) or discordant (one of the pair smoked but the other did not) with respect to the exposure variable. The data are shown in Table 6-11.

If H_0 is true, then the number of pairs in each of the two mismatched or discordant cells should be similar. That is, the number of pairs in which the HF member smoked and the other did not should be similar to the number of pairs in which the HF member did not smoke but the control did smoke. In the present example, there were 5 pairs in which the control was a smoker and the case was not a smoker, and 19 pairs in which the case was a smoker but the control was not a smoker.

McNemar's test statistic is a χ^2, computed as follows:

$$\chi^2 = \frac{(\text{Absolute value of difference of two discordant cells} - 1)^2}{\text{Sum of discordant cells}}$$

$$\chi^2 = \frac{[(19 - 5) - 1]^2}{(19 + 5)} = 7.04$$

TABLE 6-11   Data for the Calculation of McNemar's Test[a]

CASES	CONTROLS	
	SMOKER	NOT A SMOKER
Smoker	25	19
Not a Smoker	5	4

[a]Cases have heart failure; controls do not have heart failure and are matched on potentially confounding variables. Data are frequencies indicating whether cases and controls were concordant or discordant with respect to smoking status.

The probability of obtaining this value of χ^2 or a greater value by chance is determined by referring to Table B-4 (Appendix B), which lists χ^2 values with 1 df. The critical value of χ^2 with 1 df is 3.84, and the probability of obtaining values of $\chi^2 \geq 7.04$ by chance is $p < 0.05$. Therefore, the H_0 that there is no relationship between smoking and HF can be rejected.

In addition to computing a test statistic, the data in Table 6-11 can be used to calculate an odds ratio of $19/5 = 3.8$. This indicates that the odds of HF are almost 4 times greater for patients who smoked than for those who did not.

SIGN TEST

The sign test is a flexible test that is used to compare pairs of data, by computing the sign of the difference between pairs of scores. If the H_0 is true, then the number of plus (+) signs and minus (−) signs should be comparable. If the frequency of one sign is sufficiently disproportionate, it suggests that the pattern would occur rarely by chance.

Here is an example. A pharmacist wishes to test a new formulation claiming to be the best agent to reduce swelling from insect stings. So, in 15 patients with multiple insect stings, he or she treats some with the standard agent and some with the new agent. A colleague is then recruited to judge in each patient whether the areas treated with the new formulation are better (+) or worse (−) than the areas treated with the standard formulation. The data are presented in Table 6-12.

According to H_0, if there is no difference in efficacy, the probability of a plus sign is equal to the probability of a minus sign, or 0.5. There are 15 "trials" of this nature. The solution is to find the probability that 10 or more + signs would occur by chance. So this is

TABLE 6-12	Data for Calculation of the Sign Test [a]
PATIENT	OUTCOME
1	+
2	+
3	−
4	+
5	+
6	+
7	−
8	+
9	+
10	+
11	−
12	+
13	+
14	−
15	−

[a]Patients had multiple insect stings. For each patient, some stings were treated with a new formulation and some with the standard topical treatment. A + sign indicates that the new formulation was superior to the standard in reducing swelling, and a − sign indicates the opposite.

really a binomial problem with $p = 0.5$, $n = 15$, and $j = 10$. Recall from Chapter 5 that the binomial formula is

$$_nC_j\, p^j\, (1 - p)^{(n - j)}$$

where $_nC_j$ is the number of combinations of n things taken j at a time; p^j is the probability of j events, given the probability of one j event is p; $(1 - p)^{(n - j)}$ is the probability of $(n - j)$ events, given the probability of one $(n - j)$ event is $(1 - p)$. If $\alpha = 0.05$, do we reject or fail to reject H_0? What if we hypothesized that $p = 0.6$?

KAPPA (κ)

The kappa (κ) statistic is not a test statistic but an indication of the extent of agreement among two evaluators, two tests, and so on. It is an important measure because it describes the extent of agreement *beyond that expected by chance*.

Here is an example. Suppose we wish to determine how well the diagnoses of two clinicians agree. We ask both to diagnose the same patients as either positive or negative for a disease. The pairs of diagnoses are then sorted with respect to whether they are concordant or discordant. The data might look like those in Table 6-13.

What agreement between the clinicians is expected by chance? Some might contend that the probability of a positive or negative diagnosis by chance is 0.5. However, perhaps experienced diagnosticians have an expectation that more patients will be judged as negative, so the probability of a positive diagnosis is actually < 0.5.

To determine the true agreement between the clinicians that is attributable to chance, assume first that the sorting by one of the clinicians (e.g., Clinician 2) was a chance event, so that the probability of being judged a case by Clinician 2 is 229/572 or 0.4. That means that 40 of every 100 patients submitted to Clinician 2 would be judged a case. It follows that of the 240 patients diagnosed by Clinician 1 as cases (0.4×240) a total of 96 will also be diagnosed as cases by Clinician 2. This agreement, however, is by chance.

Similarly, Clinicians 1 and 2 would agree on the negative diagnoses of 199 patients (0.6×332) by chance alone. In total, Clinicians 1 and 2 would agree on the diagnoses of 96 patients as cases and 199 patients as not cases, or 295 of the 572 patients, by chance alone. The agreement expected by chance is thus 295/572, or 0.516.

The observed agreement is the sum of the concordant cells divided by the total number of patients: $(208 + 311) \div 572 = 0.907$. Therefore, the observed agreement beyond chance is equal to $0.907 - 0.516 = 0.391$, and the potential agreement beyond chance is $1 - 0.516 = 0.484$. Kappa is the ratio of these two values and is calculated accordingly:

$$\kappa = \frac{(\text{Observed agreement} - \text{Expected agreement due to chance})}{(1 - \text{Expected agreement due to chance})}$$

TABLE 6-13   **Data for calculation of κ**[a]

CLINICIAN 2	CLINICIAN 1 +	−	TOTAL
+	208	21	229
−	32	311	343
Total	240	332	572

[a]Two clinicians diagnosed the same set of patient records on a dichotomous scale. Patients with the disease were given a plus (+) and those without the disease a minus (−). Data are the frequencies of diagnoses on which the clinicians agreed and did not agree.

$$\kappa^2 = \frac{(0.907 - 0.516)}{1 - 0.516} = 0.808$$

As mentioned previously, κ is not a statistical test, so there are no associated probability values. The κ value suggests the degree of consistency between two sets of ratings beyond that expected by chance. Here are some guidelines for its interpretation.[18]

> 0.80 almost perfect agreement
>0.6–0.8 substantial agreement
>0.4–0.6 moderate agreement
< 0.4 fair or less agreement

The statistical tests reviewed to this point are used to examine the association between one exposure variable and one outcome variable. However, in many situations, these associations are contaminated by nuisance variables or confounding variables. The Mantel-Haenszel test and logistic regression analysis are used often to control for these unwanted effects.

MANTEL-HAENSZEL TEST

The Mantel-Haenszel test determines the statistical significance of an association between an exposure and an outcome variable after removing the influence of a third (confounding) variable. For example, a researcher might wish to determine the relationship between obesity and coronary heart disease (CHD) in a specific patient group. To obtain an adequate sample size, he or she includes both men and women as subjects. The researcher is not interested whether gender modifies the obesity–CHD relationship of the patients and wishes to remove its influence from the data. The Mantel-Haenszel test computes an OR to indicate the strength of this association. The statistical significance of the OR is determined by its 95% confidence interval (CI).

Notice that the Mantel-Haenszel test may also be used to study the effect of the confounding variable. A rough idea of the influence of the confounder may be obtained by comparing the results of two analyses. The first analysis, consisting of an overall analysis without regard for the confounding variable, provides a crude index of the OR. Comparing the crude to the adjusted OR suggests the role of the confounding variable.

As noted, the result of the Mantel-Haenszel test is reported as an OR with 95% CI. A statistically significant test result suggests an association between the exposure and the outcome variable, which is not dependent on the controlled variable. Computational procedures are beyond the scope of this text. The interested reader is referred to the literature.[19]

Although the Mantel-Haenszel test is useful in studying exposure–outcome associations, its inability to consider more than one confounding variable at a time is a severe limitation. As a result, statistical methods with the ability to assess and control the effects of several different variables have come into vogue. One of these methods is logistic regression analysis.

LOGISTIC REGRESSION ANALYSIS

Logistic regression analysis is a statistical method used commonly in healthcare studies to evaluate the contribution of a variety of variables (termed independent or predictor variables) to the probability that an individual belongs to a category of interest. Thus it is an example of *multivariable* or *multivariate data analysis*. The predictor variables may include factors of interest to the investigator (independent variables) and variables the investigator wishes to control (confounding variables). For example, in a study of variables associated with gastroesophageal reflux symptoms, investigators in one study were able to assess the contributions of obesity and estrogen status while isolating the potentially confounding influences of age and tobacco smoking, among other variables.[20]

Here's how logistic regression analysis works: In a case-control study, data for all study participants, both cases and controls, are assembled in one data set. The goal of the analysis is to develop a mathematical model whose output will result in the correct identification of case patients as cases and control patients as controls. The mathematical model consists of the sum of the values of the independent variables multiplied by weighting coefficients. The value of the weighting coefficient is determined to classify correctly the most cases as cases and controls as controls.

The output of the logistic regression equation is not a definitive classification of a patient as a case or a control, but the *probability* that the person is a case. The classification of the patient is the result of a decision rule. A typical rule is this: If the probability that a person is case is < 0.5, the person is judged to not be a case. Otherwise, the person is classified as a case.

The adequacy of the logistic regression equation in classifying cases and controls correctly can be expressed in several different ways, but this statistical test result almost never appears in the literature. Of major interest to the researcher, however, is the coefficient of each independent variable, because that coefficient determines the unique importance of that variable to the outcome of the classification process.

In other words, the coefficient indicates the contribution of that independent variable while controlling the effects of all other independent variables in the equation. The specific contribution is expressed as an OR and a 95% CI. In this example, the odds of gastroesophageal reflux symptoms in severely obese women were 6.3 times greater than the risk of these symptoms in normal-weight women (OR 6.3; 95% CI $4.9 - 8.0$; $p < 0.001$). Statistically significant coefficients have a 95% CI that does not include 1. A simple numerical example of this process is provided in the Extra Credit 6-2.

EXTRA CREDIT 6-2

The logistic regression equation is an extension of the basic linear regression equation:

$$Y = mx + b + E$$

where Y is the dependent variable; x is the independent variable; b is the intercept of the line, the value of Y when $x = 0$; m is the slope of the line. This equation produces a straight line by predicting values of y for different values of x. The amount y changes for a 1-unit change in x is m which is also called a coefficient of x. E is an error term.

This equation can be rewritten as follows:

$$Y = b_0 + b_1 x_1 + E$$

With b_0 substituting for b and b_1 substituting for m. It is reasonable to suggest that the precision with which the equation predicts values of y can be increased by adding other independent variables (x_2, x_3, x_4), each with a corresponding coefficient (b_2, b_3, b_4). Regression analyses with more than one independent variable are termed multivariable *analyses.*

In a logistic regression equation, the goal is to assign study participants to one of two categories of the dependent variable based on their scores on the various independent variables. This goal is accomplished in two steps. First, the probability that the person is at risk (Pr{y}) is computed based on the values of the independent variables for that individual.

Second, a classification rule is used to place the person in either the "at risk" or the "not at risk" category.

Here is a theoretical example. A researcher is interested in delineating factors that will allow him to screen new patients to determine their risk of hypertension. The first step is to identify the variables that best predict this risk. To pursue this question, the researcher obtains access to a database containing the health histories of a large number of patients, including blood pressure levels. The investigator then conducts a logistic regression analysis of the data and finds that the following equation classifies most patients correctly with respect to hypertension risk.

$$Pr\{y\} = 0.30 + (0.35)x_1 + (-0.25)x_2$$

The first item in the equation, 0.30, is a constant. Variable x_1 is smoking status. It has two levels: It is coded 1 if the person is a current smoker and 0 if the person is not a current smoker. The value of variable x_1 is modified by its coefficient, 0.35. Variable x_2 is exercise status: It is coded 1 if the person is a current exerciser or 0 if the person is not a current exerciser. The coefficient for variable x_2 is -0.25. The sign of the coefficient indicates that exercise decreases the risk of hypertension.

The probability that the person is at risk for hypertension is calculated as the sum of the constant and the products of the coefficients and variable values. For example, for a person who does not smoke and does not exercise, the probability of being hypertensive is calculated as follows:

$$Pr\{y\} = 0.30 + (0.35 \times 0) - (0.25 \times 0) = 0.30$$

In contrast, the $Pr\{y\}$ for a person who does smoke and does not exercise is 0.65.

Classification into either the "at risk" or the "not at risk" category for hypertension is based on the value of $Pr\{y\}$, the output of the logistic regression equation. If $Pr\{y\}$ is < 0.50, the person is assigned to the "not at risk" category, otherwise the person is designated "at risk." Based on the calculations given earlier, the nonsmoker/nonexerciser is classified as not at risk, whereas the smoker/nonexerciser is classified as being at risk.

The logistic regression equation also permits an estimation of an OR, or the strength of the association between each independent variable and hypertension risk.[21] This value is obtained by using the coefficient as an exponent of e, the base of the natural logarithm ($e \approx 2.718$). For current smoking status, the OR is $e^{0.35}$ or 1.42. This suggests that odds of being at risk for hypertension are 1.42 times greater for a person who smokes than for a nonsmoker. On the other hand, being a current exerciser confers a protective effect, as reflected in the OR of 0.78.

A second application of the logistic regression equation is to predict the risk status for hypertension in new patients. For example, suppose a new patient completes a survey indicating that he or she is a smoker but not an exerciser. Using the logistic regression equation, the probability of that patient's being at risk for hypertension is

$$Pr\{y\} = 0.30 + (0.35 \times 1) - (0.25 \times 0)$$
$$Pr\{y\} = 0.30 + 0.35 - 0 = 0.65$$

The patient would be classified as at risk for hypertension. In contrast, another patient who is both a smoker and an exerciser would be assigned a $Pr\{y\} = 0.40$ and would be classified as not at risk for hypertension. ■

The interpretation of the statistics for the individual variables depends on the type of logistic regression analysis conducted. One option is to include all the independent variables in the analysis. Another is to include in the equation only those independent variables that best predict the outcome variable. This method is termed a *conditional or step-wise logistic regression analysis*. There are several ways of entering and removing variables into the regression equation during a stepwise analysis. For example, variables can be entered one at a time, termed *forward stepwise logistic regression;* or all the variables can be entered into the equation and then removed selectively, which is called *backward stepwise logistic regression analysis.*

Logistic regression analyses may be applied to control the effect of independent variables in several different ways:

- As already noted, the analyses may be used to select the set of independent variables that best predict the outcome variable.
- The analysis can be used to study the interaction of several variables on the outcome variable.
- Equations can be constructed to predict the effect of individual or sets of independent variables, which can then be compared to the actual outcome.
- The equation can be used to control for the effects of potentially confounding variables.

Application of logistic regression analyses can be quite complex. For example, in a study of the risk of venous thrombosis associated with esterified estrogens versus conjugated equine estrogens in perimenopausal and postmenopausal women, multivariate logistic regression equations were used to control for group differences in the following matching factors: age, year of venous thrombosis, and treated hypertension status.[22] In addition, logistic regression analyses were used to control the confounding effects of race, body mass index, cancer history, hysterectomy status, previous oral contraceptive use, and other factors. Based on the results of preliminary conditional logistic regression analyses, the final results were adjusted only for factors that were statistically significant confounders—namely, the matching factors of race, and cancer history.

The OR for venous thrombosis comparing users of esterified estrogen to nonusers was 0.92 (95% CI 0.69–1.22; $p > 0.05$); and for conjugated equine estrogens, the OR for users compared to nonusers was 1.65 (95% CI 1.24–2.19; $p < 0.05$). When the analysis was restricted to women using estrogens, the odds for venous thrombosis were 1.78 times greater among women using conjugated equine estrogens than those using esterified estrogens (95% CI 1.11–2.84; $p < 0.05$). These data suggest an increased risk of venous thrombosis among perimenopausal and postmenopausal women who are prescribed conjugated equine estrogens compared to both nonusers and those taking esterified estrogens.

Logistic regression analysis is an essential tool in analyzing frequency data, particularly in determining factors that contribute to outcome variables such as life/death, at risk/not at risk, healthy/ill. Logistic regression analysis is flexible and is frequently used in experimental designs other than case-control studies.

An important caveat, however, is that the information provided by a logistic regression equation is unique to the data from which it is derived. Altering the original data set by adding or subtracting cases will almost surely affect the magnitude of the coefficients in the original equation and may also change the set of independent variables in the equation. Similar results are to be expected if the logistic regression equation based on one data set is applied to another data base. Although the general pattern of results may persist, the relative contribution of the different independent variables is almost certain to change.

WILCOXON TESTS FOR ORDINAL DATA

Ordinal data consist of ranks. Data in the form of ranks can arise from several sources. Often, these data are originally quantified using interval or ratio scales of measurement. However, owing to concerns that the assumptions necessary for parametric statistical testing may not be met, the data are converted to ranks and are tested with nonparametric statistical methods.

The **Wilcoxon rank-sum test** is the nonparametric equivalent of the independent-groups *t*-test. The rank-sum test is used instead of the *t*-test when there is evidence that the data, although measured on an interval or ratio scale, are not normally distributed. For example, in a study of in-hospital cardiac arrest, a rank-sum test was used to compare the amount of time devoted to cardiopulmonary resuscitation in children versus adult patients.[23] The researchers apparently determined that the time intervals would not be normally distributed.

The test statistic is developed after first converting the data to an ordinal, or rank, scale of measurement. The calculation of the test statistic is cumbersome, but results in a test statistic, z, that is referred to the standard normal distribution. Specifically, values of z that exceed either -1.96 or $+1.96$ suggest that differences between the two groups would occur by chance $< 5\%$ of the time.

The Wilcoxon signed-ranks test is designed to test data from repeated measures on the same patient, or on matched pairs of patients, much like McNemar's test. Like the rank-sum test, the signed-ranks test is often derived from interval or ratio scale data that may not be distributed normally. The test is based on statistical considerations of the behavior of the ranks of the differences among the matched pairs. Like the ranks-sum test, the computations are cumbersome and the test statistic is z, which again is referred to the standard normal distribution.

For example, in the Vascular Interaction with Age in Myocardial Infarction (VINTAGE MI) trial, the effects of a 6-month course of L-arginine vasopressin in reducing vascular wall stiffness and increasing ejection fraction were studied in patients who had suffered a myocardial infarction.[24] Changes in ejection fraction from beginning to the end of the study period were assessed using the Wilcoxon signed-ranks test. The results of this test suggested that, in contrast to current thinking, L-arginine vasopressin did not improve ejection fraction in these patients.

How to Evaluate Evidence from a Case-Control Study

To exemplify the principles described in this chapter, this section contains a critique of a case-control study by Hylek et al.[25] Your understanding of the literature evaluation points discussed here will be enhanced if you read the article before continuing with the text.

To facilitate the evaluation of evidence provided by case-control study designs, a standard reporting format, summarized in Table 6-14, is used. (This framework is also used for reporting findings from cohort study designs.) This format organizes the information contained in the research report into a number of sections that link together logically to provide a clear view of the purpose and findings of the study. The major sections and their intent are as follows:

- *Title and abstract:* Provide a snapshot and summary, respectively, of the study's content.
- *Introduction:* Provides the rationale for the research hypothesis.
- *Methods:* Indicates who was studied, how they were studied, and how the data were analyzed.
- *Results:* Presents the findings relevant to the statistical hypotheses.
- *Discussion:* Relates the findings to the general population and clinical arena and closes with implications for clinical practice.

To illustrate, the title indicates that this report is an examination of a case-control study providing evidence that acetaminophen enhances the anticoagulant properties of warfarin.

The abstract provides more detail. The research question is whether an increased risk of hemorrhage in warfarin users could be the result of the intake of acetaminophen. Hemorrhage risk was expressed in terms of the INR for warfarin. Case patients were those

TABLE 6-14	A Guide to the Evaluation of Observational Study Research Reports
SECTION	**COMMENTS**
Title and abstract	The title is a headline and should contain the intervention, outcome, study design, and patient type. It should be unbiased, brief, and accurate.
	The abstract is a brief synopsis of the study, summarizing the four main sections of the report (introduction, methods, results, and discussion/conclusion). The abstract should be written clearly and informatively and should be able to stand apart from the article. Many abstracts are truncated at 250 words (either by the journal or the indexing database) and may not present a complete depiction of the study. Thus, reading and critically evaluating the full study is imperative when making clinical decisions.
Introduction	The introduction provides the rationale for the research effort. It begins with a general statement of the research area, provides a context for the present work, and explains the need for more research. The section closes with a clear statement of the specific research hypothesis. This statement is important because it sets the goal of the research effort, which in turn determines patient selection; method; and data acquisition, analysis, and interpretation.
Methods	The methods section describes the steps taken to test the statistical hypothesis. The methods should be sufficiently detailed for a reader to replicate the study. The methods contains a description of the type of study (experimental design), who was studied (description of subjects), what was measured and how it was measured (outcomes and data collection methods), and how data were analyzed (statistical analysis).
	• Type of study (case-control, cohort, cross-sectional): Make sure the study design is appropriate for the hypothesis being tested.
	• Participants and setting: This section should identify the source of the patients and indicate whether the study was retrospective or prospective. The inclusion and exclusion criteria should be objective, standard, and based on clinically important variable levels. Evaluate how similar the participants are to those seen in your clinical practice. Be sensitive to the methods and criteria used for group assignment (definitions of cases and controls). Determine where the patients were treated and how many clinics were involved. Decide whether the standard of care in the facility is relevant to your practice. Approval by an institutional review board or other ethical board is necessary for all research performed using human beings as subjects.
	• Measurements: Determine the variables used as primary and secondary outcomes. They should be relevant to testing the research hypothesis. They should be measured and analyzed in a standard manner. Measurement intervals should also be specified.
	• Data analysis: Transformations or manipulations of the data following their initial collection should be explained. All tests of the primary and secondary outcomes should be stated explicitly a priori. The probability level for rejecting the null hypothesis, α, should be stated.
	At this point, it is good practice to predict the results. This will ensure that you understand the research hypothesis and methods. It will also provide expectations about the changes that must occur to support the research hypothesis and other evidence necessary to answer questions about bias, confounding, and other factors that might damage the internal validity of the study.
Results	The results section provides in detail the findings of the study as they relate to the statistical hypothesis. The research hypothesis gains support based on the results of statistical tests of specific null hypotheses.
	• The first step in the results section should be to present the findings for tests of differences between case and control patients. Tests should be conducted of all

(continued)

TABLE 6-14	A Guide to the Evaluation of Observational Study Research Reports
	relevant demographic, socioeconomic, health history, and physiologically important factors. Ideally, data from those who refused to participate and those who did not complete the study (dropouts) should also be examined to determine whether the volunteer effect was a source of bias. • Next, the results of analyses of primary and secondary outcome variables should be presented in clear, simple language, followed by the statistical support. Are data for all patients and all a priori defined outcomes accounted for? Be alert for results that are trends—results that are described as being meaningful even though they do not achieve statistical significance. Accept only statistically significant evidence. However, make sure the statistically significant results are also relevant clinically. Some effects, though statistically significant, may be too small or too weak to be of much clinical value in treating patients. • Third, analyses should be reported that deal with variables that might have confounded or biased the results. Their analysis should be as detailed as those for primary and secondary outcomes. • Finally, post hoc analyses, those conducted after the a priori data analyses, may be presented. These are to be considered exploratory in nature and may not be used as evidence relevant to the present hypotheses.
Discussion	The first part of the discussion section should be a straightforward description of the results and how they relate to the research hypothesis. Key evidence should be described. Next, supporting evidence should be marshaled from other studies, and differences among the studies' findings should be evaluated. This should be followed by a consideration of limitations to the study results and conclusions, including chance, bias, confounding, effect–cause, effect–effect, and/or cause–effect. Conclusions and implications should be restricted to the evidence provided by the present results. Do not accept contentions that are beyond the scope of the paper.
Other factors	Use the reputation of the authors and sponsoring organizations; the sources of funding and support provided to the authors, and the journal and its review process as indications of the quality of the paper. Editorials accompanying the paper and letters to the editor following its publication can add valuable information by providing a context for the study findings and by addressing questions raised by other experts in the field.

whose INR was > 6.0 during a routine visit, and control patients were selected randomly from a pool of patients who displayed normal, stable INR values. Analysis of information obtained from a telephone interview indicated that an INR > 6.0 was associated with use of acetaminophen and that the risk increased with the amount of acetaminophen ingested. INR was also increased by overdose of warfarin and by new medications known to potentiate the effects of warfarin. Ingesting vitamin K or low to moderate alcohol intake seemed to afford a protective effect. The authors concluded that clinicians must be aware of such drug–drug interactions and monitor such conditions in their patients more closely.

The introduction provides the rationale for the study: Warfarin is effective in preventing coagulation and, therefore, emboli. However, a drawback with the use of warfarin is the risk of hemorrhage, which increases with increasing warfarin dose. Thus it is important to keep the blood level of warfarin within a narrow therapeutic range, as indexed by the INR. In particular, an INR > 4.0 poses an excess risk for intracranial hemorrhage. Unfortunately, other factors can affect blood coagulation and therefore modify the INR independent of warfarin. The research hypothesis is stated explicitly: "to identify factors associated with an INR greater than 6.0 among outpatients whose target INR was 2.0 to 3.0. In this report, we quantify the effects of several commonly encountered risk factors, focusing on the impact of acetaminophen ingestion."[25]

LITERATURE CRITIQUE 6-1

Hylek et al. provide a clear and logical introduction to the topic of their investigation, establish the clinical relevance of the study, and provide the rationale for the research hypothesis. Because INR is a standard measure of indirectly indicating the amount of time it takes for blood to clot in patients who take warfarin, the findings of this study are pertinent to similar patients in similar clinical settings. ▪

As indicated in Table 6-14, the methods section should describe the process of testing the hypothesis. The general experimental design (a prospective case-control study) required that participants be interviewed by telephone within 24 hr of their clinic visit during the study period. Cases were patients who exhibited an INR > 6.0 at this visit after a period of normal, stable INR values. Controls were selected randomly from a pool of patients with INR values consistently within the 1.7–3.3 range. The telephone interview, conducted by trained interviewers, gathered information according to a previously tested script. Information was requested concerning newly prescribed medications, changes in medication doses, and use of over-the-counter medications. Patients were specifically asked about acetaminophen use, vitamin K intake, and alcohol consumption. Patients also provided information about compliance with warfarin dosage. Other information, such as the INR value immediately before the beginning of the study, was obtained from the clinic database.

The statistical analysis included a determination of the number of patients needed to achieve statistical power of 85% at an α level of 0.05. A variety of statistical tests was used to characterize the data, including a logistic regression analysis to determine factors associated with an INR value > 6.0.

LITERATURE CRITIQUE 6-2

The methods, which Hylek et al. present in a clear, logical manner, had been approved by the institutional review board. Assignment of cases and controls was based on objective, clinically relevant criteria. Exclusion criteria are reasonable and similar for both groups. Participation rates were high, > 90% of those eligible. The definition of cases was based on a clinically relevant threshold: INR values > 6.0.

Data were collected by trained investigators using a standardized survey tool and a standardized script to minimize interviewer bias. Specific information was sought that could be easily quantified. Although the data acquisition method depended on self-report, care was taken to limit responses to previously determined answers. Furthermore, inconclusive information was minimized by having patients confirm medication use by reading the drug label. Also, the same information was obtained several different ways, increasing the reliability of the patient answers. These data collection methods strengthen the internal validity of the study.

The plan for the data analysis is explained clearly. Notice that many of the statistical tests used by Hylek et al. have been described in this text. These are the χ^2 test, Fisher's exact test, Student's t-test, the Mantel-Haenszel test (the Cochrane-Mantel-Haenszel test for trend is a modification of the standard Mantel-Haenszel test), and the coefficient of variation. Logistic regression analyses were specifically used to "assess the independent effect of multiple clinical characteristics on the risk of having an INR greater than 6.0 and the significance of the interaction terms."[25] The statistical analyses were correctly chosen, which also lends strength to the internal validity of the study.

At this point it is useful to predict the evidence that you would expect if the research hypothesis is to receive support. This serves two purposes. First, it ensures that you have a clear understanding of the research hypothesis and methods. Second, you are more likely to recognize evidence that supports the research hypothesis and evidence that does not. In this study the expectations are is that (1) groups are shown to be comparable in all variables that might alter the exposure–outcome relationship and (2) statistical significance will be obtained for differences between cases and controls as a function of variables that affect blood coagulation properties in addition to warfarin. ▪

The results section contains several subsections. Table 1 of the report compares the demographic and pertinent health histories of cases and controls. As Hylek et al. indicate, both groups are approximately 70 years of age, about 50% are women, and almost all are white. In addition, both groups display similar disease profiles, including the condition that prompted initiation of anticoagulation therapy and duration of the treatment. The authors next confirm that both cases and controls had displayed normal INR values and INR variability before the most recent measurement, which was still normal for the controls but exceedingly high for cases (this information appears as a figure in the paper). The average warfarin dose was similar in both groups.

During the 7 days before blood was drawn for testing, 56% of the cases and 36% of controls had ingested a dose of acetaminophen. Furthermore, there was a positive relationship between the amount of acetaminophen ingested and the likelihood of exhibiting an abnormally high INR value (Table 2 of the report). Specifically, a statistically significant increase in risk of elevated INR (OR 3.5; 95% CI 1.2–10.0; $p = 0.02$) is noted at a dose of acetaminophen 2,267 mg/week and increased progressively to an OR of 10.0 (95% CI 2.6–37.9; $p = 0.001$) for acetaminophen doses exceeding 9,100 mg/week. Table 3 of the report shows other factors associated with an increased INR, such as an excessive dose of warfarin (OR 8.1; 95% CI 2.2–30; $p = 0.002$), other medications known to potentiate the effects of warfarin (OR = 8.5; 95% CI 2.9–24.7; $p < 0.001$), and advanced malignancy (OR 16.4; 95% CI 2.4–111; $p = 0.004$). A decreased INR was linked to a diet rich in vitamin K (OR 0.7; 95% CI 0.5–0.9; $p = 0.003$) and with moderate alcohol consumption of one to two drinks per day (OR 0.2; 95% CI 0.1–0.7; $p = 0.01$).

 LITERATURE CRITIQUE 6-3

The results section provides a clear picture of the findings of the study: demographic variables are similar between cases and controls and thus cannot account for group differences in INR. Major differences in disease history are not apparent, and both groups have been exposed to similar doses of warfarin for similar amounts of time. The statement that the spike in INR was of recent onset was confirmed by data. Evidence of an association between acetaminophen and elevated INR levels was provided in terms of both the proportion of cases versus controls using acetaminophen in the week before the clinic visit and the demonstration of a positive relationship between the amount of acetaminophen ingested and the increased risk of elevated INR values. From Table 2 of the report, it is apparent that doses of acetaminophen > 2,267 mg/week increase the risk of an elevated INR significantly ($p = 0.02$). The clinical significance of this finding is questionable, however, because the lower limit of the 95% CI is very close to 1.0). Doses > 9100 mg/week provided a statistically and clinically significant increased risk.

All statistical analyses were planned before the data were analyzed (a priori) and not conducted after the initial data analysis (post hoc). This lends strength to internal validity. Only statistically significant differences are discussed, differences that did not achieve statistical significance are not described as trends, for example. It is important to note that some differences that are not statistically significant provide important information. Notably, the lack of a statistically significant increase in risk of elevated INR at the two lowest acetaminophen doses suggests that acetaminophen doses < 2,267 mg/week may be safe in these patients but that doses > 2,267 mg/week may pose a risk.

Finally, the results anticipated at the end of the methods section are reported: Cases and controls are similar with respect to demographic and relevant medical history variables. Furthermore, acetaminophen is associated with dangerously elevated levels of INR, with risk increasing (as indicated by the progressive increase in ORs) as the dose of acetaminophen increases. The probability of committing a type I error in this study is below the acceptable cutoff of 5%. In fact, the probability that the monotonic increase in risk of elevated INR with increasing acetaminophen dose is the result of chance is < 0.001. Given that the internal validity of this trial is fairly strong, confidence can be placed in the significance of the findings. Such outcomes suggest a strong association between acetaminophen and elevated INR values. ■

The discussion section begins by repeating the dose response relationship between acetaminophen and excessive INR levels found in this study and points to similar findings in case reports and older clinical studies. Similar effects of malignancy and the opposite response to vitamin K and alcohol use are also explored. The discussion then turns to the most important threat to the integrity of a case-control study: bias. Evidence is marshaled to argue that minimal effects could be attributed to selection bias, different participation rates, adverse selection, self-report bias, recall bias, or interviewer bias. The authors also argue that misclassification errors could not have played a major role in the outcome.

Hylek et al. next discuss whether their findings provide evidence of a cause-and-effect relationship. The relationship "is strong, dose-dependent, and biologically plausible, follows an appropriate temporal sequence, and is supported by previous case reports and small-scale clinical experiments. In addition, the relationship persisted after control of a variety of potential confounders."[25] The authors conclude that "the current study identifies powerful risk factors for excessive anticoagulation in real-world practice. Knowledge of such risk factors should result in changes in the management of anticoagulant therapy that will reduce hemorrhagic complications."[25]

 LITERATURE CRITIQUE 6-4

The discussion section begins by relating the results of the study to the research hypothesis. Reviewed are the significance of the problem and the contribution of the present results in resolving the problem. Data from similar studies are discussed. It is important that potential sources of alternative explanations of the data—bias, confounding, and error—are considered. For example, selection bias was minimized by studying 84% of eligible case patients and a random sample of control patients. Recall bias was limited by interviewing the patient within 24 hr of the clinic visit. The potential confounding effects of other factors that might obscure the acetaminophen–INR relationship were controlled by including them in the experimental design.

In addition, evidence relating these findings to a cause-and-effect relationship is evaluated. It seems that neither the authors nor the article reviewers are familiar with the difficulties of ascribing exposure–outcome associations to cause-and-effect relationships. This is the topic of a letter to the editor that appeared after the publication of the article. Finally, implications of the results of the study, in concert with other evidence, for clinical practice are appropriately described.

In general, this study seems to have found what it reported. The hypothesis was stated clearly, and the methods were both planned and executed with rigor and forethought. Differences between the groups were based on an objective measure, the INR, which is easily reproducible and shows little variability. The explanation of the results was restricted to statistically significant findings. The discussion contained all the necessary elements and was not excessive in generalizing the results of this study to other healthcare settings. In short, the report seems to have integrity, or **internal validity.**

Having decided that the research report provides believable information, the next step is to determine whether it applies to other clinical settings. This is the **external validity** of the study. Based on the nature and characteristics of the subject population and the ubiquitous use of acetaminophen by this age group, there is little doubt that elderly patients who are using warfarin should be cautioned about their use of acetaminophen. Furthermore, elderly patients who are chronic users of acetaminophen perhaps need to undergo INR determinations more frequently.

One issue regarding the external validity of this paper is the nature of the subject pool. Particularly the advanced age of the patients (mean age = 70 years) and the fact that a high proportion of participants were white (95–98%).

The first question is, Can these data be generalized to all patients using warfarin or do they apply only to the elderly? For several reasons, the elderly might be considered to be at greater risk than younger patients. Their metabolism of drugs may be different from that of younger persons, they are more prone to drug interactions, and their synthesis and breakdown of clotting factors can be different from younger individuals.

The second question is, Can the findings of this study apply to people of different races? A search of the literature using the keywords "acetaminophen," "warfarin," and "race" identified at least one study showing some evidence that racial groups differ in the amount of warfarin necessary to maintain INR levels within a normal range, although the number of participants was small.[26] Whether this phenomenon is the result of a genetic predisposition or to cultural factors is unknown. However, it suggests that some caution may be prudent in applying these findings to other racial groups.

The last step in this process is one of the most important: Search the current issue of the journal for editorial comments on the research report and then search subsequent issues of the journal to find out if readers have commented on the research report. The paper by Hylek et al. prompted an editorial[27] and several letters. Authors are always invited to reply to these letters. Reading editorials, letters to the authors, and author replies is useful when learning literature evaluation skills.

Summary

The study of cases is a valuable source of drug information. In some applications, such knowledge is useful in itself. In other applications, the information provides the impetus for further research. Such efforts may include cohort and cross-sectional research efforts. These are the topics of the next chapter.

STUDY PROBLEMS

1. When examining the literature, why is it important to make sure that the age distributions of the groups under study are similar?

2. Read the study by Doll and Hill about carcinoma and the lung.[28] Discuss the sources of bias they identify and note the steps taken to address these sources of contamination.

3. Find a study in the literature that uses the case-control study design. Examine the paper using the criteria outlined in Table 6-14. Discuss potential sources of bias, both those identified by the authors and those overlooked. Evaluate the paper and reach a decision about the internal validity and the external validity.

4. Identify and examine observational studies reporting the use of one of the statistical tests reviewed in this chapter. What is the context of the test? Why was the test used? What were the results of the test? Was evidence marshaled from several test results to support a conclusion? Were the conclusions statistically significant and clinically significant?

REFERENCES

1. Tweed SA, Showronski DM, David ST, et al. Human illness from avian influenza H7N3, British Columbia. Emerg Infect Dis 2004;10:2196–2199.
2. Centers for Disease Control and Prevention. Outbreak of West Nile-like viral encephalitis—New York, 1999. MMWR Morb Mortal Wkly Rep 1999;48:845–849.
3. Spiller HA, Weber JA, Winter ML, et al. Multicenter case series of pediatric metformin ingestion. Ann Pharmacother 2000;34:1385–1388.
4. Carnahan RM, Kutscher EC, Obritsch MD, Rasmussen LD. Acute ethanol intoxication after consumption of hairspray. Pharmacotherapy 2005;25:1646–1650.
5. Maywald V, Schindler C, Krappweis J, Kirch W. First patient-centered drug information service in Germany—A descriptive study. Ann Pharmacother 2004;38:2154–2159.
6. Bartle WR, Blakely JA. Potentiation of warfarin anticoagulation by acetaminophen. JAMA 1991;265:1260.
7. Spigset, O. Reduced effect of warfarin caused by ubidecarenone. Lancet 1994;344:1372–1373.
8. Hylek EM, Herman H, Skates SJ, et al. Acetaminophen and other risk factors for excessive warfarin anticoagulation. JAMA 1998;279:657–662.
9. Latham RH, Kehrberg MW, Jacobson JA, et al. Toxic shock syndrome in Utah: A case-control and surveillance study. Ann Intern Med 1982;96:906 908.
10. Psaty BM, Smith NL, Lamaitre RN, et al. Hormone replacement therapy, prothrombotic mutations, and the risk of incident nonfatal myocardial infarction in postmenopausal women. JAMA 2001;285:906–913.
11. Gordis L. Epidemiology. 2nd ed. Philadelphia: Saunders, 2000.
12. Drug Digest. Cystic fibrosis. Available at: www.drugdigest.org/DD/HC/HCIntro/0,4043,851,00.html. Accessed July 2006.
13. Miller AK. Libby, Montana: Overview of asbestos exposures and health effects. Paper presented at the 101st meeting of the Cordilleran Section, Geological Society of America, San Jose, CA, April 29–May 1, 2005. Abstract available at: gsa.confex.com/gsa/2005CD/finalprogram/abstract_85952.htm. Accessed June 2006.

14. Codispoti JR, Prior MJ, Fu M, et al. Effect of nonprescription doses of ibuprofen for treating migraine headache. A randomized controlled trial. Headache 2001;41:665–679.

15. Preacher KJ, Briggs NE. Calculation for Fisher's exact test: An interactive calculation tool for Fisher's exact probability test for 2 × 2 tables [Computer software]. Available at www.quantpsy.org. Accessed Feb 2007.

16. Nuesch R. Relation between insufficient response to antihypertensive treatment and poor compliance with treatment: A prospective case-control study. Br Med J 2001;323:142–146.

17. Lebwohl M. A novel targeted T-cell modulator, efalizumab, for plaque psoriasis. N Engl J Med 2003;349:2004–2013.

18. Viera AJ, Garrett JM. Understanding interobserver agreement: The kappa statistic. Fam Med 2005;37:360–363.

19. Kuritz SJ, Landis JR, Koch GG. A general overview of Mantel-Haenszel methods: Applications and recent developments. Annu Rev Pubic Health 1988; 9:123–160.

20. Nilsson M, Johnsen R, Weimin Y, et al. Obesity and estrogen as risk factors for gastroesophageal reflux symptoms. JAMA 2003;290:66–72.

21. Wright RE. Logistic regression. In: Grimm LG, Yarnell PR, eds. Reading and Understanding Multivariate Statistics. Washington, DC: American Psychological Association, 1995.

22. Smith NL, Heckbert SR, Lamaitre RN, et al. Esterified estrogens and conjugated equine estrogens and the risk of venous thrombosis. JAMA 2004;292:1581–1587.

23. Nadkarni VM, Larkin GL, Peberdy MA, et al. First documented rhythm and clinical outcome from in-hospital cardiac arrest among children and adults. JAMA 2006;295:50–57.

24. Schulman SP, Becker LC, Kass DA, et al. L-Arginine therapy in acute myocardial infarction. The Vascular Interaction with Age in Myocardial Infarction (VINTAGE MI) randomized clinical trial. JAMA 2006;295:58–64.

25. Hylek EM, Heiman H, Skates, et al. Acetaminophen and other risk factors for excessive warfarin anticoagulation. JAMA 1998;279:657–662.

26. Blann A, Bareford D. Ethnic background is a determinant of average warfarin dose required to maintain the INR between 3.0 and 4.5. J Thromb Haemost 2004;2:525–526.

27. Bell WR. Acetaminophen and warfarin: undesirable synergy. JAMA 1998;279:702–703.

28. Doll, R, Hill AB. Smoking and carcinoma of the lung. Preliminary report. Br Med J 1950;2:739–748.

Critical Appraisal of Evidence Derived from Cohorts and Surveys

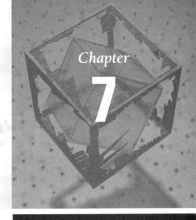

Chapter

7

CHAPTER GOALS

After studying this chapter, the student should be able to:

1. Describe cohort and cross-sectional study designs.

2. Explain the rationale for these designs.

3. Enumerate the advantages and disadvantages of each study design.

4. Evaluate the application of these study designs in the healthcare literature.

5. Describe statistical tests based on linear regression models.

6. Evaluate the application of multiple regression and analysis of variance in the healthcare literature.

In some circumstances, to understand the association between exposures and outcomes, it makes sense to study people who engage in specific behaviors or who have been exposed to specific circumstances. In other words, study participants are selected based on their exposure to a situation or condition or because they fulfill certain criteria. Then, whether these individuals have experienced or will experience a specific outcome can be determined, and the risk of exposure can be calculated.

Cohort and cross-sectional study designs incorporate such a strategy. Examples of cohort and cross-sectional study designs include:

- A study of medical and psychological symptoms and coping strategies exhibited by women whose menopausal hormone therapy has been terminated abruptly.[1]
- Examination of the effects of long-term ingestion of aspirin to reduce heart attack risk and subsequent impairment of renal function.[2]
- Investigation of the effect of folate intake on the risk of cardiovascular disease in healthy young women.[3]

Why can problems like these not be studied using other research designs like the randomized controlled trial? Three reasons are convenience, economy, and ethics. In some cases, such as an examination of the incidence of cancer in people exposed to fallout from a nuclear accident, the exposure occurs naturally. There is no experimental control over who is exposed and who is not. Second, because exposure to some interventions may be rare, a cohort design may provide the most economically efficient protocol available. Finally, it is unethical to expose people to potentially hazardous situations.

The goal of this chapter is to describe the methods of cohort and cross-sectional study designs and to indicate their contribution to the healthcare literature. As part of these studies, statistical principles and applications associated with simple and multiple linear regression and with analysis of variance will be explained.

Cohort Study Design

A cohort is a group of individuals characterized by a common bond.[*] In a cohort study, the common bond is an exposure of interest to the investigator. Cohorts might be those who smoke tobacco or those who abuse prescription drugs or those who are exposed to atmospheric chemicals. Like the case-control study, the cohort study is a type of observational study design. The cohort study design is also called a follow-up study because patients are tracked or followed-up until the outcome of interest occurs.

An overview of the cohort study design was provided in Chapter 3. Their features, summarized in Table 3-2, are as follows:

- The goal is to determine the outcome or outcomes associated with an exposure variable.
- The strategy is to assemble groups that differ only in experiencing an exposure and then to search for differences in subsequent outcome variables.
- The design is particularly prone to confounding, although factors such as bias and measurement error may also affect the exposure–outcome association.

The critical feature of a cohort study is that *the groups are defined by the presence or absence of one or more exposures.* In a **prospective cohort study design**, groups are defined at the beginning of the study period and followed until the outcome occurs. In other words, the outcome has not yet occurred when the study groups are defined. For example, after an industrial accident, workers might be followed for a number of years to detect unusually high levels of disease. In a **retrospective cohort study design**, in contrast, both exposure and outcome have already occurred when the study begins. However, because subjects are assigned to groups based on exposure and not outcome, the study design is still a valid cohort model. Such a research strategy was used to delineate the effect of thiazolidine-diones on the risk of heart failure in patients with type 2 diabetes.[4]

In a cohort study, there are three features of interest: how the cohorts are defined, how confounding variables are controlled, and how the interval between the exposure and the outcome is measured.

Cohorts may be defined in one of two basic ways. One is to assign individuals to groups based on a *specific* condition, exposure, or behavior that is of interest in the study. For example, men might be aggregated into groups based on the amount of exposure to a suspected carcinogen. The other method of designating a cohort is to define a population of individuals that will be followed for a period of time in an effort to delineate a variety of exposure–outcome associations. The Framingham Heart Study is one example of many such population-based cohort studies. Begun in 1948, the Framingham Heart Study has followed almost the entire population of Framingham, Massachusetts, and has provided much essential information about the risk factors for cardiovascular disease.[5] In 1971, the Framingham Offspring Study was initiated to carry on and extend this effort among the children of the original cohort members.[6]

---

[*]In epidemiology, the term *cohort* has two meanings. One refers to a group of people who are engaged in the same experiences or share a defining characteristic. In that sense, your graduating class is a cohort. The other use of the term cohort refers to the study design, in which a group of people with a common trait is studied. The two uses of the term are similar but not identical.

While the population-based study design is much more expensive to conduct, it enables the evaluation of a wide variety of exposure and outcome variables. Thus it is possible to examine exposure–outcome relationships that are complex or that may be modified by other factors. It also permits the identification and management of potentially confounding variables.

Although the exposure–outcome association in a cohort study can be contaminated by measurement error and bias, the primary threat to the integrity of the study is through **confounding.** Confounding variables display two characteristics:

- They are associated with the exposure stimulus.
- They are capable of causing the outcome independent of the exposure stimulus.

An example is presented in Figure 7-1. The investigator seeks the relationship between two variables: the chronic ingestion of pain relievers and subsequent compromise in renal function. However, obesity is also positively related to deficits in renal function. In addition, there is a positive relationship between the amount of pain relievers ingested and obesity.[2] As a consequence, whether alterations in renal function are the result of the pain relievers or of obesity cannot be determined precisely.

The effect of confounding variables on the exposure–outcome relationship can be controlled in one of two ways. The first method is through study design, most simply by making sure that members of both groups are matched on potentially confounding variables. For example, in the example study, subjects in both the exposed group and the unexposed group could be matched with respect to the obesity variable. This would equate the effects of obesity on renal function in both groups.

Another method of controlling confounding is to evaluate directly the effect of the suspected variable. In a study of the association of folate consumption with the incidence of hypertension in women, for example, the confounding effects of the following variables, among others, were controlled statistically: age, smoking, use of oral contraceptives, body mass index, physical activity, and family history of hypertension.[3]

Controlling confounding variables statistically is possible using either the Mantel-Haenszel test or logistic regression analysis (see Chapter 6). The Mantel-Haenszel test provides an odds ratio (OR) indicating the strength of the association between the exposure and the outcome variable after the influence of the confounding variable is removed. Because the Mantel-Haenszel test can control only one nuisance (or confounding) variable, logistic regression analysis, which can control many variables simultaneously, is more commonly used. Logistic regression analysis also provides an OR indicating the strength of association between specific exposure variables and the outcome variables absent the effect of the confounding variables. The statistical significance of the ORs provided by both these tests is indicated by a 95% confidence interval (CI).

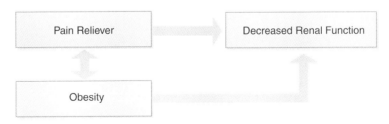

FIGURE 7-1 A Confounded Relationship. The investigator is interested in the effect of pain relievers on renal function. Obesity, however, is a confounding variable. It is positively associated with the exposure of interest and is by itself able to diminish renal function.

The third consideration of cohort studies is that the time of participation in a cohort study is often measured as person-time. As explained in Chapter 6, person-time can be determined for any unit, such as person-month and person-year. It is calculated by dividing the total participation time of a subject into segments and expressing the risk in terms of that segment. Thus risk of cardiovascular disease may be expressed in terms of person-years. Notice that this expression of the data assumes that the risk remains constant over time, as does the susceptibility of the patient to the exposure.

HOW TO EVALUATE EVIDENCE FROM A COHORT STUDY DESIGN

The principles involved in the evaluation of a cohort study are illustrated with a critique of a cohort study reported by Graham et al.[7] on rhabdomyolysis and lipid-lowering drugs. To facilitate the evaluation of evidence provided by cohort study designs, a standard reporting format is used (Table 7-1). (This framework is also used for reporting findings from case-control study designs.) The format organizes the information contained in the

TABLE 7-1	A Guide to the Evaluation of Observational Research Reports
SECTION	**COMMENTS**
Title and abstract	The title is a headline and should contain the intervention, outcome, study design, and patient type. It should be unbiased, brief, and accurate.
	The abstract is a brief synopsis of the study, summarizing the four main sections of the report (introduction, methods, results, and discussion/conclusion). The abstract should be written clearly and informatively and should be able to stand apart from the article. Many abstracts are truncated at 250 words (either by the journal or the indexing database) and may not present a complete depiction of the study. Thus, reading and critically evaluating the full study is imperative when making clinical decisions.
Introduction	The introduction provides the rationale for the research effort. It begins with a general statement of the research area, provides a context for the present work, and explains the need for more research. The section closes with a clear statement of the specific research hypothesis. This statement is important because it sets the goal of the research effort, which in turn determines patient selection; method; and data acquisition, analysis, and interpretation.
Methods	The methods section describes the steps taken to test the statistical hypothesis. The methods should be sufficiently detailed for a reader to replicate the study. The methods contains a description of the type of study (experimental design), who was studied (description of subjects), what was measured and how it was measured (outcomes and data collection methods), and how data were analyzed (statistical analysis). • Type of study (case-control, cohort, cross-sectional): Make sure the study design is appropriate for the hypothesis being tested. • Participants and setting: This section should identify the source of the patients and indicate whether the study was retrospective or prospective. The inclusion and exclusion criteria should be objective, standard, and based on clinically important variable levels. Evaluate how similar the participants are to those seen in your clinical practice. Be sensitive to the methods and criteria used for group assignment (definitions of exposure and nonexposure for cohort studies). Determine where the patients were treated and how many clinics were involved. Decide whether the standard of care in the facility is relevant to your practice. Approval by an institutional review board or other ethical board is necessary for all research performed using human beings as subjects.

TABLE 7-1	**A Guide to the Evaluation of Observational Research Reports**
	• Measurements: Determine the variables used as primary and secondary outcomes. They should be relevant to testing the research hypothesis. They should be measured and analyzed in a standard manner. Measurement intervals should also be specified. • Data analysis: Transformations or manipulations of the data following their initial collection should be explained. All tests of the primary and secondary outcomes should be stated explicitly a priori. The probability level for rejecting the null hypothesis, α, should be stated. At this point, it is good practice to predict the results. This will ensure that you understand the research hypothesis and methods. It will also provide expectations about the changes that must occur to support the research hypothesis and other evidence necessary to answer questions about bias, confounding, and other factors that might affect damage the internal validity of the study.
Results	The results section provides in detail the findings of the study as they relate to the statistical hypothesis. The research hypothesis gains support based on the results of statistical tests of specific null hypotheses. • The first step in the results section should be to present the findings for differences between exposed and nonexposed patients. Tests should be conducted of all relevant demographic, socioeconomic, health history, and physiologically important factors. Ideally, data from those who refused to participate and those who did not complete the study (dropouts) should also be examined to determine whether the volunteer effect was a source of bias. • Next, the results of analyses of primary and secondary outcome variables should be presented in clear, simple language, followed by the statistical support. Are data for all patients and all a priori defined outcomes accounted for? Be alert for results that are trends—results that are described as being meaningful even though they do not achieve statistical significance. Accept only statistically significant evidence. However, make sure the statistically significant results are also relevant clinically. Some effects, though statistically significant, may be too small or too weak to be of much clinical value in treating patients. • Third, analyses should be reported that deal with variables that might have confounded or biased the results. Their analysis should be as detailed as those for primary and secondary outcomes. • Finally, post hoc analyses, those conducted after the a priori data analyses, may be presented. These are to be considered exploratory in nature and may not be used as evidence relevant to the present outcomes.
Discussion	The first part of the discussion section should be a straightforward description of the results and how they relate to the research hypothesis. Key evidence should be described. Next, supporting evidence should be marshaled from other studies, and differences among the studies' findings should be evaluated. This should be followed by a consideration of limitations to the study results and conclusions, including chance, bias, confounding, effect–cause, effect–effect, and/or cause–effect. Conclusions and implications should be restricted to the evidence provided by the present results. Do not accept contentions that are beyond the scope of the paper.
Other factors	Use the reputation of the authors and sponsoring organizations; the sources of funding and support provided to the authors, and the journal and its review process as indications of the quality of the paper. Editorials accompanying the paper and letters to the editor following its publication can add valuable information by providing a context for the study findings and by addressing questions raised by other experts in the field.

research report into a number of sections that link together logically and provide a clear view of the purpose and findings of the study. The major sections and their intent are

- *Title and abstract:* Provide a snapshot and summary, respectively, of the study's content.
- *Introduction:* Provides the rationale for the research hypothesis.
- *Methods:* Indicates who was studied, how they were studied, and how data were analyzed.
- *Results:* Presents the findings relevant to the statistical hypotheses.
- *Discussion:* Relates the findings to the general population and clinical arena and closes with implications for clinical practice.

Refer to the cohort study by Graham et al.[7] Your understanding of the literature evaluation points discussed here will be enhanced if you read this cohort study before continuing with the chapter. A brief overview of the study is provided here. The title—"Incidence of Hospitalized Rhabdomyolysis in Patients Treated with Lipid-Lowering Drugs"—indicates clearly that the study is reporting the incidence of rhabdomyolysis in patients receiving lipid-lowering drugs. The abstract provides more detail: Lipid-lowering agents such as statins and fibrates are commonly used to lower lipid levels in adults. However, the incidence of a potentially serious side effect, rhabdomyolysis, has not been determined. Using electronic databases from 11 managed-care plans across the United States, records of more than 250,000 plan members were culled for information relating to the use of statins alone or in combination with fibrates and the incidence of rhabdomyolysis sufficiently serious to require hospitalization.

Results indicate that monotherapy with any of the currently prescribed statins is associated with an incidence of rhabdomyolysis of 0.44 per 10,000 patients, whereas the incidence rate for rhabdomyolysis owing to fibrate intake is 2.82 per 10,000 patients. Incidence increases with combined statin–fibrate therapy, particularly among older patients who have diabetes mellitus. The authors conclude that patients using only a statin drug are at low risk of rhabdomyolysis. Older patients who have diabetes mellitus, however, should be monitored carefully.

The introduction of the study report provides the rationale for the research effort: Disorders of muscle are considered to be a common adverse drug reaction to the use of statins and fibrates. However, the epidemiology of these disorders, particularly rhabdomyolysis, is based on case reports. Furthermore, estimates of the incidence of rhabdomyolysis in this patient group are few and vary widely. To clarify this situation, the authors note, "we conducted this study to estimate the incidence of rhabdomyolysis in patients treated with statins and fibrates, alone and in combination, in the ambulatory setting."[7]

LITERATURE CRITIQUE 7-1

This introduction sets the stage for the study in a straightforward manner, sketching the fact that little is known about the risk of muscle disorders associated with statin and fibrate use. Furthermore, available estimates vary widely. Questions remain concerning the incidence of rhabdomyolysis associated with statin use and fibrate use, among different formulations of statin drugs and among combinations of statin and fibrate drugs. ■

The methods section indicates that this is a retrospective cohort study in which prescription claims from 11 U.S. health plans were used to construct separate cohorts for individual statin therapies, fibrate therapies, and the combination. Person-time was used to log each patient's contribution.

Standard diagnostic codes contained in the *International Classification of Disease*, 9th revision, *Clinical Modification* (ICD-9-CM),[8] were used to flag patients who had primary or secondary diagnoses of rhabdomyolysis. Abnormal increases in muscle enzyme activity were used as well. Medical records and claims data provided demographic information as well as past history of diabetes mellitus, liver disease, or renal failure.

The flagged records were reviewed by three of the authors, and a judgment of rhabdomyolysis was made if the patient displayed muscle damage at hospital admission and had been diagnosed with rhabdomyolysis by a physician or displayed a creatinine kinase level > 10 times the upper limit of normal.

Statistical analysis of the data included relative risk (RR) estimates and calculation of 95% CI. The number needed to treat (NNT) (really, the number needed to harm; NNH) was also determined. The protocol was approved by all institutional review boards and by each participating healthcare plan.

 LITERATURE CRITIQUE 7-2

The methods section provides a clear and logical explanation of the data-gathering process. The patients are derived from a large database that is geographically diverse, contributing to the external validity of the study. The study period is indicated, along with the criteria for entering a patient into a cohort. No exclusion criteria are presented.

In a study such as this, the criteria used to define the outcome are important. In this study, standardized criteria from the ICD-9-CM provide the primary evidence of muscle disorders. The final diagnosis depends on the judgment of three of the authors. However, the specific protocol of this section is unclear. For example, did all judges review all records or did judges review different records? The preferred method is to have all judges review all records and to provide a measure of their agreement (e.g., κ statistic [see Chapter 6] or a similar measure) and a description of the steps taken to resolve disputed cases. Lack of this poses a significant threat to internal validity of this study.

The statistical analyses are based on a Poisson distribution. This probability distribution is a special case of the binomial probability distribution. It is used to characterize rare events.[9]

At this point in the critique of the paper, it is good practice to predict the results expected to confirm the research hypothesis. This ensures that you understand the intent of the study. In addition, it helps you recognize results that support the research hypothesis and results that do not. The purpose of this study is to provide estimates of the incidence of rhabdomyolysis in the U.S. population attributable to use of various statins and fibrates and their combination. Based on earlier studies, elevated incidence should be linked to fibrates compared to statins and to cerivastatin (now removed from the market) and simvastatin compared to the other statins. ■

In the total population pool of the study, 31 incident cases of rhabdomyolysis were identified from the 252,460 patients who contributed data during the study period. Of these, 13 incident cases were associated with statin monotherapy, 3 with gemfibrozil, and 8 with combined therapy. Patients with rhabdomyolysis were about 65 years of age and had been treated with one of the study drugs for an average of 6 months. About half of the study group was women.

The incident rate of rhabdomyolysis, 0.44 per 10,000 patient-years, was similar for three of the four included statins. In contrast, the incidence of rhabdomyolysis was increased among patients prescribed cerivastatin (5.34 per 10,000 patient-years) and among those prescribed the fibrate gemfibrozil (3.70 per 10,000 patient-years). The authors calculate that, after 1 year of treatment, 1 case of rhabdomyolysis can be expected for every 22,727 patients treated with atorvastatin, pravastatin, or simvastatin; 1 for every 1,873 patients treated with cerivastatin; and 1 for every 3,546 patients treated with a fibrate. The risk of rhabdomyolysis remains stable over time and does not change with length of treatment.

Treatment with combined statin–fibrate therapy exacerbates the incidence of rhabdomyolysis. For patients taking atorvastatin, pravastatin, or simvastatin, 1 case of rhabdomyolysis can be expected for every 1,672 patients treated. The NNH for cerivastatin–gemfibrozil therapy ranges between 9.7 and 12.7.

Risk is increased for patients aged 65 years or older (RR 5.4; 95% CI 1.3–21.6) and for those with diabetes mellitus (RR 2.9; 95% CI 0.7–11.8). Compared to statin monotherapy as the baseline risk, the RR for fibrate therapy is 5.5 for cerivastatin is 10. Combining risk factors exacerbates these risks substantially.

 LITERATURE CRITIQUE 7-3

The most striking data appear in Table 1 of the paper.[7] If the data for cerivastatin are not considered (because it has been removed from the market), only 7 cases of rhabdomyolysis can be attributed to monotherapy with a statin. Three cases can be attributed to a fibrate. Thus the risk of rhabdomyolysis seems to be extremely, extremely low.

The major findings are in accord with expectations: The incidence of rhabdomyolysis is low in patients prescribed statins and tends to be higher when fibrates alone or combined statin–fibrate therapies are prescribed. Risk of rhabdomyolysis increased among patients 65 years of age and older (RR 5.4; 95% CI 1.3–21.6). However, the authors' contention that the "point estimate of the RR was increased for patients with diabetes mellitus (RR 2.9; 95% CI 0.7–11.8)"[7] is not supported by the data analysis because the 95% CI for RR contains 1. As expected, other risk factors include the use of cerivastatin, combined therapy with a fibrate, and a combination of the demographic (i.e., over 65 years, of age) and health-history factors (i.e., diabetes).

The internal validity of the study seems to be rather strong. Acceptable statistical techniques were planned beforehand. A standardized definition of rhabdomyolysis was used to search a large database, and all cases were reviewed by three of the authors who were blinded with respect to the drug status of the patients. However, more detail regarding the diagnostic process, particularly with respect to the adjudication of disputed diagnoses, should have been included. Also, arguing that diabetes mellitus alone was a risk factor for rhabdomyolysis, even though the finding was not statistically significant, was inappropriate. ■

Commenting on the results, the researchers reiterate that the risk of rhabdomyolysis requiring hospitalization is low among patients using statin therapy and is increased among those taking a fibrate, those on combined statin–fibrate therapy, and older patients who have diabetes mellitus. Similar results have been observed in another study regarding the relative potency of fibrates compared to statin monotherapy.

The researchers point out that the study design, the strict definition of rhabdomyolysis, and the strategy for identifying the maximum number of cases contributed to the internal validity of the study. Limiting the findings are the small number of patients who had rhabdomyolysis, problems with the accuracy of computer prescription claims data, and patient misclassification. The authors conclude that the incidence of rhabdomyolysis is rare, even among those who may be at elevated risk.

LITERATURE CRITIQUE 7-4

The discussion is straightforward. The aim of the study—to estimate the incidence of rhabdomyolysis among ambulatory patients treated with statins and fibrates—was accomplished. Patients are at low risk for rhabdomyolysis with statin monotherapy (excluding cerivastatin). In addition, the study indicates that this risk is increased in patients taking fibrates, either alone or in addition to statins.

The paucity of cases makes it difficult to identify factors associated with increased risk of rhabdomyolysis in these patients. An increased risk of rhabdomyolysis among patients 65 years of age or older is a consistent finding. However, the role of diabetes mellitus is statistically significant only in patients 65 years of age or older who were being treated with a both a statin and a fibrate. Basically, the few incident cases of rhabdomyolysis identified make it difficult to glean more detailed information from the data.

The generalization of these findings to other clinical settings is based on the similarity of the patients, the criteria for the diagnosis of rhabdomyolysis, and the specific drugs and doses used to treat patients. The size and diversity of the database, including 11 managed-care plans and > 250,000 plan members, ensures a broad, diverse, and representative study population. Furthermore, doses of the statin and fibrate drugs are in the normal therapeutic range. Thus the study seems to have broad external validity.

An important limitation of this study is that the definition of rhabdomyolysis, although verifiable, is restricted to the most severe cases of the condition: those requiring hospitalization. The effect of statin and fibrate therapy on muscle varies in different patients and may be progressive.[10] Thus it is prudent to inquire about changes in muscle soreness or weakness during routine patient visits rather than awaiting a cataclysmic event.

In conclusion, the use of statins is associated with a risk of severe rhabdomyolysis that is extremely low. The risk is increased by combining statins and fibrates and perhaps by certain demographic and health status variables. The prudent healthcare provider will thus be vigilant in following patients on combined statin and fibrate therapy, particularly those who are older and those who exhibit compromised renal or liver function.

A letter to the editor[11] regarding this study was published. By reading the letter, the pharmacist can gain further insight to the critical evaluation of the study. ▪

In sum, cohort study designs have wide application in healthcare research. Their greatest contribution involves the evaluation of the consequences of engaging in unhealthy behaviors. However, they also provide much useful information about the beneficial effects of medications in patient populations. In evaluating cohort studies, however, the reader must be vigilant to the effects of confounding. In addition, the cohort study design is not ideal when conditions with long exposure–outcome intervals are studied or when the exposure is rare. In spite of these shortcomings, the cohort study design remains the premier study design for investigating exposures that have a negative health effect.

Relationships Among Variables

In many healthcare situations, notably in observational and cross-sectional or survey research designs, a fundamental interest is in discerning the *relationship* between an exposure variable and an outcome variable. In pharmacy, this type of information is sought quite frequently with respect to the relationship of a drug dose to its efficacy or to the frequency of adverse drug reactions or to ways this relationship may be modified by demographic, health history, environmental, and other variables. To assess the relevance of survey research designs to pharmacy practice, therefore, it is necessary to possess knowledge of the statistical principles pertaining to the expression of relationships.

The study of relationships is a different research focus from those that examine the difference between two group means or the difference in the frequency of an outcome in two groups. Regression analysis provides more information. For example, regression analyses can be used to:

- Describe the basic relationship between changes in one variable with respect to another variable
- Identify all variables involved and discard variables irrelevant to changes in the outcome variable
- Select the most important variables related to changes in the outcome variable
- Develop models to predict responses in new patients

Understanding the relationship between two variables can be visualized. Figure 7-2 is a **scatter plot** of the relationship between two *continuous* variables: an independent or an exposure variable (x) and a dependent or outcome variable (y). In this graph, 10 patients have been measured on both x and y, and these 10 data pairs have been entered into the graph. Visual inspection of the scatter plot suggests that increases in the x variable are related to increases in the y variable.

The goals of regression analysis are to:

- Provide a quantitative expression (a regression equation) of the relationship between x and y
- Test whether the information provided by the equation differs from chance
- Determine the strength of the association between x and y described by the regression equation

One notable feature of the scatter plot is that the relationship between x and y appears to be a straight line, or a linear relationship. Linear relationships are preferred in healthcare because they are relatively easy to treat mathematically and they are easier to interpret than nonlinear relationships. The mathematical formula for a straight line is

$$y = mx + b$$

where y is the dependent variable; x is the independent variable; m is the slope of the line; and b is the intercept. The intercept, b, is the value of y when $x = 0$. The slope of the

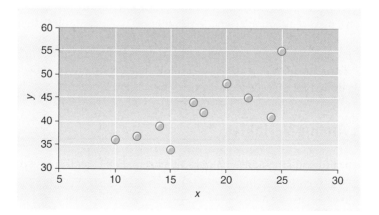

FIGURE 7-2   Scatter plot of 10 x, y pairs.

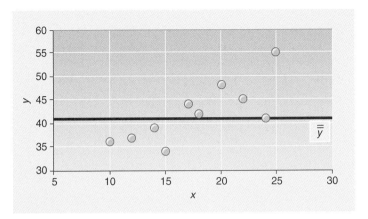

FIGURE 7-3 Scatter plot of 10 *x, y* pairs with the mean of all *y* scores ($\bar{\bar{y}}$) added.

line, *m*, is the amount of change in *y* for a one-unit change in *x*. If *y* increases as *x* increases, the relationship is termed *positive*. If *y* decreases as *x* increases, the relationship is termed *negative*. In regression analysis, the slope and intercept of the regression equation are used to predict values of *y*, termed $\hat{y}$, for each value of *x*. The regression line, therefore, consists of these $\hat{y}$ values.

To illustrate, Figure 7-3 presents the data from Figure 7-2 a plus a horizontal line labeled $\bar{\bar{y}}$. This line is equal to the mean of all the *y* values and is referred to as the grand mean of the *y* values. Because the value of the grand mean is the same for all *x, y* pairs in the scatter plot, adding the grand mean to the scatter plot results in a line that is horizontal to the *x* axis, with a slope of 0.

The usefulness of using the grand mean of the *y* values in the regression analysis may be determined by entering the slope (0) and intercept ($\bar{\bar{y}}$) of this line into the regression equation:

$$\hat{y} = (0)x + \bar{\bar{y}}$$

The difficulty is obvious: the same value of $\hat{y}$ is obtained for any value of *x* entered into the equation. Thus this equation provides no information about *changes* in *y* related to *changes* in *x*.

Figure 7-4 adds another line to the scatter plot shown in Figure 7-3. This line consists of values of $\hat{y}$ that were predicted for each *x, y* pair using the following regression equation:

$$\hat{y} = 0.96(x) + 25.08$$

This regression equation provides a much better fit of the predicted scores to the actual *y* scores than does the line with a slope of 0. That is because these $\hat{y}$ scores are much closer to the observed values of *y* than the $\hat{y}$ scores predicted from the equation using the grand mean. Put another way, the discrepancy between the actual and the predicted *y* values is much reduced with the second regression equation. This suggests that differences between *y* and $\hat{y}$ provide a measure of the error associated with the prediction of *y* based on a regression equation. This error may be the result of sampling error or of nonlinear trends in the data.

What is the difference between $\hat{y} - \bar{\bar{y}}$ In the regression equation based on the grand mean of the y scores, the slope of the regression line was 0, and the difference between $\hat{y}$ and $\bar{\bar{y}}$ was small. In the second equation, the slope of the regression line is nonzero, and

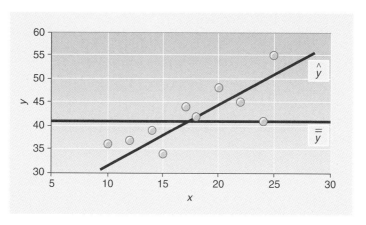

FIGURE 7-4 Scatter plot of 10 x, y pairs with the regression line ($\hat{y} = 0.96x + 25.08$) added.

discrepancies between $\hat{y}$ and $\bar{\bar{y}}$ are larger. This suggests that the difference between $\hat{y}$ and $\bar{\bar{y}}$ may be a measure of the extent to which y is predicted by the slope of the regression equation.

Finally, notice that adding $(\hat{y} - \bar{\bar{y}})$ to $(y - \hat{y})$ results in $(y - \bar{\bar{y}})$. In other words, the difference between any value y and $\bar{\bar{y}}$ is equal to the sum of the amount of information provided by the slope of the regression equation plus the amount of error associated with the regression equation. Based on this relationship, the two following propositions apply:

- If the slope of the regression equation provides a good description of the relationship between x and y, the $(\hat{y} - \bar{\bar{y}})$ differences will be greater than the $(y - \hat{y})$ differences for many of the x, y pairs.
- If the slope of the regression equation does not provide a good description of the relationship of x and y, the $(\hat{y} - \bar{\bar{y}})$ differences will not be greater than the $(y - \hat{y})$ differences for many of the x, y pairs.

Based on this reasoning, a statistical test of the slope of the regression line can be developed. A measure of the differences between y and $\hat{y}$ for the set of x values can be obtained by calculating the variance of $(y - \hat{y})$. The numerator of the variance is equal to $\Sigma(y - \hat{y})^2$, and is called the **sum of squares residual**. An unbiased estimate of the variance of $(y - \hat{y})$ is obtained by dividing this sum of squares by $(n - 2)$, where n is the number of x, y pairs. This term is called the **mean square residual**.

A measure of the differences between $\hat{y}$ and $\bar{\bar{y}}$ for the set of x values is obtained by calculating the variance of $(\hat{y} - \bar{\bar{y}})$ for each x value. The numerator is equal to $\Sigma(\hat{y} - \bar{\bar{y}})^2$, termed the **sum of squares regression**, and is divided by 1, the degrees of freedom (df), to obtain the **mean square regression**.

The total variability in the data set is obtained by adding the sum of squares residual and the sum of squares regression. For the regression line $\hat{y} = 0.96(x) + 25.08$, the sums of squares, df, and mean squares for each source of variation are presented in Table 7-2. The mean square regression equals 212.8 and the mean square residual equals 17.5. The statistical test is based on the *ratio* of these two values.

Recall that a slope of 0 provided no information about changes in $\hat{y}$ from knowledge of x. Thus H_0 is that the slope of the regression line = 0. The alternative hypothesis, H_A, is that the slope of the regression line is not 0. If the H_0 is true, the ratio of the mean square

TABLE 7-2	Components Used to Calculate the Variance Ratio[a]				
COMPONENT	SUM OF SQUARES	df	MEAN SQUARE	F	p
Regression	212.8	1	212.8	12.2	< 0.05
Residual	140.1	8	17.5		
Total	352.9	9			

[a]Data are from the regression example described in the text.

regression divided by the mean square residual should be close to 1. If the H_A is true, however, the ratio of the mean square regression divided by the mean square residual should be substantially greater than 1.

A test statistic, the variance ratio, calculated by dividing the mean square regression by the mean square residual, is presented in the column of Table 7-2 labeled "F." The value of the variance ratio is 12.2. As with other statistical tests, the next step is to determine the probability that a critical value of 12.2 or greater could occur by chance. This is determined by referring to critical values of the variance ratio, which are distributed as F, and presented in Table B-4 (Appendix B) for $\alpha = 0.05$. The critical value of F depends on the df for both the mean square regression and the mean square residual terms. In the present example, the df for mean square regression is 1 and is located under the column heading "df for numerator." The df for mean square residual is 8 and is identified in the leftmost column under the heading "df for denominator." At the intersection of the row and column indexed by the two df is the critical value of F, 5.32. Because the calculated value of the variance ratio exceeds this value, the H_0 is rejected.

An index of the *strength of the association* between x and y described by the regression equation is the **coefficient of determination**, or R^2. This is the ratio of the sums of squares regression to the total sums of squares. It can vary between 0 and 1. For these data, R^2 is equal to $212.8/352.9 = 0.60$. This suggests that 0.60 of the total variation in the data set is attributable to the linear regression function. The remaining 0.40 of the total variation is the result of nonlinear components in the data and sampling error.

Another expression of the strength of the linear relationship between two variables is the **Pearson product-moment correlation coefficient**, abbreviated r, and sometimes called the correlation coefficient. The correlation coefficient is equal to the square root of the coefficient of determination. It is further modified by assuming the same algebraic sign as the slope of the regression equation. The value of the correlation coefficient may range from -1.0 to $+1.0$. Values of r close to -1.0 or $+1.0$ indicate little error in the prediction of $\hat{y}$, and values close to 0 suggest much error of prediction.

Probabilities specifically associated with various values of r depend on the number of x, y pairs in the calculation. For this example, the probability of finding a value of r of 0.77 or greater by chance is < 5%. Thus the data analysis suggests excellent agreement between the two variables.

There is also a nonparametric equivalent of the Pearson product-moment correlation coefficient. It is the **Spearman rank correlation coefficient.** As the name implies, the test statistic is based on the correspondence of the *ranks* of data within each of two groups. The basic idea is that, for a highly positive correlation, rank values of the x variable should be paired with similar rank values of the y variable. Details can be found in any basic statistics text. Interpretation of the test statistic is the same as for the Pearson product-moment correlation coefficient.

TABLE 7-3	Ten *x, y* Pairs[a]
x	y
15	34
25	55
12	37
10	36
18	42
22	45
20	48
17	44
24	41
14	39

[a]Raw data are for the regression example described in the text.

EXTRA CREDIT 7-1

Many computer software programs, such as Microsoft Excel, are available to assist the self-learning student in exploring the different components of linear regression analysis that are beyond the scope of this summary treatment. To assist that endeavor, Table 7-3 contains the ten pairs of x, y scores used in the regression example discussed in the main text. The student is encouraged to use available software to confirm the results presented in this section and to explore how those results change as the data are manipulated. ■

In conclusion, linear regression analysis is a powerful tool and can provide information critical to appropriate healthcare decision making. Here are some guidelines to help the reader evaluate the results of linear regression analyses:

- A statistically significant relationship between *x* and *y* does not indicate that *x* causes *y*. It is possible that *y* causes *x* (i.e., effect–cause), or that both *x* and *y* are related through a third, confounding, factor that was not controlled.
- The actual numerical values of the regression equation weights the coefficient of determination and the correlation coefficient that are specific to the data used to obtain them. They are certain to change if the study is repeated with a different patient sample or if the experimental conditions change. Thus, external validity may be a problem if the results are applied too literally to different patients or settings.
- In many cases, interpolating values of *y* from values of *x* within the interval spanned by the values of *x* will provide accurate estimates of *y*. Predicting values of *y* from values of *x* not included within the measurement interval of *x*, termed extrapolation, is not a legitimate use of the regression equation.
- The regression equation describes the *linear* relationship of *x* and *y*. It is possible that there are important *nonlinear* components to the relationship.
- Outliers can distort the relationship between *x* and *y*, and these values can either foster or inhibit the finding of a linear relationship.

OTHER STATISTICAL TESTS BASED ON REGRESSION ANALYSIS

Regression analysis is not just an important topic in its own right. It also provides the basis for many other statistical tests. Two of these, analysis of variance and multivariable linear regression, appear frequently in the healthcare literature and deserve comment.

Analysis of Variance

To this point, regression models have been examined in which the relationship between two variables was quantified. However, regression analyses can also be used to examine differences between group means. In fact, regression models can be used to analyze data from a wide variety of experimental designs or models and exhibit an astonishing array of flexibility in their application to healthcare data. In this section, several basic **analysis of variance** (ANOVA) models are described.

Figure 7-5 presents hypothetical data for a drug study examining the effect of three different agents (two drug doses and a placebo) on the relief of headache pain, measured on a scale ranging from 1 to 25. A total of 15 subjects participated in the study, 5 being assigned randomly to each group. Notice the similarity between this scatter plot and that the one presented in Figure 7-2. One difference between the plots is that the y scores are clustered around specific x values in Figure 7-5. Even so, we can apply a similar analytic strategy to these data as was used for regression analysis: y scores still indicate actual data values and the mean of all the y scores is $\bar{\bar{y}}$, but $\hat{y}$ scores are replaced by group means, $\bar{y}$.

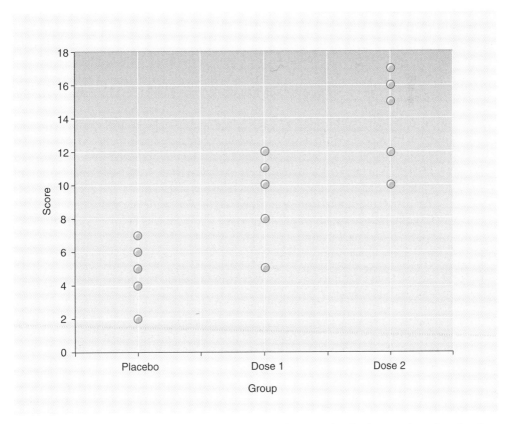

FIGURE 7-5 Scatter Plot: Pain-Relief Scores. Data from patients administered a placebo, one dose of a pain reliever (*Dose 1*), or a larger dose of the pain reliever (*Dose 2*). See Table 7-4 for an analysis of variance of these data.

TABLE 7-4	Analysis of Variance of the Efficacy of Two Drug Doses vs. Placebo in Providing Headache Pain Relief.				
SOURCE	SUM OF SQUARES	df	MEAN SQUARE	F	p
Treatment	211.7	2	105.9	16.0	< 0.05
Error	79.6	12	6.6		
Total	291.3	14			

Differences among group means, reflecting an effect of the pain relief treatment, are measured in terms of the difference between each group mean and the grand mean. Differences between each y value and its group mean, $\bar{y}$, index the experimental error in the study.

Such computations are usually carried out using computer software that provides the output presented in Table 7-4. Notice that the ANOVA table contains the sums of squares, df, and mean square values for both treatment and error sources of variation. The ratio of mean square treatment to mean square error is termed the F statistic.

The rationale for the statistical test of the association between the drug doses and the amount of pain relief is similar to that used for regression analysis. That is, if there is a treatment effect, differences among the group means will be larger than differences within the groups. If treatment effects are small or owing to chance, however, then treatment effect differences among the group means and within the groups will be similar. In the example, the mean square for the treatment group is 105.9, the mean square for the error is 6.6; thus and $F = 105.9/6.6 = 16.0$. From Table B-4 (Appendix B), the critical value of F for 2 and 14 df is 4.75 for $\alpha = 0.05$. Because the calculated value of F exceeds the critical value, the H_0 that there is no difference in pain relief owing to the drug doses can be rejected.

The results of this ANOVA indicate that there is a difference between the means of the three groups but does not indicate which specific means differed. For example, it is possible that only drug dose 2 was effective, in which case the means of the dose 2 and placebo groups would differ, but the means of the dose 1 and placebo groups would be similar.

Thus further testing is necessary to detect mean differences between specific groups using *post hoc analyses*. Currently, the Bonferroni test is preferred for post hoc analysis testing because it preserves the overall level of α even though multiple tests are conducted on the same data. Thus it reduces the chances of a type I error.

The results of the Bonferroni procedure for this example are presented in Table 7-5. The table contains the means of all three groups. Differences between pairs of means are

TABLE 7-5	Bonferroni Post Hoc Test of Headache Pain Relief Provided by Two Drug Doses and Placebo[a]		
	TREATMENT		
DIFFERENCE BETWEEN THE MEANS	PLACEBO	DOSE 1	DOSE 2
Means	4.8	9.2	14.0
Placebo		4.4	9.2*
Dose 1			4.8*

[a]Data are differences between pairs of means. Differences that are statistically significant at $p < .05$ for the set of the three comparisons are indicated with an asterisk (*). The results indicate that, although little pain relief was obtained with drug dose 1 compared to placebo, pain relief associated with drug dose 2 exceeded that of both placebo and drug dose 1.

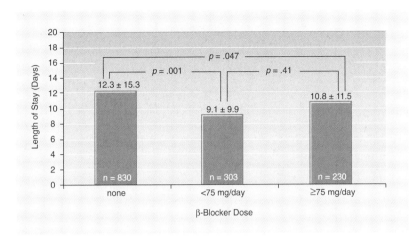

FIGURE 7-6 Analysis of Variance and Bonferroni Post Hoc Tests: Length of Hospitalization vs. Administration of β-Blockers after Cardiothoracic Surgery. Adapted with permission from Coleman C, Perkerson KA, Gillespie EL, et al. Impact of prophylactic postoperative β-blockade on post-cardiothoracic surgery length of stay and atrial fibrillation. Ann Pharmacother 2004;38:2012–2106.

located within appropriate cells. An asterisk (*) indicates the differences between mean pairs that were statistically significant. The results of this analysis indicate that pain relief provided by drug dose 1 was similar to placebo, but the pain relief provided by dose 2 was superior to that provided by both placebo and drug dose 1.

Application of ANOVA with Bonferroni post hoc tests is illustrated by an investigation of differences in length of hospitalization and incidence of atrial fibrillation in patients who underwent cardiothoracic surgery.[12] Specifically, the authors studied the effects of two doses of β-blocking drugs in reducing length of hospitalization compared to placebo. Figure 7-6 presents the results of a Bonferroni analysis of the differences between the means. In the figure, lines above the bars are used to show the specific mean comparison being evaluated and the probability that the difference was owing to chance. The results of this analysis indicated that the low drug dose, but not the high drug dose, reduced length of stay for patients.

The authors concluded, somewhat speciously, that length of stay was reduced by the lower drug dose but that no further reduction in length of stay was observed with the higher dose of β-blocking drug. The interpretation of these data would have been facilitated if a measure of the strength of association between drug dose and length of stay had been reported.

The ANOVA is not one statistical test, but a general template for many different analyses. For example, ANOVA models can be used to study the effect of several different independent variables, or factors, on a dependent variable. ANOVA models can also be used to analyze repeated measures obtained from the same patients. Both of these applications are illustrated by a study that examined the effects of hormone-replacement therapy and alendronate in preventing bone loss in postmenopausal women.[13] Based on data in younger women, an enhanced effect of combination therapy was expected compared to either drug administered alone.

Results of this trial are presented in Figure 7-7. The percent change in total hip bone mineral density for each of the four groups is presented: placebo, alendronate, hormone-replacement therapy, and combined therapy. Notice first that the data display repeated measurements on the same patients, so this is a repeated-measures design.

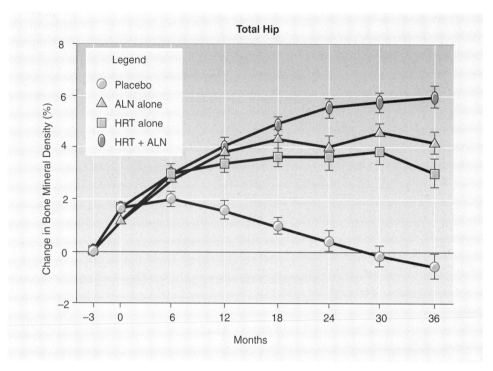

FIGURE 7-7 Change in Bone Mineral Density of the Hip over 36 Months of Treatment. Data indicate that the combined treatment of alendronate (ALN) plus hormone-replacement therapy (HRT) increased bone-mineral density scores more than either agent alone from 12 months of treatment to the end of the study period. Adapted with permission from Greenspan SL, Resnick NM, Parker RA. Combination therapy with hormone replacement and alendronate for prevention of bone loss in elderly women. A randomized controlled trial. JAMA 2003;289:2525–2533.

Furthermore, changes in bone mineral density differ between the groups over time. This is an example of an **interaction**, or an effect modification. That is, the effect of one variable is modified by another variable. In this case, bone mineral density changes are temporary with placebo, modest with either hormone-replacement therapy or alendronate alone, and greatest with combined drug therapy. Analyses of these differences at each time interval indicate that the difference between combined and individual therapies emerge at the 12-month measurement period and persist for the remaining months. An interaction, then, suggests information about two variables acting together that is not available from a study of each variable alone.

When is an ANOVA appropriate? ANOVA *may* be used instead of a *t*-test to compare differences between two group means. The ANOVA *must* be used when comparing more than two group means. This is because calculating more than one *t* statistic from the same set of data increases the probability of committing a type I error. With four treatment means, for example, six different *t*-tests would be necessary to compare all two-way combinations of means. Although the α level might be set at 0.05 for each test, the actual α level would be substantially higher. With six *t*-tests α is 0.26. (The general formula for this calculation is $[1 - (1 - \alpha)^k]$, where α is the probability of rejecting the H_0 on one test of significance, and k is the number of tests. For the example, $1 - 0.95^6 = 0.26$.) In other words, there is a greater than 1 in 4 chance that a type I error would be committed during this sequence of *t*-tests.

The ANOVA avoids the problem of multiple testing by using a two-step process. The first is to provide a statistical test indicating whether any of group means differ from each other. If such differences are found, then a series of post hoc tests can be used to detect which specific means differ from each other.

Multivariable Linear Regression

Multivariable linear regression is an extension of the simple linear regression described previously. Like logistic regression analysis, multivariable linear regression seeks to develop an additive model of independent variables that describe changes in a dependent variable. Unlike logistic regression analysis, however, the dependent variable is continuous rather than dichotomous.

For example, suppose we wanted to quantify an index of patient satisfaction with pharmacist-provided influenza immunization. The dependent variable, patient satisfaction, is measured as a continuous variable that is free to vary on a scale between -100 (indicating maximum dissatisfaction) through 0 (neutral) to $+100$ (maximum satisfaction). Independent variables may include any number of factors that characterize the pharmacist, the therapeutic setting, and the patient. For illustrative purposes, let's use one variable from each category.

Multivariable linear regression is an extension of simple linear regression. The simple linear regression equation describes the relationship of the independent (x) variable to the dependent variable (y) in terms of the slope of the regression equation. This slope is also considered to be a *coefficient* that modifies the value of x to enhance the accuracy of its prediction of y, termed $\hat{y}$.

Multivariable linear regression includes more than one independent variable to enhance the precision of the prediction of the y variable—that is, an equation is developed in which each of a series of independent variables is modified by a coefficient, with the result being the description of the dependent variable, y.

So the multivariable linear regression equation might be

$$\hat{y} = b_0 + b_1x_1 + b_2x_2 + b_3x_3 + E$$

where $\hat{y}$ is the predicted dependent variable, patient satisfaction; x_1, x_2, and x_3 are the independent variables; b_0 is the intercept; and b_1, b_2, and b_3 are the coefficients of the independent variables; and E is the error term. The patient satisfaction score for any individual can be predicted by entering into the equation that individual's scores on variables x_1 through x_3.

Multivariable linear regression analysis, available in many statistical analysis software packages, can be used in several ways. One is to determine the coefficients that best predict the dependent variable using all the independent variables in the equation. Coefficients that bear a relationship to the dependent variable beyond that owing to chance are deemed to be statistically significant. This application of the regression model is illustrated later in this chapter.

Another form of multivariable linear regression is termed *stepwise multiple linear regression analysis*. In this version, only the independent variables having statistically significant coefficients are entered into the regression equation. The result is that the total set of independent variables is reduced to include only those that contribute to the determination of the value of the independent variable.

For example, stepwise multiple regression analysis was used to identify a set of variables that were associated with medication adherence by patients who have asthma.[14] The original set of variables included a wide array of information, including demographic, health history, health status, health belief, and quality of life. In the final model, adherence to asthma medications was related to a much-reduced set of variables: greater perceived severity of asthma, greater interval since diagnosis, a greater number of metered dose inhaler instructors, stronger beliefs in the importance of treatment and avoidance of asthma triggers, and the mental component measure of the Medical Outcomes Study (MOS) 36-item short-form health survey (SF-36).[15] However, the R^2 was 0.26, suggesting that the adequacy of the model was moderate at best.

Cross-Sectional Study Design

The purpose of cross-sectional or survey research is to obtain information about an issue in healthcare in a way that allows quantification of the answer. In other words, surveys provide a means of measuring knowledge, attitudes, emotions, experiences, intentions, and so on. Cross-sectional or survey research serves not only as an independent paradigm in healthcare studies but is often an essential component of observational studies and randomized controlled trials. Therefore, it is important to understand the basic principles underlying survey research.

An overview of the major features of the cross-sectional or survey research design was provided in Chapter 3. The major points follow:

- *Goal*: To obtain evidence of exposures, outcomes, and their associations
- *Strategy*: To gather information on exposure and outcome at a single point in time
- *Major weaknesses*: Several sources of bias and the problem of drawing cause-effect conclusions

A survey is a questionnaire consisting of a set of items. Participants are asked to respond to the items in a variety of ways. For some items, an essay response is requested. In other cases, subjects may be asked to rank some attribute of a list of items. Subjects may also be asked to indicate the degree to which they agree with a statement.

To have value as a measuring tool, questionnaires must be shown to display three properties: validity, reliability, and sensitivity. **Validity** means that the survey tool measures what it is intended to measure. There are many ways to validate a survey. One is to demonstrate that the new survey provides information similar to that of a standard index of the effect. For example, a new survey tool assessing healthy lifestyles might be compared to the SF-36[15] (described later in the chapter). Another way to validate a survey is to obtain the opinion of likely respondents on whether the survey measures what it is intended to measure. This is **face validity**.

In addition to validity, the output of the survey tool must exhibit reliability—that is, it must provide the same answers every time the same subject completes the survey under the same test conditions. This is another way of saying that answers to the test items must be stable and that the error of measurement is small. A common strategy to assess reliability is to compare responses to survey items administered to the same subjects on two separate occasions. This type of reliability is termed **test–retest reliability**.

Finally, the items in the test instrument must display **sensitivity** to changes in test conditions. Ideally, the responses to the test items are sensitive to changes in variables relevant to the exposure–outcome relationship but resistant to change when irrelevant variables change. For example, a test instrument designed to index risk of cardiovascular disease based on physical-conditioning behavior must exhibit changes in risk to meaningful change in behaviors designed to reduce risk.

Although several methods exist for the quantification of responses to a survey item, a common approach is to measure responses on a **Likert scale**. In this type of scale, responses to test items include several alternatives (usually five) that describe the range of possible answers. For example, to the test item "Biostatistics is my favorite class" the response items might include "strongly agree," "somewhat agree," "neither agree nor disagree," "somewhat disagree," and "strongly disagree." Respondents select one response item, which has been assigned a numerical value. For example, "strongly agree" might be assigned a value of 5, and "strongly disagree" a value of 1.

In some surveys, responses to questions are combined to quantify a concept. For example, an attitude toward drug information might be quantified as the sum of the responses for the following items: "Biostatistics is my favorite class," "I like to search the literature to find answers to healthcare questions," "I don't accept the conclusions of research studies uncritically," and "Knowing how to evaluate research articles is an important part of being a competent pharmacist." Assigning a score of 5 to the answer "strongly agree" and a 1 to "strongly disagree" for each of the four questions, researchers could determine that respondents who valued quantitative literacy would score about 20, people who disagree totally would score about 4, and those who were neutral would score about 12.

Surveys are of two general types. Some surveys are standardized, whereas others are custom designed for specific situations. Examples of standardized surveys are the following:

- *SF-36:*[15] A general survey of health attitudes that quantifies eight health concepts—(1) limitations on physical activities owing to health problems, (2) limitations on social activities owing to physical or emotional problems, (3) physical health limitations on usual activities, (4) physical pain, (5) general mental health, (6) emotional problems, (7) vitality, and (8) general health perceptions—and has been adapted to many different cultural and clinical settings.
- *Mini Mental State Examination (MMSE):*[16] A brief, rapid tool to assess cognitive functioning—orientation, attention, short-term recall, and the capacity to respond appropriately to verbal and written instructions—and provide a total score that can be used to categorize the global cognitive functioning of the patient.

Custom surveys are ubiquitous in healthcare research. For example, they have been used to:

- Estimate the use of herbal drugs in a large metropolitan area.[17] The authors of the study describe a portion of the questionnaire as follows:

    The survey included a section designed to document prevalence of use of any herbal product and use of 13 specific herbs. This section also included questions to assess issues related to use of herbs (rationale for use, perceived efficacy, and source of product information). Another section included questions to collect demographic information and to assess use of multivitamin and individual nutritional supplements.

- Assess factors that promote adherence to drug regimen in patients diagnosed with asthma.[14] The study combined custom questions with a standardized survey:

    The Behavioral Model of Health Services Utilization was used as a framework to identify significant predictor variables and their relationship to the outcome of adherence. The model consists of predisposing, enabling, and illness level (need) factors, which are hypothesized to be the primary determinants of health services utilization. . . . Illness level or need variables were operationalized using measures of asthma severity and health-related quality of life. Patient-perceived severity was measured using a survey item with a 5 point scale that ranged from very mild to very severe. Evaluated severity was measured using a symptom-derived scale based on symptom frequency during the previous 4 weeks.

Problems with cross-sectional studies include both volunteer bias and recall bias. Volunteer bias occurs when participation is not mandatory. The fact that some people are willing to participate in surveys but others are not indicates that a difference exists between the two types of respondents. Another source of bias is recall bias, which is the tendency for individuals to have different recollections of the same event.

Another potential problem with survey data is that it is often difficult to discern the cause from the effect. Are healthy patients healthy because they comply with their drug regimens, or does compliance with drug regimens make them healthy? It's like the chicken and the egg question: Which came first? The chicken or the egg? Because information about both variables is obtained at the same time, a time interval between the two variables cannot be used to discriminate the cause from the effect.

On the other hand, data can be collected quickly and economically using cross-sectional research tools. Furthermore, groups of interest can be targeted quite precisely, decreasing wasted effort. Finally, the increased application of Internet technology to survey research is certain to increase its use if not its value as a research tool.

In summary, cross-sectional survey research provides valuable information not only in its own right but as an essential tool used in many observational studies and randomized controlled trials. In the next section, many of these points are illustrated in an evaluation of a cross-sectional study to identify variables that promote adherence to medication after cardiothoracic surgery.

HOW TO EVALUATE A CROSS-SECTIONAL STUDY

The evaluation of a cross-sectional study design is illustrated using a report by Sud et al.[18] (reprinted in Appendix C).

To facilitate the evaluation of evidence provided by cross-sectional study designs, the standard reporting format for observational studies is used (Table 7-1). (This framework is also used for reporting findings from case-control and cohort study designs.) The format organizes the information contained in the research report into a number of sections that link together logically and provide a clear view of the purpose and findings of the study. The major sections and their intent are:

- *Title and abstract*: Provides a snapshot and summary, respectively, of the study's content.
- *Introduction*: Provides the rationale for the research hypothesis.
- *Methods*: Indicates who was studied, how they were studied, and how data were analyzed.
- *Results*: Presents the findings relevant to the statistical hypotheses.
- *Discussion*: Relates the findings to the general population and clinical arena and closes with implications for clinical practice.

Refer to the cross-sectional study by Sud et al.[18] Your understanding of the literature evaluation points discussed here will be enhanced if you read this cohort study before continuing with the chapter. A brief overview of the study is provided here. The title—"Adherence to Medications by Patients after Acute Coronary Syndrome"—and abstract provide an overview of the study purpose, methodology, and findings. Briefly, 10 months after surgery for acute coronary syndrome, patients were contacted by telephone to obtain information about their level of adherence to medications and reasons for termination. Lack of adherence with medications was a function of the type of drug. The most common reason for lack of adherence was that discontinuance was based on the advice of a physician. Adherence was related positively to self-perceived heart health and to the perception that medications were important to continued good health.

Cardiovascular disease is the leading cause of death in the United States, largely owing to morbidity attributable to acute coronary syndrome (ACS). Although several organizations have provided evidence-based guidelines for postsurgical treatment of ACS with β-blockers, angiotensin-converting enzyme (ACE) inhibitors, aspirin and other antiplatelet agents, and lipid-lowering drugs, nonadherence to medication regimens is common. Variables associated with nonadherence include demographic, socioeconomic, and medical factors. Another important class of factors relating to adherence, however, involves beliefs about health behaviors and the use of drugs in initiating and maintaining health. The goal of the report by Sud et al.[18] was to determine "the relationship between patient, disease and treatment variables with adherence to the 4 classes of medications."

 LITERATURE CRITIQUE 7-5

The introduction is well written and describes the research area, indicates the value of the present effort, and specifically states the research goals of the investigation. Cardiovascular disease, including ACS, is a major cause of mortality in the United States. Although medications have been demonstrated to reduce mortality after surgery to treat ACS, adherence to the drug regimen is less than ideal, increasing mortality and morbidity in this population. Much effort has been expended to understand this lack of adherence, and many different variables have been identified. One neglected area of study, however, is the patient's beliefs about the value of drug therapy. ▪

The methods section indicates that a cross-sectional telephone survey was conducted among all patients discharged from the study hospital with a diagnosis of unstable angina or acute myocardial infarction from January 2002 to May 2003. To participate in the study, patients were required to be able to communicate in English using a telephone.

Patients were identified from electronic medical records by trained cardiac fellows using standard data-collection forms. Between 6 and 12 months after discharge, patients were contacted by telephone by trained interviewers who gathered the data for the study using a standardized form and interview script. Data collected were reviewed by nurses for quality.

Data collection instruments included health status ratings and completion of two standardized tools, the Beliefs about Medicines Questionnaire (BMQ)[19] and the Medication Adherence Scale (MAS).[20]

> Overall and cardiac-related health status were determined by asking the patient to rate his/her status on a 5-point Likert scale (1 = excellent, 2 = very good, 3 = good, 4 = fair, 5 = poor). To determine beliefs toward medication, patients were administered the previously validated BMQ. The BMQ consists of 18 items that generate 4 scale scores: Specific Necessity, Specific Concerns, General Harm, and General Overuse. Each BMQ item uses a 5-point Likert scale (from 1 = strongly agree to 5 = strongly disagree). Each scale score is derived from the mean of the scale items, with a possible score range from 1 to 5. Lower BMQ scale scores indicate stronger agreement with the belief scale. A question regarding self-perceived health status was also included. The MAS was used to explore reasons for discontinuance of drugs.[18]

Changes in drug use were assessed "by comparing the list of drugs obtained at discharge for the index ACS event to the list of drugs reported by the patient at the time of the telephone survey."[18] Discrepancies were resolved by obtaining a reason for discontinuation from a set of preselected response possibilities.

Examination of the data is primarily descriptive. A multivariate (i.e., multivariable) regression analysis was used to express the relationship between selected variables and drug compliance as measured by the MAS.

LITERATURE CRITIQUE 7-6

The study was conducted carefully. Identification of participants was carried out by expert personnel using standardized criteria and supervised by personnel with clinical experience. The criteria for selecting patients are explicit: all patients 18 years of age or older with a documented diagnosis of unstable angina or acute myocardial infarction during the study period who could converse in English using a telephone. Exclusion criteria are not provided.

Data were collected by trained personnel using standardized scripts and standardized testing instruments (BMQ and MAS). Other data were obtained from medical records. MAS data were further processed to define "less than perfect adherence" as a scale score > 1.0. This means that *any* missed dose was scored as nonadherent. This is a stringent criterion, given that the width of the scale was from 1 to 5, and suggests that patients were for the most part adherent with respect to their medications.

Data analysis was primarily descriptive. The choice of multiple linear regression analysis was correct for providing information critical to understanding the relationship among the variables.

The internal validity of the study is questionable. Strengths include that participants were identified in a standardized manner and the interview process was carried out according to a defined protocol. In addition, other data were obtained from medical records. However, validity is weakened by the definition of nonadherence as a MAS score of > 1; that the width of the scale is from 1 to 5 hints that most patients were still totally adherent to their medications at the time of the interview. In addition, the study is prone to volunteer bias and recall bias. Efforts to corroborate respondents' answers are not described. ■

The results section indicates that of 563 patients eligible to participate in the study, 39% refused to participate and only 37% completed the interview. These individuals were approximately 65 years of age, 60% were men, and 96% were white. Respondents were reported not to differ from nonrespondents in regard to age, gender, or race. Most patients viewed their current health status as good to very good, valued their medications, and disagreed that the medications were harmful.

Of the four classes of postsurgical medications, the greatest percent decrease in adherence was found with β-blockers (−12%) and the least with aspirin (−7%). The most frequent reason for discontinuation was that the physician had indicated that the medication was unnecessary. The next most frequent response relates to adverse effects of the drug. Adherence did not seem related to type of medication.

The findings from the multiple regression analysis revealed that continued adherence to a drug regimen for ACS is related positively to a belief that medications are important to continued good health and a positive self-perception of heart-related health status.

 LITERATURE CRITIQUE 7-7

The results of the study have two major limitations. One is the lack of participation by many potential study subjects. Only 37% of the eligible patients agreed to the interview. The major reason for discontinuing the survey was refusal to respond to adherence-related items. The study thus suffers from volunteer bias—only the most compliant patients completed the survey. In addition, the results may be the result of a healthy subject effect—an increased tendency of the healthier patients to participate in the study. Evidence for this is provided by the patient satisfaction scores.

There are two consequences of this bias. First, the descriptive data are relevant only to the most adherent patients. Almost all respondents indicated that they "always" complied with medication directives; the mean adherence score is 1.3 and the median score is 1.1. The descriptive data thus provide little information about potential variables that might be related to differences in adherence.

A second consequence of the homogeneity of the participant pool is that the data demonstrate little variability. This increases the difficulty of identifying relationships among independent variables and adherence. If everyone is adherent, it is difficult to identify variables related to a lack of adherence. In the multivariable regression analysis, for example, only two factors were statistically significant. Furthermore, the regression equation explained only 13.2% of the variability in the data set.

In summary, the bane of this study is volunteer bias, which resulted in a data set with so few differences in adherence that it is difficult to identify relationships among the independent variables studied and differences in adherence to prescribed drugs. Thus, although the study was planned relatively carefully and carried out well, the findings provide little information regarding the research hypotheses. ∎

The discussion places the findings in perspective. The participation rates in the present study were high compared to other reports, owing perhaps to the cohort studied or to the efficiency of the healthcare delivery system. The reason given most often for discontinuation of a drug—that the physician decided it was unnecessary—is puzzling and is not resolved by the current data. However, the multiple regression results remind pharmacists of the importance of reinforcing patient attitudes concerning the need for continued self-medication and a positive attitude toward heart health.

 LITERATURE CRITIQUE 7-8

This study illustrates the effect that bias can exert on a study protocol that is otherwise well conceived and conducted. Owing perhaps to the nature of the study topic and variables affecting a lack of adherence to prescribed medications, only those who were adherent to the drug regimen participated.

There are two consequences of this volunteer bias. The first is the similarity of participants with respect to health status ratings and adherence to medications. Because of this, there was little evidence of discontinuation of drug regimens and few clues to variables that might account for a lack of adherence. Second, because of the greater tendency for healthy patients to participate in interviews, it is difficult to determine whether the adherence to medications was the result of the health status of the patients or if the health status of the patients was the result of the adherence to the medication program—a common shortcoming of survey research. Little guidance is offered on this topic in the study report.

The most striking finding in the study is that discontinuance of medications is based on physician advice that continued use of the drug was not necessary. This statement is most remarkable, given evidence of misunderstandings related to patient–physician communications and certainly merits pursuit.

In summary, the external validity of the study is limited to the subject pool actually studied: patients 10 months after treatment for acute coronary syndrome. Even here, little evidence is offered to explain the adherence—patients who are most adherent (none is not adherent) value heart health and the role of drugs in that endeavor.

Although the findings are limited, these data could be used as baseline information for a longitudinal study of these patients that could mark the timing of discontinuance of medications and capture the reasons for that discontinuance in initially compliant patients. The results of such a study would assist healthcare providers, including pharmacists, in planning measures to counter nonadherence.

Furthermore, as noted, the notion that patients were told by their physicians to discontinue medication is certainly surprising and deserves to be pursued. Perhaps the suggestion here is for pharmacists to be alert to the premature discontinuance of drugs for chronic conditions and to follow up with the patient regarding a change in medication. ■

Summary

In this chapter, basic cohort and cross-sectional research paradigms are described. In both research paradigms, study participants are grouped together based on a common characteristic or exposure experience. Both cohort studies and survey research paradigms provide much unique, valuable information about the association among events and outcomes. Thus they are valuable tools in providing drug information, particularly when adverse events are studied.

Exploring associations among variables using regression analyses was also explained somewhat extensively because it is important to understand the rationale for its use. In addition to the applications described here, the regression model is the basis for more complex statistical analyses, such as multivariable regression and logistic regression

Finally, a powerful analytical tool, the analysis of variance, was described and illustrated with examples. The ANOVA is not one test, but a family of analytical models. The ANOVA is the preeminent statistic for detecting differences among more than two group means, for examining the effects of more than one independent variable, and for elucidating the relationship among independent variables as they interact to produce effects.

STUDY PROBLEMS

1. Discuss with your classmates the advantages and disadvantages of using the research designs in this chapter to study the effects of Agent Orange among Vietnam War veterans. Be sure to search the literature for published studies. Critique these papers so that your study design corrects for any flaws you might find. Be particularly sensitive to recall and volunteer bias.

2. Select one of the papers cited in this chapter that was not critiqued. Evaluate its internal and external validity. What are the major characteristics that define each? How does the external validity change as a function of your practice setting?

3. Search the Internet for information about the SF-36, MMSE, or a similar survey tool. Identify efforts taken to validate the survey in different populations or for different research applications.

4. You receive the following drug information question from an internal medicine resident who is spending the month training in the dialysis unit of a community hospital. He says, "I know that β-blockers, ACE inhibitors, statins, and aspirin provide cardiovascular

protection in the general population and are widely used. Because cardiovascular disease is the leading cause of mortality in patients with renal failure, I'm wondering if you can provide me with information on how often these medications are used for patients on hemodialysis. I'm wondering if there is any good evidence to support a lack of use of these medications in patients on hemodialysis, as I would like to propose the establishment of a protocol in the dialysis unit for screening patient medication profiles to ensure they are prescribed these medications." Read and critically evaluate the cross-sectional study by Miller et al.[21] and provide a response the resident's question.

REFERENCES

1. Ockene JK, Barad DH, Cochrane BB, et al. Symptom experience after discontinuing use of estrogen plus progestin. JAMA 2005;294:183–193.
2. Rexrode KM, Buring JE, Glynn RJ, et al. Analgesic use and renal function in man. JAMA 2001;286:315–321.
3. Forman JP, Rimm EB, Stampfer MJ, Curhan GC. Folate intake and the risk of incident hypertension among U.S. women. JAMA 2005;293:320–329.
4. Delea TE. Use of thiazolidinediones and risk of heart failure in people with type 2 diabetes. A retrospective cohort study. Diabetes Care 2003;26:2983–2989.
5. Kannel WB, Dawber TR, Kagan A, et al. Factors of risk in the development of coronary heart disease—Six year follow-up experience. The Framingham Heart Study. Ann Intern Med 1961;55:33–50.
6. Kannel WB, Feinleib M, McNamara PM, et al. An investigation of coronary heart disease in families: The Framingham offspring study. Am J Epidemiol 1979;110:281–290.
7. Graham DJ, Staffa JA, Shatin D, et al. Incidence of hospitalized rhabdomyolysis in patients treated with lipid-lowering drugs. JAMA 2004;292:2585–2590.
8. American Medical Association. *International Classification of Disease, 9th revision, Clinical Modification: physician ICD-9-CM, 2005.* AMA Press. 2005.
9. Kachigan SK. Statistical Analysis. New York: Radius, 1986.
10. Rhabdomyolysis with statins. Bandolier [serial online] Jan 2005. Available at: www.jr2.ox.ac.uk/bandolier/band131/b131–2.html. Accessed July 2006.
11. Tenenbaum A, Fisman EZ, Motro M. Rhabdomyolysis and lipid-lowering drugs [Letter]. JAMA 2005:293:1448.
12. Coleman C, Perkerson KA, Gillespie EL, et al. Impact of prophylactic postoperative β-blockade on post-cardiothoracic surgery length of stay and atrial fibrillation. Ann Pharmacother 2004;38:2012–2016.
13. Greenspan SL, Resnick NM, Parker RA. Combination therapy with hormone replacement and alendronate for prevention of bone loss in elderly women. A randomized controlled trial. JAMA 2003;289:2525–2533.
14. De Smet BD, Erickson SR, Kirking DM. Self-reported adherence in patients with asthma. Ann Pharmacother 2006;40:414–420.
15. Ware JE, Sherbourne CD. The MOS 36-Item Short-Form Health Survey (SF-36). I. Conceptual framework and item selection. Med Care 1992;30:473–483.
16. Tufts-New England Medical Center, Department of Psychiatry. The Mini Mental State Examination. Tufts University School of Medicine, Boston. Available at: hwww.nemc.org/psych/mmse.asp. Accessed July 2006.
17. Harnack LJ. Prevalence of use of herbal products by adults in the Minneapolis/St Paul, Minn, Metropolitan area. Mayo Clin Proc 2001;76:688–694.
18. Sud A, Kline-Rogers EM, Eagle KA, et al. Adherence to medications by patients after acute coronary syndrome. Ann Pharmacother 2005;39:1792–1797.
19. Horne R, Weinman J, Hankins M. The Beliefs about Medicines Questionnaire: The development and evaluation of a new method for assessing the cognitive representation of medication. Psychol Health 1996;14:1–24.
20. Morisky DE, Green LW, Levine DM. Concurrent predictive validity of a self-reported measure of medication adherence. Med Care 1986;24:67–74.
21. Miller LM, Hopman WM, Garland JS, et al. Cardioprotective medication use in hemodialysis patients. Can J Cardiol 2006;22:755–760.

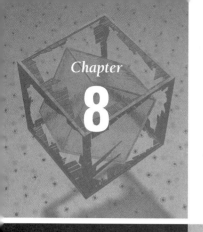

Critical Appraisal of Evidence Derived from Randomized Controlled Clinical Trials

CHAPTER GOALS

After studying this chapter, the student should be able to:

1. Describe placebo and active control study designs.

2. Explain the rationale for these study designs.

3. Enumerate the advantages and disadvantages of each study design.

4. Evaluate applications of these study designs to clinical practice.

5. Interpret statistical test results that characterize the pattern of change in outcome variables over time.

For many healthcare professionals, the most credible evidence regarding cause-and-effect relationships between independent and dependent variables is derived from randomized controlled trials (RCTs). The study design consists of two or more study groups that are, theoretically, identical at the beginning of the experiment. Members of one group receive a new treatment, and members of the other group receive either a placebo or a standard treatment. Because the groups are equal in all respects before the treatments are administered, differences between the groups in the dependent variable are attributed to the treatment (or independent) variable.

Example RCTs reviewed in this chapter include:

- Evaluation of antiresorptive therapy in preventing bone loss in elderly women.
- Treatment of benign prostatic hyperplasia with saw palmetto.
- The role of statins in reducing and preventing myocardial infarction.

The ability to infer that changes in the outcome (or dependent) variable are caused by the treatment (or independent) variable is the result of two features of the RCT. The first is the amount of control the investigator exerts over almost all aspects of the experimental situation. For example, the investigator characterizes subjects to be examined by defining inclusion and exclusion criteria and determines the experimental and control treatments in terms of amount, duration, and other factors. In addition, the investigator chooses the setting in which the study will take place, the variables used to measure the outcomes, the methods used to analyze the data, and the vehicle used to report the results.

Another crucial aspect of the RCT is *randomization of participants to the different study groups*. Randomization is a method of group assignment that is not under the control of the investigator. Therefore, group membership cannot be affected by selection or other forms of bias. One strength of randomization is that the study groups are similar in variables known to contaminate the treatment–outcome relationship. Difference in outcome, therefore, cannot be attributed to these variables.

An added benefit of randomization is an increased probability that study groups are matched on many other variables that the investigator does not control or of which he or she may be ignorant but that nevertheless may affect the results.[1] For example, Table 8-1

TABLE 8-1	Randomized Controlled Trial: Baseline Characteristics of Patients in the Prevention of Bone Loss[a]				
CHARACTERISTIC	PLACEBO (n = 93)	HRT (n = 93)	ALN (n = 93)	HRT + ALN (n = 94)	p VALUE[b]
Age (years)	72 (5)	71 (5)	71 (4)	72 (6)	.24
Height (cm)	159 (7)	158 (5)	159 (6)	158 (6)	.38
Weight (kg)	69 (18)	69 (12)	71 (17)	70 (15)	.84
BMI (kg/m^2)	27 (6)	28 (5)	28 (7)	27 (5)	.83
Dietary calcium (mg/day)	969 (456)	859 (416)	856 (421)	877 (452)	.31
Dietary vitamin D (IU/day)	258 (193)	234 (180)	264 (320)	252 (201)	.82
Number of medications	3 (2)	3 (2)	3 (2)	3 (2)	.61
Number of participants (%)					
Taking NSAIDs or aspirin	29 (31)	34 (37)	31 (33)	26 (28)	.62
Hysterectomy	31 (33)	33 (35)	33 (35)	33 (35)	.99
Currently smoking	5 (5)	7 (8)	7 (8)	7 (7)	.92
Currently drinking alcohol[c]	34 (37)	35 (38)	39 (42)	32 (34)	.73
Adult fracture[d]	31 (33)	35 (38)	36 (39)	44 (47)	.29
IADL score (9–27)	26.9 (0.5)	26.9 (0.5)	26.8 (0.8)	26.9 (0.6)	.40
FMMS score (0–30)	28.9 (1.7)	29.3 (1.0)	28.9 (2.4)	29.3 (0.9)	.24
Serum calcium (mg/dL)[e]	9.1 (0.4)	9.1 (0.4)	9.1 (0.4)	9.1 (0.3)	.56
Serum albumin (g/dL)[e]	4.4 (0.3)	4.4 (0.3)	4.4 (0.3)	4.5 (0.3)	.64
Serum PTH (pg/mL)[e]	37.9 (16.1)	39.5 (19.4)	36.1 (15.8)	36.6 (14.9)	.56
Serum 25-hydroxyvitamin D (ng/mL)[e]	17.9 (7.2)	18.2 (8.2)	17.1 (9.0)	19.4 (9.3)	.54
Serum hematocrit (%)	39.5 (2.8)	39.7 (2.7)	39.9 (3.0)	40.4 (2.8)	.13
Bone mineral density, mean (SD)					
Total hip (g/cm^2)	0.787 (0.125)	0.805 (0.112)	0.786 (0.138)	0.787 (0.118)	78
Total hip T-score[f]	−1.3 (1.0)	−1.1 (0.9)	−1.3 (1.1)	−1.3 (1.0)	.78
Femoral neck (g/cm^2)	0.655 (0.102)	0.663 (0.098)	0.658 (0.103)	0.650 (0.094)	.96
Femoral neck T-score[f]	−1.7 (0.9)	−1.7 (0.9)	−1.7 (0.9)	−1.8 (0.8)	.96
Posteroanterior lumbar spine (g/cm^2)	0.889 (0.166)	0.901 (0.184)	0.888 (0.178)	0.882 (0.137)	.98

(continued)

TABLE 8-1	Randomized Controlled Trial: Baseline Characteristics of Patients in the Prevention of Bone Loss[a], cont.				
Posteroanterior lumbar spine T-score[f]	−1.4 (1.5)	−1.3 (1.7)	−1.4 (1.6)	−1.5 (1.2)	.98
Lateral lumbar spine (g/cm²)	0.639 (0.131)	0.644 (0.129)	0.645 (0.115)	0.612 (0.102)	.29
Lateral lumbar spine T-score[f]	−2.2 (1.6)	−2.1 (1.5)	−2.1 (1.4)	−2.5 (1.2)	.29

[a]Values expressed as mean (standard deviation), unless otherwise noted.

[b]Overall comparison across groups.

[c]At least 1 drink per week

[d]Fracture after age 50 years

[e]SI conversion factors: to convert serum calcium mg/L to mmol/L, multiply by 0.25; serum albumin from g/dL to g/L multiply by 10; serum PTH from pg/L to mg/L, multiply by 1.0; to convert serum 25-hydroxyvitamin D from ng/mL to nmol/L, multiply by 2.496.

[f]T-score is the standard deviations below young adult peak bone mass.

ALN, alendronate; BMI, body mass index; FMMS, Folstein Mini-Mental Status; HRT, hormone-replacement therapy; IADL, instrumental activities of daily living; NSAID, nonsteroidal anti-inflammatory drugs; PTH, parathyroid hormone.

Adapted with permission from Greenspan SL, Resnick NM, Parker RA, Combination therapy with hormone replacement and alendronate for prevention of bone loss in elderly women. A randomized controlled trial. JAMA 2003;289:2525–2533.

displays baseline demographic and clinical data for patients in a study of antiresorptive therapy on bone loss in elderly women. The four treatments consisted of placebo, hormone-replacement therapy (HRT) as conjugated equine estrogen 0.625 mg/day with or without medroxyprogesterone 2.5 mg/day, alendronate (ALN) 10 mg daily, and the combination of HRT and ALN. Data are presented as means and standard deviations.

The comparability of the baseline values among the groups is striking. The far right column of the table lists the p values for the overall comparison between treatment groups. Each p value is > 0.05, indicating that no statistically significant differences appear to exist between the groups. Notice particularly the comparability of variable values that were not restricted in the patient selection process, like serum hematocrit and baseline bone mineral density. Randomization helps ensure that the values of all variables, both those to be measured by the investigator and those not assessed as part of the experiment, are comparable among the study groups. The result is a study design that maximizes the initial similarities between study groups.

The goal of this chapter is to provide guidelines for evaluating evidence presented in RCTs. Included is an examination of clinical trial experimental designs and methods used to acquire, analyze, and report healthcare information.

Types of Randomized Controlled Clinical Trials

The basic experimental designs for a randomized controlled clinical trial are presented in Figures 3-4 and 3-6. These designs include at least one treatment group and one comparison group. In a *placebo controlled trial*, the comparison group receives an intervention identical to the treatment except for the active ingredient. In an *active controlled trial*, the placebo treatment is replaced by another treatment. Typically, the active control treatment is a standard intervention. The goal of both study designs is to gauge the efficacy and safety of the new treatment.

PLACEBO CONTROLLED TRIALS

In placebo controlled trials, the placebo control group is used to index changes in dependent outcome variables owing to factors other than the treatment. These may include patient expectations regarding the efficacy or side effects of the treatment or may reflect changes in the dependent variable that occur naturally over time. A **placebo effect** is a change in the dependent outcome variable attributable to factors other than those associated with the treatment.

An effect similar to the placebo effect is the **Hawthorne effect**, a tendency of study subjects to increase performance simply because they have been chosen to participate in a study. This phenomenon was discovered in a series of investigations conducted at a Western Electric plant in Cicero, Illinois, that was intended to delineate environmental and psychological factors affecting productivity. The researchers discovered, however, that almost any change in environment (e.g., raising or lowering workshop illumination) increased productivity. They concluded that the workers were increasing productivity because they had been singled out and were being treated differently.

However, there are some examples of using the Hawthorne effect to increase compliance. For example, a sample of orthodontic patients with a history of poor oral hygiene was assigned to an experimental or a control group. The experimental group members were treated as if they were in an experiment, signing a consent form and being instructed in the use of an "experimental" toothpaste formulated specifically for orthodontic patients.[2] A control group received usual care. After 3 and 6 months, the oral hygiene measures had not changed for the control group but had improved significantly in the experimental group. Since the experimental toothpaste was actually one of several commercially available products, this change in oral hygiene habits was attributed to a Hawthorne effect—the patients were practicing improved oral hygiene because they were being studied.

ACTIVE CONTROLLED TRIALS

Increasingly, research designs are appearing in the literature that compare two active agents in terms of efficacy and safety without the benefit of a placebo control group. One reason for the emergence of this design is the desire of pharmaceutical companies to demonstrate that their product is equivalent to, not inferior to, or superior to, another product, often the currently accepted, standard therapy. A second reason for the **active controlled trial** design is that a placebo control group may be unethical. This is often the case for an established disease when there is an accepted therapy in place. It makes sense, then from a practical and an ethical standpoint, to compare two active agents.

As noted earlier, there are three basic applications of the active controlled trial design. One is the demonstration that two agents are *equivalent* or similar in efficacy and/or safety. In some cases, it may be sufficient to demonstrate that one agent is no worse than, or *noninferior* to, another drug. Finally, a *superiority trial* is used to test whether one agent is better than another in terms of efficacy and/or safety.

Equivalence Trials

The purpose of an **equivalence trial** is to establish the *absence* of a meaningful difference in the efficacy or safety of a standard treatment (T_S) and an alternative treatment (T_A). This seems to demand a proof of no difference, which conflicts with the dictum "Absence of proof does not constitute proof of absence." However, the method of hypothesis testing makes this possible. Here's how. First, assume that all possible differences between T_S and T_A are normally distributed with a mean of 0. Within this distribution, there is a range of differences between the treatments that is so small as to be meaningless, which is

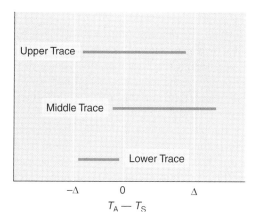

FIGURE 8-1   Evidence for the Equivalence of Treatment A (T_A) with Respect to Treatment S (T_S). The criteria for equivalence are (1) the 95% CI (*horizontal line*) of the difference between the means lies between the lower ($-\Delta$) and the upper ($+\Delta$) equivalence limits and (2) the 95% CI includes 0, as indicated by the *Upper Trace*. If the 95% CI extends beyond the lower or the upper equivalence limits, the criteria for equivalence are not met, as in the *Middle Trace*. If the 95% CI does not include 0, as in the *Lower Trace*, the criteria for equivalence are not met because the analysis indicates the superiority of one treatment over the other. The abscissa displays the mean difference between T_A and T_S.

indicated by an interval from a minimum difference of $-\Delta$ to a maximum difference of $+\Delta$. Note that the values of Δ do not have to be the same. The H_0 is that the two treatment means differ, which is assessed by the 95% confidence interval (CI) of the difference between T_S and T_A. Specifically, evidence favoring the H_0 is indicated if the 95% CI of $(T_S - T_A)$ includes either $-\Delta$ or $+\Delta$. To reject H_0 the entire 95% CI of $(T_S - T_A)$ must be located entirely within the $-\Delta$ to $+\Delta$ interval *and* must include the null value, 0.

The decision process used in equivalence trials is given in Figure 8-1. The abscissa consists of all possible differences between the mean T_S and the mean T_A. These mean differences are normally distributed, with an average value of 0. The abscissa also contains limits of the difference between the means that are clinically important (i.e., $-\Delta$ and $+\Delta$). The Upper Trace represents a 95% CI that includes 0 and is contained within the $-\Delta$ to $+\Delta$ interval, demonstrating equivalence. The Middle Trace, in which the 95% CI extends beyond the $+\Delta$ margin, does not permit rejection of the H_0. In the Lower Trace, the 95% CI is located within the $-\Delta$ to $+\Delta$ margin but does not include 0 and does not permit the inference of equivalence. Note: If the mean difference were expressed as a ratio, such as an odds ratio (OR) or relative risk (RR), the criteria for equivalence would be that the 95% CI be located entirely within the $-\Delta$ to $+\Delta$ interval, and include 1.

An example of an equivalence trial is provided by a study in which head louse infestation was treated with either two applications 7 days apart of a 4% dimeticone solution applied for 8 hr or overnight, or of a 0.5% *d*-phenothrin liquid used for 12 hr or overnight.[3] The study "was structured to detect equivalence to within 20% between treatment groups on the basis of 95% confidence limits."[3] This interval is displayed in Figure 8-2, along with the results of the per-protocol analysis. Positive outcomes were observed in 69% of the children treated with dimeticone and 78% of the children treated with phenothrin. Thus the point estimate for the differences in efficacy was -9%. The 95% CI of the difference extended from -19% to $+3\%$, suggesting equivalence.

Equivalence trials are often used by pharmaceutical companies to examine the bioactivity of two agents, generally a standard agent and a new, perhaps generic competitor. In these cases, a 90% CI is considered appropriate for most comparisons. Does this CI increase or decrease the probability of rejecting the H_0?

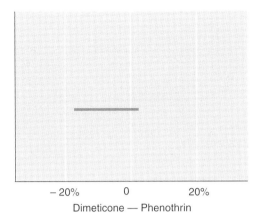

- 20%   0   20%
Dimeticone — Phenothrin

FIGURE 8-2 Evidence for the Equivalence of Dimeticone with respect to Phenothrin. Equivalence margins were set so differences in the efficacy of the two treatments could not exceed ± 20%. The difference in efficacy was 8%, favoring phenothrin, with a 95% CI from −19% to +3%. Because the 95% CI did not include either equivalence margin but did include 0, the two drugs were considered equivalent.

One factor that is critical to the outcome of the hypothesis test for equivalence trials is the setting of $-\Delta$ and $+\Delta$. These margins should be derived from *clinically significant criteria* with respect to patient outcomes. Similarly, departures from these margins should be accompanied by a difference in the manner in which the patient is treated. Unfortunately, the clinical bases of the equivalence limits used in the head lice study were not stated in the research paper.

Another issue is the sample population analysis used to evaluate equivalence trials. There is some evidence that intention-to-treat analyses may be biased when applied to superiority and equivalence trials. Furthermore, in contrast to placebo controlled trials, the vector of the bias may increase or decrease the probability of the H_0 being rejected. To remedy this, these trials should be assessed using per-protocol analysis of sample populations.[4]

A basic assumption in equivalence trials is that both agents are efficacious with respect to a placebo control group. However, this cannot be tested directly because a placebo control group is not included in the trial design. In some cases, it may be possible to compare data indirectly using a historical placebo control group. However, the validity of this comparison assumes that *all other factors*, including advancements in treatment and pharmacy practice, have not changed meaningfully during the interval between the two data collection periods. Such is rarely the case, and the use of historical control groups is discouraged.

Finally, if two treatments are equivalent, how is one to choose between them? According to some experts, the basis for selection should be addressed explicitly and directly in the equivalence trial.[5] In the report on head lice, in addition to the major finding of equivalence in efficacy, it was also reported that significantly fewer side effects were reported from subjects using demeticone than from those using phenothrin. This difference in safety, then, provides the rationale for the choice between the two treatments.

Noninferiority Trials

Noninferiority trials seek to establish that one treatment (e.g., a novel intervention) is no worse than another (e.g., the current standard of care). As such, they represent a kind of equivalence trial in which only a $-\Delta$ value, termed a *noninferiority margin*, is considered.

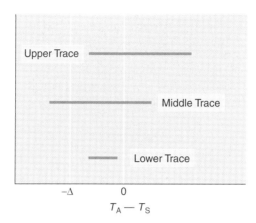

FIGURE 8-3 Evidence for the Noninferiority of Treatment A (T_A) with Respect to Treatment S (T_S). The criteria for non-inferiority are (1) the 95% CI (*horizontal line*) of the difference between the means lies above the noninferiority margin $(-\Delta)$ and (2) the 95% CI includes 0, as indicated by the *Upper Trace*. If the 95% CI includes the noninferiority margin, the criteria for noninferiority are not met, as shown by the *Middle Trace*. If the 95% CI does not include 0, the criteria for noninferiority are not met, as shown by the *Lower Trace*.

In such an analysis, two treatments are noninferior if the 95% CI of their difference does not include the noninferiority margin $(-\Delta)$ but does include the null value (0).[6] When differences between the treatments are expressed as ratios, such as OR, the criteria for noninferiority are that the 95% CI not include $-\Delta$ but include the null value, 1.

The statistical decision process for a noninferiority trial is presented in Figure 8-3. The figure provides the probability distributions of the differences between all possible standard treatment means (T_S) and alternative treatment means (T_A). The probability distribution is assumed to be normally distributed with a mean of 0. The H_0 is that T_A is inferior to T_S and is indicated by a 95% CI of $(T_A - T_S)$ that includes $-\Delta$, the noninferiority margin. If the 95% CI lies to the right of $-\Delta$ and includes 0, the H_0 is rejected and the conclusion is reached that the two treatments are noninferior, as indicated by the Upper Trace. In the Middle Trace, the 95% CI includes the noninferiority margin; thus the H_0 is not rejected. In the Lower Trace, although the 95% CI does not include the noninferiority margin, it does not include 0 and thus does not permit rejection of H_0.

A noninferiority trial design was used by the Thrombin Inhibitor in Venous Thromboembolism (THRIVE) treatment study investigators to compare the efficacy and safety of ximelagatran against the standard treatments for the prevention of recurrent venous thrombosis: enoxaparin and warfarin.[7] The study was prompted by problems associated with the standard therapy, particularly the need to monitor drug dosages frequently. Patients were treated for 6 months with either ximelagatran 36 mg twice daily or subcutaneous enoxaparin 1 mg/kg twice daily for 5–20 days followed by warfarin in doses sufficient to maintain an international normalized ratio (INR) between 2.0 and 3.0. The prespecified primary end point was the incidence of recurrent thromboembolism; secondary end points assessed adverse events, notably bleeding. The protocol, including diagnosis and treatment, was conducted according to current standard clinical practices.

The noninferiority margin was set at -4%, which means that noninferiority would be demonstrated if the 95% CI for the difference between enoxaparin (T_S) and ximelagatran (T_A) did not include -4%. In other words, the incidence of thromboembolism in the ximelagatran group could be worse than the incidence in the enoxaparin group by no more than 4%.

TABLE 8-2	**Efficacy of Ximelagatran and Enoxaparin in Reducing Thromboembolic Events: Intention-to-Treat vs On-Treatment Populations**		
	NUMBER (%)[a]		
EVENT	XIMELAGATRAN (n = 1240)[b]	ENOXAPARIN/WARFARIN (n = 1249)[b]	DIFFERENCE (95% CI)[c]
Intention-to-treat population			
Total recurrent venous thromboembolism	26 (2.1)[d]	24 (2.0)[d]	0.2 (−1.0 to 1.3)
Deep vein thrombosis	15	17	
Pulmonary embolism	11	7	
On-treatment population			
Total recurrent venous thromboembolism	23 (2.0)[e]	17 (1.5)	0.5 (−0.6 to 1.6)
Deep vein thrombosis	14[e]	12	
Pulmonary embolism	9	5	

[a]Number of patients in each group with a recurrence (estimated cumulative risk)

[b]Same number of patients for both types of analysis; censoring of data in the on-treatment analysis as described in the original paper.

[c]Observed difference and corresponding 95% CI for ximelagatran – enoxaparin/warfarin; predefined noninferiority margin set at 4%

[d]Numbers indicate centrally adjudicated events; locally confirmed venous thromboembolism events were reported in 43 and 42 patients in the ximelagatran and enoxaparin/warfarin groups, respectively

[e]One patient in the ximelagatran group with a recurrence of deep vein thrombosis erroneously received only placebo treatment.

CI, confidence interval.

Reprinted with permission from Fiessinger J, Hiusman MV, Davidson BL, et al. Ximelagatran vs low-molecular-weight heparin and warfarin for the treatment of deep vein thrombosis. A randomized trial. JAMA 2005;293:681–689.

Results from the primary outcome of the study are shown in Table 8-2. For the on-treatment (i.e., per-protocol) analysis of the sample population, the ximelagatran group experienced 23 events and the enoxaparin/warfarin group experienced 17 events during the 6-month study period. The resulting 95% CI ranged from −0.6% to 1.6%. Because the 95% CI interval did not include −4%, noninferiority was demonstrated.

Given that the two treatments are comparably efficacious, a decision between the two would be based on another criterion, such as safety, cost, or ease of administration. The evaluation of safety in the THRIVE study included a census of the number of patients with above-normal levels of alanine aminotransferase. This liver enzyme level was 9.6% in the ximelagatran group and 2.0% in the enoxaparin/warfarin group. Enzyme levels were reported to return to normal with continued treatment with ximelagatran. Furthermore, in a post hoc analysis, there were more serious coronary events in patients assigned to the ximelagatran group.

The investigators concluded that although the efficacy of ximelagatran seemed adequate, the potential damage owing to the side effects warranted further investigation. Indeed, additional concerns regarding the hepatic effects of ximelagatran emerged, leading to rejection of its new drug application by the U.S. Food and Drug Administration (FDA) and the subsequent withdrawal of ximelagatran from the world market.[8,9]

A problem involving noninferiority trials arises because the experimental design does not include a placebo control group. Therefore, there is no benchmark against which to judge the absolute treatment effect of a new, noninferior treatment. For example, imagine that the efficacy of a standard treatment has been established in a placebo controlled trial. A subsequent study demonstrates that a novel treatment is noninferior to the standard treatment, although the mean difference between the treatments favors the standard treatment A. This demonstration of noninferiority, however, does not indicate whether the novel treatment is better than the original placebo condition. Indeed, based on this evidence, an investigator may conclude that the novel treatment is not worse than a standard treatment, when in fact the novel treatment may be no better than placebo. The erosion of the magnitude of the original treatment versus placebo effect through noninferiority trials is termed **biocreep**.[10]

Superiority Trials

The goal of a **superiority trial** is to examine whether the efficacy or safety of one treatment (e.g., T_A) is better than a standard treatment (i.e., T_S). For illustration purposes, assume that the superiority of T_A compared to T_S is measured with respect to their mean difference. The H_0 for the comparison is that the difference between the two means is zero. (If the difference between the means were expressed as a ratio, the H_0 for the comparison would be that the ratio = 1.) Because of measurement error, chance, and other factors, however, it is likely that the difference between the two means will not be exactly zero. However, if it is assumed that the difference between the means is normally distributed with a mean of 0, then the criteria to reject H_0 could be defined in terms of the 95% CI of $(T_A - T_S)$. Specifically, the H_0 is rejected if the 95% CI for $(T_A - T_S)$ does not include 0. An additional requirement is that the difference between T_A and T_S is positive—that is, the mean of T_A is greater than that of T_S.

This approach is presented in Figure 8-4. Treatment mean differences are arranged on the abscissa along a continuum, with 0 (or the point of no difference) at the center. Mean differences are expressed as $(T_A - T_S)$. Two 95% CIs are indicated for $(T_A - T_S)$. For the Upper Trace, the 95% CI for $(T_A - T_S)$ meets both criteria for superiority: The 95% CI does not include 0, and the difference between $(T_A - T_S)$ favors T_A. For the Lower Trace, the 95% CI does include 0; therefore, the H_0 cannot be rejected.

Note that failure to reject H_0 does not justify the conclusion that T_S and T_A are equivalent or that one is inferior to the other. This is because failing to reject H_0 differs from accepting H_0. In a sense, failure to reject H_0 can be interpreted as having insufficient evidence to reject H_0.

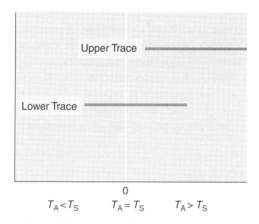

FIGURE 8-4   Evidence for the Superiority of Treatment A (T_A) with Respect to Treatment S (T_S). The criteria for the superiority of T_A are (1) the 95% CI (*horizontal line*) of the difference between the means does not include 0 and (2) the mean value of T_A exceeds that for T_S, as indicated in the *Upper Trace*. If the 95% CI includes 0 or if the mean value of T_A is less than that for T_S, the criteria for superiority are not met, as shown by the *Lower Trace*.

Superiority analyses are commonly used after the failure to demonstrate noninferiority. Such a method was to test the efficacy of the use of hypericum extract St. John's wort 900 mg/day three times per day or paroxetine 20 mg once per day in ameliorating symptoms of moderate and severe depression as indicated by Hamilton depression scores.[11] After 6 weeks of treatment, the depression scores in the St. John's wort group decreased by 57% compared to 34% in the standard treatment group. The 95% CI for the average group difference in Hamilton depression scores displayed a lower limit of 1.5. Because this value is > 0, the findings indicate the superiority of St. John's wort compared to the standard treatment. Supporting evidence was derived from scores on the Montgomery-Asberg Depression Rating Scale (MADRS), which evidenced a difference in average values of 3.3 and a 95% CI from 1.1 to 6.5, with the advantage for St. John's wort.

Sometimes investigators switch between active controlled trial study designs. For example, imagine a study in which the investigators, failing to find evidence of superiority, reexamined the data using a noninferiority analysis. Is that appropriate? To answer this question, consider that the results of a noninferiority analysis depend critically on the noninferiority margin, $-\Delta$. Recall that the margin must be *prespecified* and must be meaningful clinically.[12]

Switching from a superiority trial design to a noninferior trial design is appropriate, therefore, only if the noninferiority margin has been established *before* the superiority trial analysis takes place. Such a regimen was followed in the Valsartan in Acute Myocardial Infarction (VALIANT) trial comparing the angiotensin-converting enzyme (ACE) inhibitor captopril (goal dose of 25 mg three times a day) to the angiotensin receptor blocker valsartan (goal dose of 80 mg two times a day) in patients at high risk for recurrent cardiovascular events.[13] "If valsartan did not prove to be superior to captopril, the noninferiority of valsartan with respect to captopril was to be assessed. . . . The threshold considered to indicate noninferiority . . . was prespecified."[13]

The opposite transition, from a noninferiority to a superiority trial, presents no such problems, because the criteria for rejecting the H_0 using a superiority design are not established by the investigator; one criterion is the H_0 is rejected if the 95% CI includes 0. Such an approach is exemplified by a report from the Pravastatin or Atorvastatin Evaluation and Infection Therapy—Thrombolysis in Myocardial Infarction 22 (PROVE IT–TIMI 22) researchers, who compared intensive lipid lowering with atorvastatin 80 mg/day to moderate lipid lowering with pravastatin 20 mg/day on the recurrence of acute coronary events.[14] The median low-density lipoprotein (LDL) levels during the study were ~ 100 mg/dL with pravastatin and ~ 60 mg/dL with atorvastatin. Associated with these differences was a 16% reduction in incidence of the primary end point in the atorvastatin group. The 95% CI for the difference in risk between the two treatments (95% CI = 5–26%) met the criteria for concluding that atorvastatin 80 mg was superior to pravastatin 20 mg in preventing the primary outcome. The difference in efficacy was attributed to the extent of lipid lowering.

Active controlled trials are valuable study designs for comparing the efficacy and safety of similar treatments or when ethical considerations preclude the inclusion of a placebo control group. However, care must be taken in applying these study designs to healthcare data and in interpreting the results of these investigations.

Methodological Considerations

As indicated in Chapter 5, a *research* hypothesis is a statement about the way nature works. A *statistical* hypothesis is a statement that provides evidence regarding the veracity of a research hypothesis. An experiment is a controlled test of the statistical hypothesis. In this section, several important aspects of such experimental control are considered: patient selection, assignment of patients to experimental conditions, attrition and adherence, and statistical analysis. Although these topics are discussed within the context of a RCT, they also apply to observational studies.

PATIENT SELECTION

Critical steps in planning an RCT are defining the study population and then selecting a portion or sample of this population for the study. For example, an investigator may wish to probe the efficacy and safety of a drug combination on reducing decreases in bone mineral density (BMD) in elderly women. However, the drugs cannot be tested in all elderly women because patients may refuse to volunteer, be undiagnosed, or be unavailable for study for reasons unrelated to either the condition or the treatments. Still other patients may already be treated with the study drugs or with drugs that modify BMD as a side effect. Selection of the study population, therefore, entails both the recruitment and the screening of those who volunteer.

Volunteers are recruited using a variety of formats. In many studies, patients are recruited when first diagnosed in clinics, hospitals, and other healthcare venues. This may occur at one center or at many centers located in different countries. Patients may be identified from medical records and be recruited via telephone. Other recruitment tactics include advertisements in doctors' offices, newspapers, and magazines as well as via radio and television commercials.

Some investigators offer compensation for participating in the study. This may raise concerns that the investigators attract subjects who are more strongly motivated than patients in the general population. For example, such patients may be more apt to exhibit positive effects on self-reported variables in order to perform well and receive payment. These concerns can indicate selection bias in the study.

Not all volunteers are admitted into the experiment, however, because potential participants are screened using inclusion and exclusion criteria. **Inclusion criteria** are a set of characteristics desired in a study subject, and **exclusion criteria** are used to disqualify patients with nuisance or confounding characteristics. Inclusion criteria describe the population the study sample represents and specifically identify patient subsets to which study results may be extrapolated. Exclusion criteria help ensure the study sample is as homogenous as possible, specifically identify patient subsets to which study results should not be extrapolated, and ensure patient safety by excluding individuals for whom some aspect of the study would be dangerous or contraindicated.

Inclusion and exclusion criteria should be defined precisely, providing explicit detail so the reader can appreciate the subject attributes. For example, it is not sufficient to list an inclusion criterion such as this: "Patients were included in the study if they had hypertension." The investigator should define hypertension; in the example, was it defined as a blood pressure > 140/90 mmHg (the diagnostic level for the general population) or > 130/80 mmHg (the diagnostic blood pressure level for diabetic patients)? Other specifications for inclusion and exclusion criteria might include the following: (1) are the patients newly diagnosed, (2) have standard diagnostic methods and criteria been used, and (3) have the patients been exposed to any other treatments or procedures that might affect the current treatment–outcome association?

These considerations can be illustrated by a report of bone loss prevention in elderly women using antiresorptive therapy.[15] The researchers stated the following (ideal) research hypothesis: "our study was designed to examine the efficacy and safety of combination therapy with hormone replacement and alendronate, compared with each agent alone."[15] in preventing bone loss in community-dwelling elderly women.

The trial profile for this study is presented in Figure 8-5. Of 573 women eligible for participation in the study, 25 were excluded for medical reasons. These included

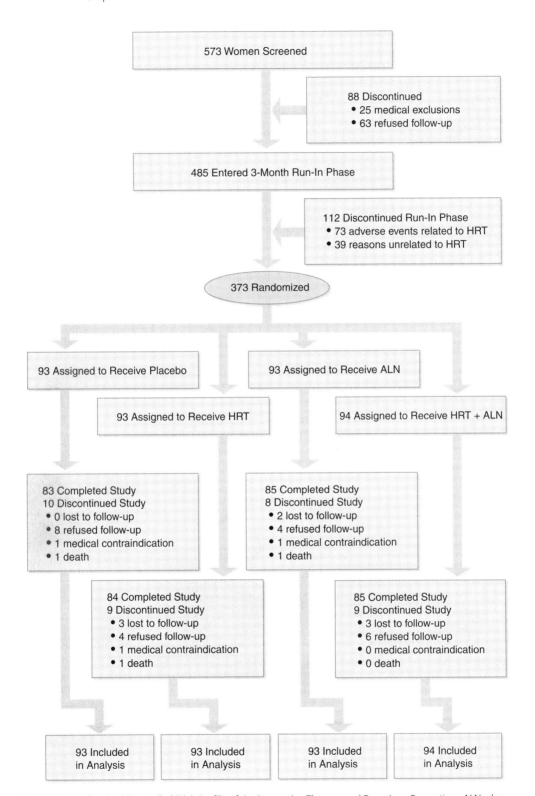

FIGURE 8-5   Randomized Controlled Trial: Profile of Antiresorptive Therapy and Bone Loss Prevention. *ALN*, alendronate; *HRT*, hormone-replacement therapy. Adapted with permission from Greenspan SL, Resnick NM, Parker RA, Combination therapy with hormone replacement and alendronate for prevention of bone loss in elderly women. A randomized controlled trial. JAMA 2003;289:2525–2533.

concomitant conditions known to affect BMD, use of drugs that affected BMD, or treatment with anti-osteoporosis medications within a year of screening. A total of 63 other potential participants refused to comply with the study protocol and were disqualified.

Those who passed muster were then enrolled in a run-in phase. This is a period in which those who will comply with the medication protocol are winnowed from those who will not. The strategy is used to increase the number of patients who comply with the study protocol by eliminating those who will be noncompliant before the study begins. A total of 112 subjects were eliminated during the run-in phase, leaving 373 to be assigned to the four study groups.

In summary, the recruitment and selection of study subjects are critical parts of the RCT. Although these steps help define a study group in which the treatment–outcome association can be assessed accurately, they also limit the external validity the results enjoy. For example, although the run-in phase of the BMD trial ensured that only women who complied with the drug regimen would be included in the study (and therefore enhance the chances of finding a positive result), it also restricted the findings of the study to that population. Thus, careful determination and assessment of inclusion and exclusion criteria are an essential part of any study evaluation. The next challenge is assigning patients to study groups in an objective manner.

ASSIGNMENT OF PARTICIPANTS TO STUDY GROUPS

After determining the subjects eligible to participate in the study, researchers must assign participants to treatment and control groups in a manner that is free from bias. Three strategies are used to achieve this goal. The first is the random assignment of participants to treatment and control groups. The second, **concealed allocation**, means that the group to which the individual is assigned is not disclosed until after a patient is selected for inclusion in the study. Third, **blinding** refers to the fact that a person is unaware of a patient's group assignment. Each of these strategies are discussed in the following paragraphs.

Although there are many different randomization protocols, several general formats are used commonly. The first is **simple random assignment**. Simple random assignment uses the outcome of a random event to determine the allocation of patients to experimental or control groups. Recall that a random event is an event whose outcome cannot be determined until the event occurs. Usually, the random event is obtained from a table of random numbers found in a biostatistics text or generated by a computer.

Here's how assignment of patients to conditions works using simple random assignment. Assume that the investigator has assembled a pool of eligible patients for a study and has ordered them in some sequence. Perhaps the investigator places all patient codes in a hat and then selects one name at a time. The result is a list of patients whose selection sequence was determined by a random process.

The next step is to assign each patient to one of two study groups using a table of random numbers. Table 8-3 contains a set of random numbers between 1 and 50. The general strategy is to associate each patient with a random number. The random numbers are coded before the study so that even numbers signify assignment to the placebo group and odd numbers signify assignment to the treatment group. The investigator begins by placing a finger (eyes closed) on the random number table, and reading the number above the finger. Say this process identifies number 9 in the second column. Because this is an odd number, the first patient drawn from the hat would be assigned to the treatment condition. The second person is assigned according to the next number in the random number table. For example, if the investigator had decided beforehand to proceed down the column, the next number 46, being an even number would assign the

TABLE 8-3	Table of Random Numbers between 1 and 50.	
16	33	38
32	30	35
42	18	29
29	8	50
37	10	8
20	44	8
21	9	31
20	46	1
46	18	49
3	33	31
44	47	34
12	10	38
18	9	28
6	17	39
40	15	11
9	38	7
10	19	44
8	26	5

second patient to the control group. This process continues until all subject placements are complete.

The simple random assignment protocol is given in Figure 8-6A, in which a population of individuals eligible for the study has been assigned to a treatment or a placebo condition. Note that there are no restrictions on the assignment of participants to conditions. As a result, groups may not be balanced with respect to certain variables. In the figure, for example, the treatment and placebo groups are not balanced on the "smiling face/frowning face" variable—that is, the treatment group contains 9 smiling faces and 1 frowning face, whereas the placebo group is composed of 7 smiling faces and 3 frowning faces.

One advantage of the simple random assignment protocol is that it is simple to carry out. Furthermore, the use of a table of random numbers to allocate patients to conditions helps minimize selection bias. However, simple random assignment does have several drawbacks. The most serious of these is that simple random assignment relies on the laws of probability, which depend on large numbers of patients and thus may not provide a sufficient level of control of all important variables. A solution is to assign patients to groups using a restricted random assignment method.

One method of randomization used to control for the effects of a potentially confounding factor is to make sure that each group contains similar proportions of the different levels of the confounding variable. For example, if the investigators were concerned about the effects of dietary calcium on BMD, patients could be randomized so that each group contained similar proportions of patients with low, medium, and high in calcium intake.

This method of group assignment is termed **stratification** (Fig. 8.6B). In this group assignment protocol, assignment was random, with the restriction that the treatment and

Panel A

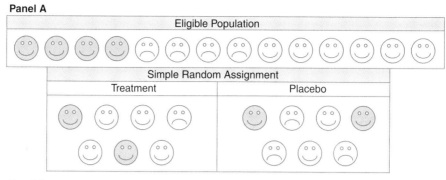

Panel B

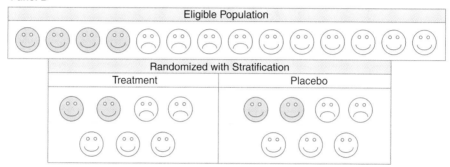

Panel C

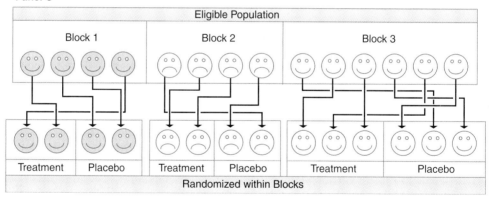

FIGURE 8-6   Methods of Assigning Eligible Participants to Specific Study Conditions. **A.** In a simple random assignment method, the group assignments are made without regard to other variables; thus the composition of groups may vary in one or more variables. In this example, the sampling method resulted in an imbalance of smiling and frowning faces in the two groups. **B.** The stratification method randomly assigns participants to conditions with the restriction that the variable of interest be represented in equal proportions in both study groups. Here, the sampling method resulted in an equal proportion of smiling and frowning faces in both groups. **C.** In the blocking method, participants are aggregated into groups, termed blocks, based on differences in a variable—for example, the clinic at which they receive treatment. Patients are then assigned to study groups within each block using a simple or stratified random assignment method. This method ensures that the blocking variable is equally represented in each study group.

placebo groups have the same proportion of dark/smiling faces, light/frowning faces, and light/smiling faces.

By stratifying groups based on different levels of a variable, changes in the dependent measure can be examined as a function of differences in the stratified variable. For example, because of the care taken to stratify women in the BMD study on the dietary calcium variable, changes in BMD as a function of differences in that variable can be assessed. Note also that the investigator could have decided to study patients at only one level of the calcium intake variable. This is in fact the strategy adopted in the BMD study: both calcium and vitamin D supplements were provided to all patients to ensure adequate levels of these variables. The patients were said to be matched on these variables.

Another randomization strategy is termed **block randomization**. This strategy is used commonly when the study is carried out at different clinical sites. To control for differences in treatment and other factors at the different sites, random assignment of patients is carried out at each individual site to make sure that the proportion of treatment and control patients is similar at each site.

The block randomization strategy is demonstrated in Figure 8-6C. The eligible population is composed of three blocks: dark/smiling faces, light/frowning faces, and light/smiling faces. Within each block, a random assignment is carried out. The final study groups have the same composition as the stratified groups.

Although clinical sites are commonly used as a blocking variable, virtually any variable can be used to form blocks. For example, the study of a novel treatment to prevent recurrence of breast cancer may entail first aggregating patients with similar treatment histories into blocks and then assigning the patients to intervention and nonintervention conditions.

Blocking is an important consideration in multisite clinical trials. First, blocking ensures that similar proportions of treatment and control patients are present in each of the blocks. Second, statistical analyses can be used to examine differences in the dependent variable as a function of the blocking variable. This would indicate whether the treatment effects occurred in some blocks but not others.

In summary, the random assignment of participants to study groups is important for two reasons: it is a condition that must be met to obtain valid results from many statistical tests and it helps ensure that investigator and patient bias do not influence the treatment assignment and, therefore, the study results. Successful randomization is achieved when every subject has an equal chance of receiving any available study intervention. Even when variables are stratified or blocked, the final assignment of participants is a random event. Randomly assigning patients to treatment groups tends to create groups that are comparable in key baseline or concurrent variables, especially when large sample sizes are involved.

In addition to randomization schemes, two other maneuvers are used to control bias. One of these is concealed allocation. This means that the investigator is not made aware of group assignments until after the patient selection process. If the investigator were aware, for example, that the next patient would be assigned to a placebo group, he or she might be tempted to selectively exclude a seriously ill patient.

Another tactic to make the assignment of patients to groups impartial is blinding—that is, concealing the treatment status of a patient throughout the trial. **Single-blind studies** are those in which the patient is unaware of treatment status. **Double-blind studies** are those in which neither the patient nor the investigator are aware of the treatment status of the patient. **Triple-blind studies** are those in which the patient, the investigator, and all other individuals associated with the study are unaware of the treatment group assignment. **Open-label studies**, in contrast, are those in which there is no attempt to conceal treatment status of the patient.

Sometimes, use of a **double-dummy technique** is needed to maintain blinding. This technique employs the use of two or more dummy treatments. For example, investigators wish to compare the effectiveness of inhaled albuterol to oral albuterol for asthma control. By virtue of the dosage form—inhaler versus pill—the patient and investigator would be aware of treatment group assignment. To negate this information, the investigator uses a dummy inhaler and a dummy pill, both of which contain a placebo. So subjects assigned to the albuterol inhaler group receive the drug-containing inhaler plus the dummy pill, and subjects assigned to the oral albuterol group receive the active albuterol tablet plus the dummy inhaler. This way, all patients are using both dosage forms and blinding is maintained.

The necessity of blinding is determined somewhat by the nature of the dependent variables. If the dependent variables are objective and easy to determine, like death, blinding is not as critical. If the dependent variable is based on clinical judgment or a self-reported measure such as a visual analog pain scale, blinding procedures become much more important to control placebo effects and observer bias.

The process of patient assignment in the RCT of bone loss prevention illustrates many of these points. In the following description, find evidence of these methods: blinding, concealed allocation, randomized allocation to groups with stratification, and blocking. According to the study protocol, once the patient agreed to participate, "the study coordinator entered the participant's data into a computer program and received a randomization number."[15] This number had been determined by a statistician and was used by the pharmacist to prepare drug regimens. "Use of this computer program ensured that participants were randomized only after procedures were completed and that participants were randomized in strict sequential order. . . . Randomization was stratified by prior history of hysterectomy and 3 levels of total hip BMD. . . . Within each strata, randomization was blocked using block sizes of 4, 8, or 12 (block size randomly determined) to reduce the chances that study staff could deduce the treatment assignment."[15]

OUTCOMES/DATA COLLECTION

Once subject selection and assignment to treatment groups have been addressed, the next consideration is an evaluation of the outcome variables. A critical feature of literature evaluation is an assessment of the appropriateness of the outcome variables.

As discussed in Chapter 3, the investigator designates a **primary outcome** and possibly one or more **secondary outcomes**. The best evidence is provided by outcomes that are objective, quantitative measurements that display validity, reliability, and sensitivity. Less desirable are self-reports, and not acceptable are outcomes based solely on the professional experience of the study investigators.

Measurement methods must be described in sufficient detail so that the study could be replicated by the reader. Methods of gathering, analyzing, and summarizing data should be standardized if more than one performance site is involved. Bioassays used should be described in detail or be referenced.

In addition, time points for obtaining measurements should be clinically relevant. For example, if testing the efficacy of a new antidiabetic medication in lowering hemoglobin A_{1c} (HbA1$_c$), at least 90 days should elapse between treatment onset and the first the HbA1$_c$ measurement. This interval is necessary to achieve complete total red blood cell turnover and thus provide a stable measure of the change in HbA1$_c$.

In some RCTs, a **composite outcome** is created by combining individual component outcomes. This is encountered commonly in studies with cardiovascular-dependent variables. For example, the composite outcome in the PROVE IT–TIMI 22 study included death from any cause, death from myocardial infarction, documented unstable angina requiring rehospitalization, revascularization (performed at least 30 days after randomization), and stroke.[13]

Component outcomes of the composite outcome should be related in some manner. In the PROVE IT–TIMI 22 study, the component outcomes were all frequent manifestations of cardiovascular disease. In contrast, grouping the occurrence of stroke and pneumonia with changes in bone mineral density does not make sense because these individual outcomes are not related clinically.

The evaluation of composite outcome should include an assessment of each of the component outcomes because the composite outcome has a greater probability of achieving statistical significance. In addition, although the composite outcome provides a big picture of the treatment effect, differences among individual components may have greater consequences for clinical decision making. For example, in the PROVE IT–TIMI 22 trial, although the composite outcome reached statistical significance, only the revascularization component of the composite outcome was statistically significant. Other component outcomes that might have been more salient clinically, such as all-cause mortality, did not attain statistical significance. Thus the clinical significance of the composite outcome is weakened.

ATTRITION AND ADHERENCE

Once the study is under way, the challenges are to prevent participants from dropping out and ensure that participants adhere to the protocol. A major task is to retain patients in the study, because patients who drop out alter the composition of the study groups, disrupting the balance afforded by the randomization process. One strategy used to lessen the effect of dropping out is to overstock the study groups at the beginning of the trial. In the antiresorptive treatment of bone density study, for example, the investigators assigned more patients to the groups than were needed for the analysis in anticipation of an 8% attrition rate annually. However, there is evidence that those who drop out of a study are different from those who do not drop out, questioning the effectiveness of this strategy.[16]

A related challenge is to maintain patients' adherence to the treatment regimens. Failure to adhere to the study protocol reduces the treatment effect, increasing the probability of a type II error. Lack of adherence includes not only discontinuation of the active treatment but also switching a patient from the placebo group to a treatment group or from one treatment group to another. Evidence of patient compliance is usually based on self-report or the number of unused treatments. Both of these measures depend on the veracity of the patient. Occasionally, investigators will measure blood levels of the drug, which supplies more objective evidence of compliance. However, this practice is more invasive for the patient and more expensive for the investigators.

In summary, a major challenge is to preserve the original composition of the study groups and to maintain adherence to the study protocol. Failure to do so diminishes the internal validity of the study.

DATA ANALYSIS

The overall goals of the study are to provide information regarding the efficacy and safety of the treatment. To attain these goals, data are analyzed to:

- Provide evidence that the groups were similar on baseline demographic, physiologic, and potentially confounding variables
- Provide statistics on attrition and adherence
- Describe changes in the primary outcome variable that relate to efficacy and safety
- Explain supporting evidence provided by the secondary outcome variables
- Carry out other preplanned analyses

For the data analysis to be convincing, two parameters need to be defined. One is the number of subjects needed in each study group to achieve a desired level of statistical power; the other is the designation of the type of statistical analysis to be carried out.

Statistical power is the probability that a predefined difference between the groups will be detected by a test of statistical significance. It is determined as the complement of β, the probability that a predefined group difference is not determined to be statistically significant. As described in Chapter 5, factors that affect β are the true difference between the group means (*d*), the standard deviations of the groups (*s*), the level of α, and the sample size (*n*). Two of these variables, the level of α and *n*, are under the control of the investigator. The level of α is typically set at a maximum level of 0.05, so the major control of power is exercised by setting sample size. The values of the other variables are obtained from preliminary studies or from previously published work.

Equations to calculate sample size per group are available from statistics textbooks. These functions indicate that the number of subjects per group increases with the size of the standard deviations and decreases as the true difference between the groups increases, the level of α decreases, or the level of β is reduced (and thus power increased).

The number of subjects needed, as indicated by these calculations, is really an estimate of the *optimal* number of subjects required to detect a statistically significant effect. Studying fewer patients than indicated increases the probability of a type II error—a real difference may not be detected. Using too many patients may result in the statistical significance of a difference that is trivial clinically. In addition, an excess of study patients is a waste of time, money, and effort.

One factor affecting the availability of study subjects is the prevalence of the disease. Although it is generally true that larger sample sizes provide more accurate population estimates and thus are preferred when extrapolating the study findings to clinical practice, rarer diseases necessarily provide a smaller patient pool. Thus, for example, although it may be very reasonable to find 10,000 patients to study a novel antidiabetic medication, enrolling a similar number of patients suffering from a rare form of brain cancer might be out of the question.

So what does statistical power mean? For example, the investigators in the antiresorptive bone density study "specified that the study needed to randomize 92 participants to each treatment group (total 368 patients) to provide 80% power to detect a difference of 3% . . . between each treatment group and the placebo group, with α = 0.05 [2-sided]."[15] This suggests that, in 8 out of 10 studies, a real difference of at least 3% between a treatment group and the placebo group will be detected if 92 participants populate each of the four groups and the primary outcome is the dependent variable.

A second aspect of the data analysis is whether the statistical analysis is to be based on an intention-to-treat (ITT) or on a per-protocol regimen (see Chapter 5). The ITT protocol is once randomized, always analyzed. In other words, data for every subject assigned to a treatment group are retained for data analysis. Because it is based on data from compliers, noncompliers, and drop outs, the ITT analysis is thought to reflect more accurately a typical outcome in the target population. The per-protocol or on-treatment method, in contrast, includes only those who do not drop out of the study. Thus it likely reflects the best-case outcome. The data analysis for the antiresorptive bone density study was an ITT analysis.

In the antiresorptive bone density study, statistical comparison of baseline characteristics involved a number of different tests, depending on the scale of the dependent measure. For example, tests of between group differences involving frequency variables were calculated using χ^2 and Fisher exact tests. Rank data were analyzed with Kruskal-Wallis analysis of variance by ranks and the Wilcoxon rank-sums test. Differences among groups were characterized using analysis of variance (ANOVA). These statistical tests were described in previous chapters.

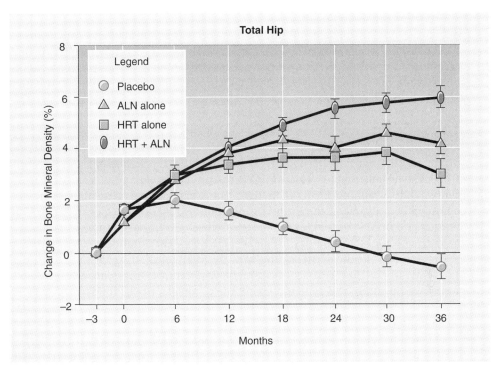

FIGURE 8-7   Changes in Total Hip Bone Mineral Density over 36 months of Treatment. *ALN,* alendronate; *HRT,* hormone-replacement therapy. Adapted with permission from Greenspan SL, Resnick NM, Parker RA, Combination therapy with hormone replacement and alendronate for prevention of bone loss in elderly women. A randomized controlled trial. JAMA 2003;289:2525–2533.

Examination of baseline data indicates that the four groups displayed similar levels of all variables (Table 8-1). Notice that all four groups also met the criterion of the power calculation—a minimum of 92 per group. In addition, "Compliance and retention were similar in all groups. Fifty-one percent (48/94) of participants were adherent, which was defined as taking 80% of both medications during the study. . . . Retention was 90% (337/373) for all participants after 3 years."[15]

The efficacy of the combined treatment versus the individual treatments for the total hip is given in Figure 8-7. Changes were similar for most sites at which BMD was measured: BMD remained fairly stable in the placebo group and increased in the two single treatment conditions. An enhanced increase in BMD, however, was found with combined HRT and ALN therapy. The difference between the combined therapy and the single therapies was statistically significant at the 36-month measurement period. Further analyses indicated that "the changes in BMD were not consistently related to baseline BMD, age, BMI, dietary calcium or vitamin D, or baseline serum vitamin D. The changes in BMD were related to adherence."[15]

The incidence of adverse events was predictable: "Women receiving hormone replacement (with or without alendronate) had the expected increased incidence of menstrual spotting, cramps, and breast tenderness when compared to the 2 groups of women not receiving hormone replacement. . . . The number of hospitalizations, falls, and clinical fractures was similar in all four groups."[15]

The authors conclude that, for many elderly women who can tolerate HRT therapy, the rewards of combined HRT and ALN therapy in terms of increasing BMD outweigh the risk of adverse events attributable to HRT.

Evaluation of the four methodological areas that have been examined in this section— patient selection, assignment to groups, attrition and adherence, and data analysis—are essential for the proper critical assessment of a RCT. Patient selection relates principally to the external validity of the study, whereas group assignment and attrition and adherence contribute to internal validity. Data analysis provides information germane to both internal and external validity.

SURVIVAL ANALYSES

In many studies of drug effects, interest is in studying the *pattern of change* over time in the dependent outcome, comparing patterns of change among placebo and treatment groups, and examining changes in time-based patterns as a function of preexisting conditions. For example, the Fifth Organization to Assess Strategies in Acute Ischemic Syndromes (OASIS-5) trial examined the efficacy of fondaparinux 2.5 mg/day and enoxaparin 1 mg/kg twice a day for an average treatment duration of 6 days in reducing the number of ischemic events, along with the safety of these agents in reducing bleeding events, in patients with acute coronary syndrome at 9 days after diagnosis.[17] The purpose of the study was to demonstrate the noninferiority of fondaparinux to enoxaparin with respect to efficacy and the superiority of fondaparinux to enoxaparin with respect to safety.

Statistical techniques discussed thus far are not adequate to describe or analyze these types of data. For example, some patients may withdraw from the study for a variety of reasons. As a consequence, the data are incomplete because the patients' fates are unknown; they are said to be lost to follow-up. Still other patients will not display an outcome during the study period. In both cases, the patients have contributed important information to the investigation. Because the outcome was not observed in these patients, their data is said to be censored, or more specifically, right censored.

Studying patterns of change in outcome variables over time is termed **survival analysis**. In pharmaceutical studies, two common analytical models are the Kaplan-Meier survival curve and the Cox proportional hazards model. The **Kaplan-Meier survival curve** is often used to depict the survival of a group of patients, to compare the rates of change in two survival curves, and to associate differences in survival with the presence of independent variables. The **Cox proportional hazards model** is used to assess the effects of preexisting conditions on the survival of patients. Often, the complete characterization of drug effects involves use of both statistical tools.

The Kaplan-Meier Survival Curve

Figure 8-8 presents the results of the primary efficacy and safety analyses of the OASIS-5 trial in terms of Kaplan-Meier survival curves. The total time period of the study is displayed in days on the abscissa of the graph, and the cumulative incidence rate for the primary outcome (here termed a hazard rate) is presented on the ordinate. The two lines labeled *enoxaparin* and *fondaparinux* demonstrate the pattern of change in the primary outcome over time in the two study groups.

Although the total time period of the study is indicated on the abscissa, 0 is not absolute time. Time 0 begins for each participant when he or she is enrolled in the study. Furthermore, because patients may experience the outcome event or be lost to follow-up, the number of individuals at risk differs at each measurement period. These values are indicated in the tabulation below the abscissa. For example, on the fourth day, 9,724 patients receiving enoxaparin and 9,752 patients receiving fondaparinux were at risk for a primary event.

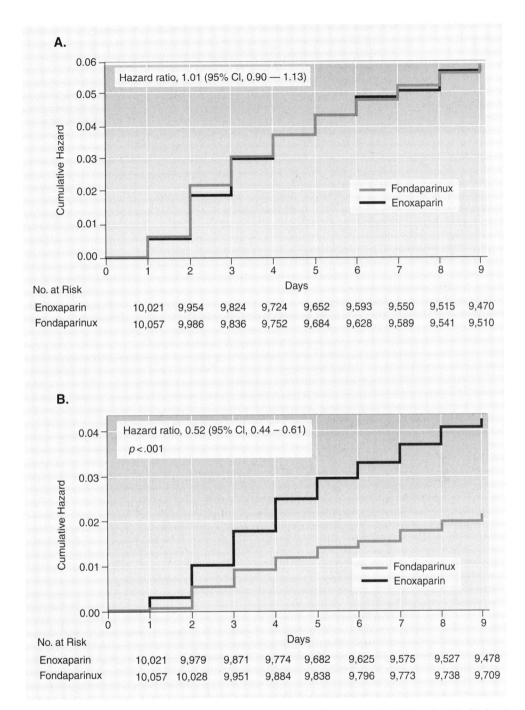

FIGURE 8-8 Kaplan-Meier survival curves comparing fondaparinux and enoxaparin in reducing the risk of ischemic events over 9 days of treatment with respect to the primary efficacy outcomes of death, myocardial infarction, or refractory ischemia. **(A)**, and the major safety outcome of major bleeding events **(B)**.[17] Adapted with permission from The Fifth Organization to Assess Strategies in Acute Ischemic Syndromes Investigators. Comparison of fondaparinux and enoxaparin in acute coronary syndromes. N Engl J Med 2006;354:1464–1476.

The ordinate registers the cumulative incidence of the primary end point. At time 0, no patients are affected, so the cumulative incidence is 0%. Each time a primary outcome occurs; the cumulative incidence is recalculated, and an upward deflection of the survival curve is observed. In the OASIS-5 study, the data are presented as a hazard ratio. A **hazard** is a measure of risk. A **hazard ratio** (HR) is the ratio of the hazard in one group divided by the hazard in another group and is an index of relative risk.

Several methods are used to test the statistical significance of the difference between two Kaplan-Meier survival curves. One method is to use the *log-rank statistic*, sometimes called the Mantel-Cox statistic. A statistically significant log-rank value indicates that the two survival functions came from different populations. An alternative method is to examine the 95% CI of the statistic, such as the hazard ratio.

Figure 8-8A provides the Kaplan-Meier survival curves for the efficacy outcome of the OASIS-5 trial. Visual inspection of the data suggests that the curves virtually overlap. This is confirmed by the results of the data analysis: the hazard ratio = 1.02, and the 95% CI = 0.90–1.13. Furthermore, the 95% CI is below the prespecified noninferiority margin of 1.185, suggesting the noninferiority of fondaparinux to enoxaparin.

Figure 8-8B provides the Kaplan-Meier survival curves for the safety outcome of bleeding, along with the results of the statistical analysis: hazard ratio = 0.52; 95% CI = 0.44–0.61. Because the 95% CI does not include 1, the hypothesis that fondaparinux is superior to enoxaparin in reducing bleeding events is accepted.

Cox Proportional Hazards Model

In addition to detecting differences in the rates of events in two groups, it is often informative to examine the association of the outcomes to *preexisting variables* like gender, disease severity, or concomitant conditions. This type of information is obtained using another survival model, the Cox proportional hazards survival analysis model. This model is much like the logistic regression models discussed in Chapter 6. The model calculates a weighting coefficient for each independent variable in a multivariable equation. The weighting coefficient can be used to generate a hazard, or an index of risk. The hazard ratio expresses how much more likely an outcome is with the factor than without it.

A Cox proportional hazards model was used in the OASIS-5 trial to explore associations between levels of preexisting variables (e.g., age, sex, creatinine level) and the primary and secondary outcomes. Results are presented in Figures 8-9 and 8-10. Specific subgroup designations are indicated in the leftmost column. The next columns indicate the number of patients in each subgroup and the percent in each subgroup exhibiting the primary event. The hazard ratio and the 95% CI for each subgroup are also provided. Hazard ratios < 1.0 favor fondaparinux, whereas hazard ratios > 1.0 favor enoxaparin. Statistical significance effects are indicated by the failure of the 95% CI to include the null value, 1.0.

In addition, the figures permit comparison of the interaction of subgroup levels with the primary efficacy and safety outcomes. This comparison involves an examination of the 95% CIs of the two subgroups. If the 95% CIs overlap, both subgroups are affected similarly by the treatments. Disparity in the 95% CIs suggests an interaction. The statistical significance of the interaction effect is indicated in the rightmost column of the figures.

The results of the efficacy analysis are congruent with the Kaplan-Meier results indicating noninferiority: The 95% CI for each variable level contains the null value (Fig. 8-9). In addition, none of the subgroup comparisons suggests an interaction.

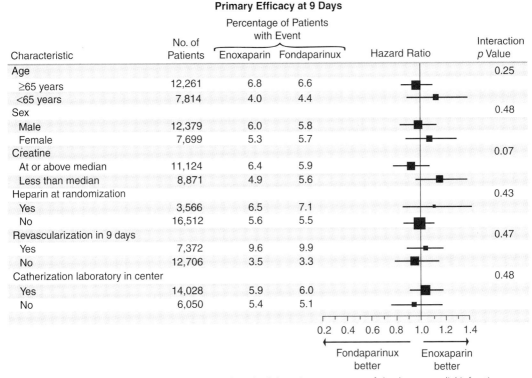

Characteristic	No. of Patients	Percentage of Patients with Event		Hazard Ratio	Interaction p Value
		Enoxaparin	Fondaparinux		
Age					0.25
≥65 years	12,261	6.8	6.6		
<65 years	7,814	4.0	4.4		
Sex					0.48
Male	12,379	6.0	5.8		
Female	7,699	5.3	5.7		
Creatine					0.07
At or above median	11,124	6.4	5.9		
Less than median	8,871	4.9	5.6		
Heparin at randomization					0.43
Yes	3,566	6.5	7.1		
No	16,512	5.6	5.5		
Revascularization in 9 days					0.47
Yes	7,372	9.6	9.9		
No	12,706	3.5	3.3		
Catherization laboratory in center					0.48
Yes	14,028	5.9	6.0		
No	6,050	5.4	5.1		

Primary Efficacy at 9 Days

0.2 0.4 0.6 0.8 1.0 1.2 1.4

Fondaparinux better ← → Enoxaparin better

FIGURE 8-9   Cox Proportional Hazards Analysis. The risk of the primary outcome of death, myocardial infarction, or refractory ischemia in subgroups participating in the OASIS-5 Trial is expressed in terms of 95% CIs of the hazard ratio. CIs that intersect the vertical line are not statistically significant; differences between subgroup values are statistically significant if their 95% CIs do not overlap. The probability that subgroup differences are the result of chance is indicated in the rightmost column. Adapted with permission from The Fifth Organization to Assess Strategies in Acute Ischemic Syndromes Investigators. Comparison of fondaparinux and enoxaparin in acute coronary syndromes. N Engl J Med 2006;354:1464–1476.

As for the results of the subgroup analysis for safety (Fig. 8-10), the 95% CIs of all subgroups contained values < 1.0, reinforcing the statistical evidence of the superiority of fondaparinux compared to enoxaparin in reducing bleeding events. In addition, the group undergoing revascularization in 9 days exhibited an enhanced reduction in bleeding events compared to the subgroup that was not revascularized. This is indicated by the lack of overlap in the two 95% CIs, and the p value for interaction.

In summary, survival analyses can divulge much information about the time course of an event, compare two or more event rates, and identify baseline variables that are associated with changes in the rates of change. In evaluating the results of survival analyses, however, keep the following factors in mind:

- The groups must be derived from random samples obtained from large, virtually infinite, populations.
- Each observation is independent of the others.
- It is important to assume that the risk of the outcomes remains constant throughout the study period (statistical tests are available to test this assumption).
- The time of censoring is assumed to be unrelated to time of survival, which might occur, for example, if a patient became too ill to continue participation owing to untoward factors preceding the primary event.

Major Bleeding at 9 Days

Characteristic	No. of Patients	Percentage of Patients with Event		Hazard Ratio	Interaction p Value
		Enoxaparin	Fondaparinux		
Age					0.11
≥65 years	12,261	5.5	2.7		
<65 years	7,814	2.1	1.4		
Sex					0.07
Male	12,379	3.3	2.0		
Female	7,699	5.5	2.5		
Creatine					0.71
At or above median	11,124	4.7	2.4		
Less than median	8,871	3.4	1.9		
Heparin at randomization					0.35
Yes	3,566	5.0	3.0		
No	16,512	4.0	2.0		
Revascularization in 9 days					<0.001
Yes	7,372	6.0	4.2		
No	12,706	3.0	1.0		
Catherization laboratory in center					0.88
Yes	14,028	5.0	2.6		
No	6,050	2.3	1.2		

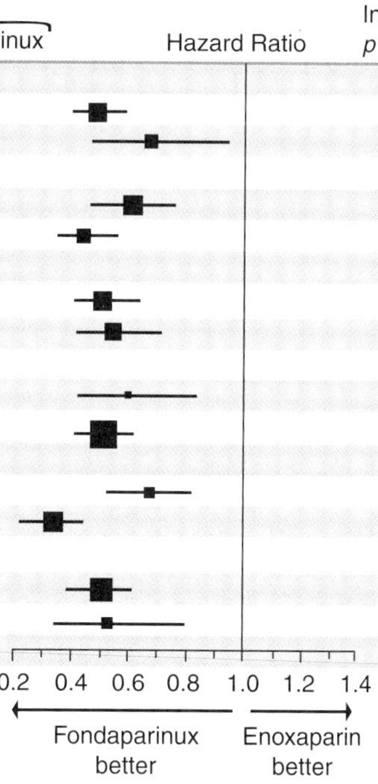

0.2   0.4   0.6   0.8   1.0   1.2   1.4

Fondaparinux better   Enoxaparin better

FIGURE 8-10   Cox Proportional Hazards Analysis. The risk of major bleeding events in subgroups participating in the OASIS-5 Trial is expressed in terms of 95% CIs of the hazard ratio. CIs that intersect the vertical line are not statistically significant; differences between subgroup values are statistically significant if their 95% CIs do not overlap. The probability that subgroup differences are the result of chance is indicated in the rightmost column. Adapted with permission from The Fifth Organization to Assess Strategies in Acute Ischemic Syndromes Investigators. Comparison of fondaparinux and enoxaparin in acute coronary syndromes. N Engl J Med 2006;354:1464–1476.

How to Evaluate Evidence from a Clinical Trial Design

Many guidelines for evaluating clinical trials have appeared in the literature. One basic method of evaluating a clinical trial is to follow the guidelines established by the Consolidated Standards of Reporting Trials (CONSORT) group, termed the CONSORT statement. The original CONSORT statement was intended to standardize the reporting of clinical trials to increase the quality of the design and conduct of such investigations, to promote the adoption of evidence-based practices and principles, and to enhance the transparency of the published reports.[18] The adoption of the original CONSORT statement by major healthcare journals was accompanied by empirical evidence of improvement in clinical trial design and reporting.[19] Based on this success, the CONSORT statement has been refined and revised for parallel-group randomized trials and extended to noninferiority and superiority active controlled trials.[20,21]

The CONSORT recommendations are presented as checklists. Table 8-4 presents the list for parallel-group randomized trials. The table provides the information that should be presented for each topic or section of the study paper and provides a space to enter the page number of the journal on which the information appears. Electronic versions of the CONSORT checklists are available on the Internet.[22] The online lists include hyperlinks to documents with explanations, elaborations, and examples of the information considered for each item.

The application of the CONSORT recommendations in evaluating a RCT is illustrated here by critiquing a study using parallel-groups trials to evaluate the use of saw palmetto for the treatment of benign prostatic hyperplasia.[23] This study was selected because the research hypothesis is not supported (see Appendix C for a copy of the study report). Reading this study before continuing with this chapter will greatly enhance your understanding of the literature evaluation concepts discussed here.

TITLE AND ABSTRACT (ITEM 1)

The title of the paper should list sufficient information to attract an interested reader's attention. It should contain an indication of the intervention, outcome, and patient population and be nonbiased. The abstract should be a nonbiased summary of the study, providing enough pertinent information for the reader to judge if the article pertains to his or her research question. It should contain the study design, major subject characteristics, interventions, outcome measures, findings, conclusions, and implications. The findings, conclusions, and implications noted in the abstract should be contained in the paper itself. The CONSORT recommendation is to state explicitly that patients were randomly assigned to conditions; this ensures the study's inclusion as an RCT in electronic databases.[24]

 LITERATURE CRITIQUE 8-1

The title indicates that the study will deal with the efficacy and safety of saw palmetto as a treatment for benign prostatic hyperplasia. The abstract is divided into background, methods, results, and conclusion sections, making it easy to distinguish the topic of each paragraph. Note that the background provides an idea of the rationale and purpose of the study. The methods contain a clear description of the intervention, including the study design (with randomization explicitly stated) and the primary and secondary end points. The results are provided for all primary and secondary end points, and the conclusion is straightforward. ■

INTRODUCTION (ITEM 2)

The introduction should provide the scientific background and rationale for the study. This often consists of a description of the general problem, including its epidemiologic and economic characteristics. Using evidence from published literature, the focus of the introduction is then narrowed to the specific question posed by the investigators. The introduction concludes with a formal statement of the research hypothesis or objective: "we conducted a randomized double-blind trial to determine the efficacy of saw palmetto for the treatment of benign prostatic hyperplasia."[23]

 LITERATURE CRITIQUE 8-2

The introduction provides the rationale for the study: although benign prostatic hyperplasia (BPH) is widespread and many of those afflicted use saw palmetto for treatment, evidence supporting this intervention is flawed by methodologic considerations. The present study was undertaken to examine the beneficial effects of saw palmetto using a careful methodology. ■

TABLE 8-4 Consort Group Checklist for Parallel-Group Randomized Trials

PAPER SECTION AND TOPIC	ITEM NO.	DESCRIPTION	REPORTED (PAGE NO.)
Title and abstract	1	How participants were allocated to interventions (e.g., random allocation, randomized, or randomly assigned)	
Introduction: background	2	Scientific background and explanation of rationale	
Methods			
Participants	3	Eligibility criteria for participants and the settings and locations where the data were collected	
Interventions	4	Precise details of the interventions intended for each group and how and when they were actually administered	
Objectives	5	Specific objectives and hypotheses	
Outcomes	6	Clearly defined primary and secondary outcome measures and, when applicable, any methods used to enhance the quality of measurements (e.g., multiple observations, training of assessors)	
Sample size	7	How sample size was determined and, when applicable, explanation of any interim analyses and stopping rules	
Randomization: sequence generation	8	Method used to generate the random allocation sequence, including details of any restrictions (e.g., blocking, stratification)	
Randomization: allocation concealment	9	Method used to implement the random allocation sequence (e.g., numbered containers or central telephone), clarifying whether the sequence was concealed until interventions were assigned	
Randomization: implementation	10	Who generated the allocation sequence, who enrolled participants, and who assigned participants to their groups	
Blinding (masking)	11	Whether or not participants, those administering the interventions, and those assessing the outcomes were blinded to group assignment; when relevant, how the success of blinding was evaluated	
Statistical methods	12	Statistical methods used to compare groups for primary outcome(s); methods for additional analyses, such as subgroup analyses and adjusted analyses	
Results			
Participant flow	13	Flow of participants through each stage (a diagram is strongly recommended); specifically, for each group report the numbers of participants randomly assigned,	

TABLE 8-4 Consort Group Checklist for Parallel-Group Randomized Trials, con't.

		receiving intended treatment, completing the study protocol, and analyzed for the primary outcome; describe protocol deviations from study as planned, together with reasons
Recruitment	14	Dates defining the periods of recruitment and follow-up
Baseline data	15	Baseline demographic and clinical characteristics of each group
Numbers analyzed	16	Number of participants (denominator) in each group included in each analysis and whether the analysis was by intention-to-treat; state the results in absolute numbers when feasible (e.g., 10/20, not 50%)
Outcomes and estimation	17	For each primary and secondary outcome, a summary of results for each group and the estimated effect size and its precision (e.g., 95% confidence interval)
Ancillary analyses	18	Address multiplicity by reporting any other analyses performed, including subgroup analyses and adjusted analyses, indicating those prespecified and those exploratory
Adverse events	19	All important adverse events or side effects in each intervention group
Discussion		
Interpretation	20	Interpretation of the results, taking into account study hypotheses, sources of potential bias or imprecision, and the dangers associated with multiplicity of analyses and outcomes
Generalizability	21	Generalizability (external validity) of the trial findings
Overall evidence	22	General interpretation of the results in the context of current evidence

Adapted with permission Moher D, Schulz KF, Altman D, et al. The CONSORT statement: Revised recommendations for improving the quality of reports of parallel-group randomized trials. JAMA 2001;285:1987–1991.

METHODS (ITEMS 3–12)

The methods section should contain a sufficient amount of information so that the reader may replicate the study. This includes descriptions of the participants, the setting, the interventions, method of assigning patients to treatments, the primary and secondary outcomes, and the data collection methods. Details of laboratory procedures are either referenced or described in detail, as are calculated measures like body mass index.

The description of the data analyses should include the sample size calculation needed to achieve statistical power, interim analyses and stopping rules, planned analyses of primary and secondary outcomes, and subgroup analyses. Note that only hypotheses stated a priori, or before the analysis, can be used as evidence in the present study. Data analyses carried out after the data have been examined, or post hoc, cannot be used as evidence in the present study, although they may provide a hypothesis for future studies.

 LITERATURE CRITIQUE 8-3

The description of the methods follows the recommended format of the CONSORT statement. The following aspects of the methods section merit special notice:

- *Participants:* Eligibility criteria are based on well-defined, objective, quantitative, and standard clinical criteria. For example, a peak urinary flow rate of < 15 mL/sec was used as part of the inclusion process as was a designated score on a validated index of BPH: the American Urological Association Symptom Index (AUASI). Severely affected subjects were excluded according to appropriate and objective criteria. A run-in period was used to reduce to the threat of noncompliance.
- *Intervention:* The dose of saw palmetto (160 mg twice daily) is similar to that used in other studies. Steps were taken to ensure the quality control of saw palmetto during the study and to maintain the blinding of the patients with respect to the intervention. The study plan is to follow each patient during a 12-month period of treatment.
- *Objectives and outcomes:* The primary objective of the study is to examine improvement in urinary peak flow or AUASI scores attributable to the saw palmetto intervention. Secondary objectives include measurement of prostate size, residual volume after voiding, and several self-reported quality of life measures. Once again, notice that many of the measures are objective and quantitative.
- *Randomization:* Subjects were assigned to treatment conditions only after completing the run-in period successfully. Randomization was stratified according to AUASI score and blocked using a computerized software package. The study medication was provided by the manufacturer and neither the investigator, the patient, nor any other study personnel were aware of the treatment assignment.
- *Statistical methods:* The study is designed to detect a minimum difference of 3 units in AUASI score with a power of 90% by studying 89 men in each group. To compensate for dropouts, 112 men were assigned to each condition. Statistical analyses of primary and secondary outcomes were based on regression analyses. The precise model used (linear versus nonlinear) depended on the effect of time within each study group. Baseline variables were tested using univariate statistical tests. All tests used intention-to-treat populations. Finally, several a priori subgroup analyses were carried out.

At this point, it seems that the internal validity of the study is quite strong. The study plan is well thought out, including criteria for diagnosis of the condition. The dependent measures are standard, and many have been used in previous studies of BPH. Methods for allocation of patients, concealment of treatments and blinding are exceptional. Finally, critical statistical analyses are chosen appropriately and presented well, with care being taken so the model fits the data. Finally, what changes in the primary and secondary outcomes would support the research hypothesis? ■

RESULTS (ITEMS 13–19)

The results section begins with a trial profile, which illustrates the flow of participants through the study protocol and accounts for the progress of all participants who were assessed for eligibility. An ideal flow chart for the trial profile appears in the CONSORT statement (Figure 8-11). The results section then compares the study groups on baseline variables and presents efficacy analyses of the major and minor outcomes, subgroup analyses, and analyses of variables reflecting adverse effects.

 LITERATURE CRITIQUE 8-4

The findings of the study are presented according to the CONSORT recommendations:

- *Participant flow:* The trial profile is presented in Figure 1 of the report and, according to CONSORT recommendations, consists of information from four stages of the trial: enrollment, allocation, follow-up, and analysis. Reasons for exclusion, loss to follow-up, and withdrawal from the study are detailed. Of the 225 men assigned to study groups, 19 were lost to follow-up or withdrew, so that 206 completed the study.
- *Recruitment:* The men were screened and assigned to groups between July 2002 and May 2003.
- *Baseline data:* At baseline (Table 1 of the report), the men in both groups were ~ 63 years old, predominantly white, college educated, and exhibited mean AUASI scores in the middle of the possible score range (suggesting a moderate level of benign prostatic hyperplasia). Average baseline values were similar among the groups for all variables except the BPH Impact Index Score. Differences in this variable, however, are not important because the averages of both groups indicate few symptoms.
- *Numbers analyzed:* It is stated elsewhere that an intention-to-treat analysis was used and that 96% of those randomized completed the study.
- *Efficacy—outcome and estimation and ancillary analyses:* During the 12-month study period, saw palmetto neither decreased AUASI scores nor increased peak urinary flow compared to the placebo group. Similarly, no group differences were detected in any secondary outcome or in any preplanned subgroup analysis. Effect sizes were not estimated because the findings were not statistically significant.
- *Safety—adverse events:* A total of 26 serious adverse events occurred in 17 men—6 men in the saw palmetto group and 11 men in the placebo control group. However, there were no group differences in the risk of a serious adverse events or nonserious adverse events.

At the end of the study, the adequacy of the study protocol in hiding group assignment from participants was assessed by asking subjects to guess the contents of their capsules. About 40% of the saw palmetto group and 46% of the placebo group believed they had been taking the active ingredient.

The data analysis is well-reported. The description of the baseline characteristics is comprehensive and relevant to BPH. The analyses of efficacy and safety data are also well conducted. Because the number of patients in each group met the minimum required for a power of 90%, it is quite likely that this finding of no difference is real. Additional evidence supporting the veracity of these findings is presented in the next section of the paper. ■

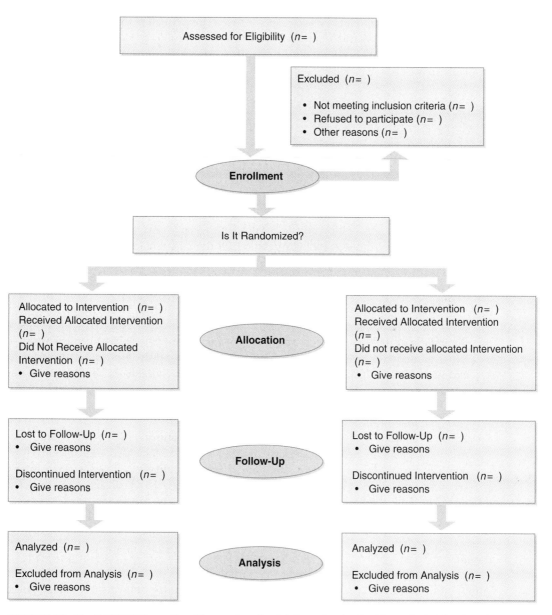

FIGURE 8-11   The CONSORT Group Flow Diagram for a Parallel-Group Randomized Controlled Trial. Adapted with permission from Moher D, Schulz KF, Altman D, et al. The CONSORT statement: Revised recommendations for improving the quality of reports of parallel-group randomized trials. JAMA 2001;285:1987–1991.

COMMENT (ITEMS 20–22)

The comment or discussion section should be organized to describe the major findings of the RCT in plain language. Other elements normally treated in this section include similarity and differences between these findings and other studies, a comment on discrepancies in the present data, implications for the interpretation of the intervention–exposure association as cause and effect. The section concludes with a statement of the external validity of the study and the significance of the findings to the provision of healthcare.

 LITERATURE CRITIQUE 8-5

The discussion section of the study follows the CONSORT recommendations:

INTERPRETATION

The findings of the study did not support the research hypothesis. However, because there were no changes in any of the study variables, the lack of support for the research hypothesis is based on the absence of evidence. Is absence of evidence, evidence of absence?

One question is whether a difference would have been detected if indeed it had been present. This revolves around statistical power. The power of the study to detect a change was set at 90% for the primary outcome of AUASI score and was based on a clinically important minimum change of 3 units in AUASI values. Establishment of a 3-unit change in AUASI score as clinically important was based on other literature.

Another issue is whether the primary outcomes were sensitive to changes that did occur. That the AUASI is sensitive is based on its use in other studies of urinary function. In addition, within-group changes in AUASI scores were detected in the interval from screening to baseline determinations. Thus, sensitivity of the test instrument seems adequate.

The authors go on to provide additional evidence regarding their findings. They state that the 95% CIs for the primary outcomes were narrow, suggesting that the lack of an effect was not the result of measurement error. In addition, the outcomes were consistent in providing no evidence of efficacy. The consistently negative findings extends to subgroups based on prostate size or symptom severity. However, remember that the study was not powered based on the subgroup analyses, so the evidence they provide may not be convincing.

The present finding seems to be at variance with other reports. However, the authors suggest several reasons for this discrepancy. One is the inadequacy of blinding techniques in previous studies compared to the present study. Another is the amount of the active ingredient provided for the saw palmetto group, pointing out that the contents were similar to saw palmetto products available in the United States.

GENERALIZABILITY

The authors do not comment on the external validity of the study. There are suggestions that the effect may depend on an active ingredient in saw palmetto preparations that to date has escaped detection. There do not seem to be any demographic factors that would restrict the findings of the study, although evidence is scanty.[25] However, the study results should be restricted to relatively healthy men who are not experiencing severe BPH symptoms.

OVERALL EVIDENCE

"In summary, we found that 160 mg of saw palmetto given twice daily for one year does not improve lower urinary tract symptoms caused by benign prostatic hyperplasia."[23] The authors' conclusions seem to be well supported by the study because internal validity is strong and type II error is unlikely. Clinicians should bear this new evidence in mind when discussing the use of natural supplements for the treatment of moderately severe BPH with their patients. However, care should be used in generalizing these results to nonwhite patients, different severities of BPH, or different formulations of saw palmetto. ■

How a Pharmacist Might Use Critical Evaluation of RCTs to Provide Drug Information

Since RCTs provide the best evidence of the efficacy and safety of treatments that promote health and treat disease, they provide information essential to the provision of effective healthcare. This section provides an example of the clinical application of the information derived from an RCT.

Assume a pharmacist working in a hospital is asked to write an article for the hospital newsletter, which is circulated to physicians. The physician editor of the newsletter poses the following drug information question to the pharmacist: "Is aspirin plus warfarin better than aspirin alone for preventing myocardial infarctions?" Upon executing the systematic approach (see Chapter 2), the pharmacist expands the question to derive the true question, classifies the question, searches for and evaluates literature, and formulates and communicates the following written response (to be published in a newsletter) to the editor.

REQUEST

Does combined antithrombotic therapy (aspirin plus warfarin) offer advantages over aspirin alone when used for secondary prevention after acute myocardial infarction (AMI) and if so, is the combination safe?

RESPONSE

Background

Current treatment guidelines for secondary prevention support the use of antithrombotic therapy but recommend warfarin only in patients unable to tolerate aspirin.[26] The use of aspirin 75–325 mg daily after an AMI has been shown to conclusively reduce subsequent AMI, stroke, and death.[27] High-intensity warfarin (INR 2.8–4.8) has also been proven effective in secondary prevention by decreasing mortality and cardiovascular events but was accompanied by a higher risk of hemorrhagic complications.[28–30] However, moderate-intensity warfarin (INR 2.0–2.5) was not shown to be superior to low-dose aspirin for prevention of recurrent ischemic events in patients with acute coronary syndrome (ACS) in one recent study.[31]

The hypothesis that both platelet-dependent and non-platelet-mediated coagulation mechanisms contribute to thrombosis after AMI has resulted in trials of dual antithrombotic therapy (aspirin plus warfarin) for secondary prevention. Recently published data, taken together with the results of previous clinical trials, provide further insight into the most rational approach to secondary prevention after myocardial infarction.

Primary Literature Analyzed

Four long-term randomized, controlled studies have looked specifically at efficacy and safety of combination low-dose aspirin with warfarin for secondary prevention after AMI and are here synthesized to provide an evidence-based recommendation for the proposed question.[32–35] Other related studies are available but are not included in this summary because they were short term (< 6 months), used small sample sizes with inadequate power (< 80%), or evaluated secondary prevention after other types of acute coronary syndromes.

Almost 18,500 post-myocardial infarction patients were evaluated in these four trials and followed for an average of 2.2 years—12 months in the Antithrombotics in the Secondary Prevention of Events in Coronary Thrombosis 2 (ASPECT-2) study to 48 months in the Warfarin Aspirin, Reinfarction Study (WARIS-II)[34,35]. Combined antithrombotic therapy in each trial consisted of low-dose aspirin (75–81 mg/day) plus either fixed-dose or moderate intensity warfarin (target INR = 1.5–2.5 or 2.0–2.5).[32–36] Patient-oriented outcomes evaluated in these studies included mortality and various morbidity factors, such as another nonfatal myocardial infarction (MI), stroke, cardiovascular death, and hemorrhage.

Evidence-Based Conclusions and Recommendations

Despite the positive results in reducing the primary composite outcome (i.e., death, non-fatal MI, and thromboembolic strokes) obtained with dual warfarin (INR 2.0–2.5) plus aspirin 75 mg/day versus low-dose aspirin monotherapy (29% risk reduction, $p = 0.001$) in WARIS-II,[35] the benefit seen was mainly the result of a reduction in the component outcomes of non-fatal MI and strokes. No mortality benefit was found with dual therapy over aspirin alone. However, increased rates of major hemorrhage were three times more likely with combination therapy than with aspirin alone (0.57% per year with combination vs. 0.17% per year with low-dose aspirin alone; statistical significance not reported in trial).[35] This finding makes it difficult to recommend dual therapy over low-dose aspirin alone at this time.

In agreement with the WARIS-II trial, results from the Coumadin Aspirin Reinfarction Study (CARS) and Combination Hemotherapy and Mortality Prevention (CHAMP) study did not indicate significantly greater benefit with dual antithrombotic therapy over aspirin alone. However, the subtherapeutic INR values obtained in these trials (mean INR 1.2 and 1.8, respectively) suggest that the drug doses were inadequate to provide valid data.[32,33] Despite subtherapeutic INRs, however, bleeding risk was increased with combination therapy versus aspirin alone in each of these trials.[32,33]

In a report of the ASPECT-2 trial, dual warfarin (INR 2.0–2.5) plus aspirin 80 mg/day was significantly more effective than aspirin alone in reducing a combined incidence of death, MI, and stroke (HR 0.50, 95% CI 0.27–0.92; p 0.03).[34] However, further scrutiny of the results of this composite outcome shows nonsignificant differences when the components are analyzed separately. This may be in part the result of ASPECT-2 having a smaller study sample and a shorter duration of follow-up than the other trials synthesized here. Although the risk for hemorrhage was low in ASPECT-2, major bleeding was two times greater ($p = 0.20$) and the risk for minor bleeding was three times greater ($p < 0.0001$) with combination therapy versus aspirin monotherapy.[34]

Although in theory dual antithrombotic therapy may provide additional benefit in reducing subsequent coronary events, risk of bleeding is increased. Until further evidence is accumulated from well-designed, long-term ($\geq$ 4 years), randomized controlled trials that firmly conclude benefit of dual antithrombotic therapy over aspirin alone for reducing mortality and morbidity without increasing hemorrhagic risk, aspirin 75–325 mg/day should remain first-line therapy for secondary prevention after an MI. Combination moderate-intensity warfarin (INR 2.0–2.5) plus aspirin (75–81 mg/day) should be considered only for patients at greatly increased risk for thromboembolic events—those who have experienced events while on aspirin or warfarin monotherapy.

Added caution should be exercised if using combination therapy in high-risk elderly patients ($>$ 75 years of age) because this population was not well represented in current trials. Complexities of monitoring and potential compliance issues may also serve as noteworthy deterrents to the use of combination therapy as first-line treatment. If dual antithrombotic therapy is used, rigorous monitoring is needed to ensure that moderate-intensity INR levels are maintained and bleeding events minimized.

Summary

Randomized controlled designs and active controlled designs have a special place in healthcare research because they alone can provide evidence of cause-and-effect relationships. To do so, however, requires quality in the design, analysis, and reporting phases of the research process. This chapter highlights some of the issues important in the evaluation of these study designs, discusses statistical evaluation of the data using survival analysis, and provides and exemplifies a framework for the evaluation of published research. In addition, an example is provided to show how pharmacists might use primary literature evaluation skills to render drug information. To be sure, literature evaluation skills need to be practiced to be mastered. Reading and evaluating RCTs offers great opportunity to hone these skills.

STUDY PROBLEMS

1. Select a recent randomized placebo controlled trial from the literature, and provide a critique using the CONSORT guidelines. Based on the outcome, comment on the internal and external validity of the research report.

2. Repeat question 1 using a report of an active control trial. Use the CONSORT guidelines for active controlled trials to guide your assessment.[22]

3. Review the factors detailed in the analysis of the saw palmetto data that support the conclusion that the lack of statistical significance was a real effect. Apply these criteria to evaluate the findings of another study in which statistical significance was not obtained for the efficacy measures.

4. Describe ethical considerations that apply to each of the study designs described in this chapter and discuss the consequences for patient care.

5. Develop your own checklist for evaluating RCTs. Compare your items with those of other students. What items and principles can be extended to case-control and cohort study designs? Which cannot?

REFERENCES

1. Gordis L. Epidemiology. New York: Saunders, 2000.
2. Feil PH, Grauer JS, Gadbury-Arnyot CC, et al. Intentional use of the Hawthorne effect to improve oral hygiene compliance in orthodontic patients. J Dent Educ 2002;66:1029–1035.
3. Burgess IF, Brown CM, Lee PN. Treatment of head louse infestation with 4% dimeticone solution: A randomized controlled trial. Br Med J 2005;330:1423–1426.
4. Hauck WW, Anderson S. Some issues in the design and analysis of equivalence trials. Drug Inf J 1999;33:109–118.
5. Djudbegovic B, Clarke, M. Scientific and ethical issues in equivalence trials. JAMA 2001;285:1206–1208.
6. Piaggio G, Elbourne DR, Altman D, et al. Reporting of noninferiority and equivalence randomized trials. An extension of the CONSORT statement. JAMA 2006;295:1152–1160.
7. Fiessinger J, Hiusman MV, Davidson BL, et al. Ximelagatran vs low-molecular-weight heparin and warfarin for the treatment of deep vein thrombosis. A randomized trial. JAMA 2005;293:681–689.
8. AstraZeneca International. AstraZeneca receives action letter from FDA for Exantra (ximelagatran) [Press Release]. Oct 11, 2004. Available at www.astrazeneca.com/pressrelease/3285.aspx. Accessed July 2006.
9. Wood S. FDA opts not to approve ximelagatran. Medscape Medical News, Oct 11, 2004. Available at www.medscape.com/viewarticle/537950. Accessed July 2006.
10. D'Agostino RB Sr, Massaro JM, Sullian LM. Non-inferiority trials: Design concepts and issues—The encounters of academic consultants in statistics. Stat Med 2003;22:169–186.
11. Szegedi A, Kohnen R, Dienel A, Kieser M. Acute treatment of moderate to severe depression with hypericum extract WS 5570 (St John's wort): Randomized controlled double blind non-inferiority trial versus paroxetine. Br Med J 2005;330:503–507.
12. Committee for Proprietary Medicinal Products. Points to consider when switching between superiority and non-inferiority. Clin Pharmacol 2000;52:223–228.
13. Pfeffer MA, McMurray JJV, Velazquez EJ, et al. Valsartan, captopril or both in myocardial infarction complicated by heart failure, left ventricular dysfunction, or both. New Engl J Med 2003;349:1893–1906.
14. Cannon CP, Braunwald E, McCabe CH, et al. Intensive versus moderate lipid lowering with statins after acute coronary syndromes. New Engl J Med 2004;350:1495–1504.
15. Greenspan SL, Resnick NM, Parker RA, Combination therapy with hormone replacement and alendronate for prevention of bone loss in elderly women. A randomized controlled trial. JAMA 2003;289:2525–2533.
16. Masuda Y, Kubo A, Kokaze A, et al. Personal features and dropout from diabetic care. Environ Health Prev Med 2006;11:115–119.
17. The Fifth Organization to Assess Strategies in Acute Ischemic Syndromes Investigators. Comparison of fondaparinux and enoxaparin in acute coronary syndromes. N Engl J Med 2006;354:1464–1476.
18. Begg C, Cho M, Eastwood S, et al. Improving the quality of reporting of randomized controlled trials: The CONSORT statement. JAMA 1996;276:637–639.
19. Moher D, Jones A, Lepage L, et al. Use of the CONSORT statement and quality of reports of randomized trials: A comparative before-and-after evaluation. JAMA 2001;285:1992–1995.
20. Moher D, Schulz KF, Altman D, et al. The CONSORT statement: Revised recommendations for improving the quality of reports of parallel-group randomized trials. JAMA 2001;285:1987–1991.
21. Piaggio G, Elbourne DR, Altman D, et al. Reporting of noninferiority and equivalence randomized trials. An extension of the CONSORT statement. JAMA 2006;295:1152–1160.
22. CONSORT. E-checklist and -flowchart. Available at: www.consort-statement.org/Downloads/download.htm. Accessed August 2006.
23. Bent S, Kane D, Shinohara K, et al. Saw palmetto for benign prostatic hyperplasia. N Engl J Med 2006;354:557–566.
24. CONSORT. Checklist item 1. Available at: www.consort-statement.org/examples1.htm. Accessed August 2006.
25. Guess HA. Epidemiology and natural history of benign prostatic hyperplasia. Urol Clin North Am 1995;22:247–261.
26. Ryan TJ, Antman EM, Brooks NH, et al. 1999 update: ACC/AHA guidelines for the management of patients with acute myocardial infarction: A report of the American College of Cardiology/American Heart Association Task Force on Practice Guidelines (Committee on Management of Acute Myocardial Infarction). J Am Coll Cardiol 1999;34:890–911. Available at www.acc.org. Accessed Nov 2002.
27. Antiplatelet Trialists' Collaboration. Collaborative overview of randomized trials of antiplatelet therapy—I: Prevention of death, myocardial infarction, and stroke by prolonged antiplatelet therapy in various categories of patients. Br Med J 1994;308:81–106.
28. Smith P, Arnesen H, Holme I. The effect of warfarin on mortality and reinfarction after myocardial infarction. N Engl J Med 1990;323:147–152.

29. Meijer A, Verheugt FWA, Werter CJ, et al. Aspirin versus Coumadin in the prevention of reocclusion and recurrent ischemia after successful thrombolysis: A prospective placebo-controlled angiographic study. Results of the APRICOT study. Circulation 1993;87:1524–1530.

30. ASPECT Research Group. Effect of long-term oral anticoagulant treatment on mortality and cardiovascular mortality after myocardial infarction: Anticoagulants in the Secondary Prevention of Events In Coronary Thrombosis (ASPECT) Research Group. Lancet 1994;90:499–533.

31. Huynh T, Theroux P, Bogaty P, et al. Aspirin, warfarin, or the combination for secondary prevention of coronary events in patients with acute coronary syndromes and prior coronary artery bypass surgery. Circulation 2001;103:3069–3074.

32. Coumadin Aspirin Reinfarction Study (CARS) investigators. Randomized double-blind trial of fixed low-dose warfarin with aspirin after myocardial infarction. Lancet 1997;350:389–396.

33. Fiore LD, Ezekowitz MD, Brophy MT, et al. Department of Veterans Affairs cooperative studies program clinical trial comparing combined warfarin and aspirin with aspirin alone in survivors of acute myocardial infarction: Primary results from the CHAMP study. Circulation 2002;105:557–563.

34. Van Es RF, Jonker JJ, Verheugt FWA, et al. Aspirin and Coumadin after acute coronary syndromes (the ASPECT-2 study): A randomised controlled trial. Lancet 2002;360:109–113.

35. Hurlen M, Abdelnoor M, Smith P, et al. Warfarin, aspirin, or both after myocardial infarction. N Engl J Med 2002;347:969–974.

Critical Appraisal of Evidence Derived from Pharmacoeconomics Studies

Kem P. Krueger and Linda Gore Martin

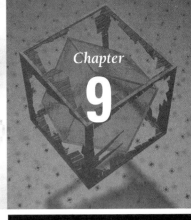

After studying this chapter, the student should be able to:

1. Evaluate a pharmacoeconomics study by identifying the type of analysis, sources of data, and outcomes used in the study.

2. Determine whether the article will help answer the pharmacoeconomics question.

3. Apply the results of a relevant pharmacoeconomics study to answer a pharmaco-economics question.

Many of the chapters in this book have involved the concept of health as "being without disease" and emphasized the individual. For healthcare to be available to and used optimally by the individual, the study of healthcare for populations is important. Pharmacoeconomics encompasses a set of tools to help evaluate healthcare use at the population level.

Healthcare is an interesting economics system, especially in the United States. As with all resources, healthcare funding is limited and the needs are seemingly infinite. However, often different groups of people make, pay for, and reap the benefits of healthcare decisions. In addition, healthcare is frequently needed regardless of the ability or desire to purchase it. The changes in the U.S. market leading to fewer employers providing full insurance coverage and the drive to create consumer-directed healthcare (such as health savings accounts) are resulting in a redistribution of payment. Still, patients cannot, in actuality, spend more than they have even if they are willing to do so.

Pharmacoeconomics is the subdivision of outcomes research or health economics that focuses on pharmaceuticals or pharmacy services. Medications and pharmacy services may be compared to other therapies, such as medical devices, counseling, and surgery, or to other professionals providing similar services. Therefore, by definition, comparative analysis of two or more alternatives must always be done. One of the alternatives is typically more effective and more costly. Therefore, decision makers use pharmacoeconomics analyses to help them deal with uncertainty—that is, determining if the additional **benefits** are worth the extra cost.

The Pharmacoeconomics Question

The following scenario and question are used to guide the reader through the evaluation of a pharmacoeconomics study.

OVERVIEW

Plains HealthCare is a staff-model health maintenance organization (HMO) established in 1982 that has 10 clinics in two states (Kansas and Missouri). Of these, 4 clinics are affiliated with the HMO-run hospital. The HMO has 94,000 covered individuals through contracts with area employers. Currently, only 1,500 of the enrollees are over age 65. The HMO employs 450 people, contracts with local hospitals for inpatient care and local pharmacies for pharmacy services, and maintains a single formulary for the hospital and all clinics. A central pharmacy and therapeutics (P&T) committee is composed of medical directors from each clinic, the vice president for pharmacy services, and the pharmacy clinical coordinator. In addition to maintaining the formulary, the P&T committee is responsible for developing treatment and diagnostics guidelines for the entire HMO.

- *Situation under consideration*: The HMO has decided to contract as a Medicare Advantage program, which would enroll people age 65 and over and some younger people with disabilities.
- *Patient population with potential for disease*: According to the U.S. Bureau of the Census estimate for 2005 (newest available) the population > 65 years of age for Kansas is 330,128 (286,814 females). For Missouri, the estimate is 721,138 (409,640 females).[1] The committee estimates that 10,000 people age 65 years and older will enroll (67% from Missouri).
- *The decision to be made*: Mammograms (optional under Medicare) cost the HMO $110 per person. The HMO is trying to decide whether to cover mammograms under the Medicare Advantage plan.
- *The pharmacoeconomics question*: Are mammography screenings for women over the age of 65 years cost-effective?

This question is really asking if the benefits of this procedure outweigh the costs in this specific population. A MEDLINE search was conducted using this expression: "(mammography OR breast cancer screening) AND cost-benefit analysis." "Cost-benefit analysis" is PubMed's medical subject heading (MeSH) term covering cost–benefit analyses, cost-effectiveness analyses, and cost-utility analyses.

LITERATURE SEARCH

Among the articles identified from the literature search, three are used to illustrate the concepts addressed in this chapter. The first two are used as examples throughout the chapter and the third article is used for the study questions. (See Appendix C for copies of articles 1 and 2.)

Article 1

The first article by Boer et al., "A Longer Breast Carcinoma Screening Interval for Women Age Older Than 65 Years?"[2] The abstract follows.

> BACKGROUND: The observed increase in sojourn time for preclinical breast carcinoma raises the question of whether women age $>/= 65$ years can be screened less frequently than younger women. METHODS: A cost-utility analysis using a computer model that simulates the demography, epidemiology, and natural history of breast carcinoma to

estimate expected life-years gained, extra incidence, extra life-years with disease, and costs incurred by different breast carcinoma screening programs in the general population was conducted. RESULTS: The estimated ratio of favorable/unfavorable effects was lower for longer screening intervals compared with shorter screening intervals. The cost-effectiveness ratio was much less favorable in shorter screening intervals. CONCLUSIONS: The results of the current analysis showed that although a longer sojourn time for preclinical breast carcinoma should not necessarily be accompanied by a longer screening interval, a shorter screening interval was not very efficient.

Article 2

The second article by Ostbye et al., "Screening Mammography and Pap Tests among Older American Women 1996–2000: Results from the Health and Retirement Study (HRS) and Asset and Health Dynamics among the Oldest Old (AHEAD)."[3] The abstract follows.

BACKGROUND: We wanted to determine the frequency of self-reported receipt of screening mammography and Papanicolaou (Pap) tests in older women and investigate important predictors of utilization, based on 2 national longitudinal surveys. METHODS: This cohort study includes participants from 4 waves (1994–2000) of the Health and Retirement Study (HRS)—5,942 women aged 50 to 61 years, and 4 waves (1993–2000) of the Asset and Health Dynamics Among the Oldest Old (AHEAD) survey—4,543 women aged 70 years and older. The self-reported receipt of screening mammograms and Pap smears in the most recent 2 years were reported in 1996 and 2000 for HRS, with predictors of receipt measured in 1994 and 1998. In AHEAD, the self-reported receipt of screening mammograms and Pap smears in the most recent 2 years were reported in 1995 and 2000, with predictors of receipt measured in 1993 and 1998. RESULTS: Receipt of mammography is stable at 70% to 80% among women aged 50 to 64 years, then declines to around 40% among those aged 85 to 90 years. For Pap tests there is a decline from 75% among women aged 50 to 54 years to 25% in those aged 85 to 90 years. For both mammography and Pap tests, the rates increased in all groups from 1995/1996 to 2000. Higher education, being married, higher income, not smoking, and vigorous exercise were consistently associated with higher rates of receipt. CONCLUSIONS: Although the use of mammography and Pap tests for screening declines into old age, use has been increasing recently. The large and increasing number of tests performed might not be justified given the lack of evidence of effect in older age-groups.

Article 3

The third article by Kerlikowske et al., "Continuing Screening Mammography in Women aged 70 to 79 Years: Impact on Life Expectancy and Cost-Effectiveness."[4] The abstract follows.

CONTEXT: Mammography is recommended and is cost-effective for women aged 50 to 69 years, but the value of continuing screening mammography after age 69 years is not known. In particular, older women with low bone mineral density (BMD) have a lower risk of breast cancer and may benefit less from continued screening. OBJECTIVE: To compare life expectancy and cost-effectiveness of screening mammography in elderly women based on 3 screening strategies. DESIGN: Decision analysis and cost-effectiveness analysis using a Markov model. PATIENTS: General population of women aged 65 years or older. INTERVENTIONS: The analysis compared 3 strategies: (1) Undergoing biennial mammography from age 65 to 69 years; (2) undergoing biennial mammography from age 65 to 69 years, measurement of distal radial BMD at age 65 years, discontinuing screening at age 69 years in women in the lowest BMD quartile for age, and continuing biennial mammography to age 79 years in those in the top 3 quartiles of distal radius BMD; and (3) undergoing biennial mammography from age 65 to 79 years. MAIN OUTCOME MEASURES: Deaths due to breast cancer averted, life expectancy, and incremental cost-effectiveness ratios. RESULTS: Compared with discontinuing mammography screening at age 69 years, measuring BMD at age 65 years in 10000 women and continuing mammography to age 79 years only in women with BMD in the top 3 quartiles would prevent 9.4 deaths and add, on average, 2.1 days to life expectancy at an incremental cost of $66773 per year of life saved. Continuing mammography to age 79 years in all 10000 elderly women would prevent 1.4 additional breast cancer deaths and add only 7.2 hours to life expectancy at an incremental cost of $117,689 per year of life saved compared with only continuing mammography to age 79 years in women with BMD in the top 3 quartiles. CONCLUSIONS: This analysis suggests that continuing mammography screening after age 69 years results in a small gain in life expectancy and is moderately cost-effective in those with high BMD and more costly in those with low BMD. Women's preferences for a small gain in life expectancy and the potential harms of screening mammography should play an important role when elderly women are deciding about screening.

Numerous guidelines for conducting and evaluating outcomes studies are available. This chapter uses a modified version of the evaluation guidelines developed by Chandramouli and Tyler,[5] who reviewed many published guidelines for conducting outcomes studies. The guidelines provide a basic outline for evaluating pharmacoeconomics and outcomes studies. Table 9-1 can be used to lead the reader through the general concepts addressed

TABLE 9-1	Criteria for Evaluating a Pharmacoeconomics or Outcomes Study
SECTION OF ARTICLE	**QUESTIONS TO ASK[a]**
Introduction	Is the reason for conducting the study discussed (what is the problem)?
	Are the study objectives well defined and address the problem?
Methodology and results	Were the methods transparent?
Perspective	Whose perspective is considered?
	How would a different perspective change the study?
Alternatives	What alternatives are compared?
	Are the comparators reasonable?
	Are all the relevant alternatives included?
	Is the do-nothing alternative relevant and included?
Costs	Are all relevant costs and consequences considered?
	Were the considered costs relevant to the perspective?
Outcomes	Are the selected outcomes appropriate? Do they make sense relative to the perspective?
	Are the selected outcomes measurable?
	Are intermediate outcomes used appropriately?
	Is the length of the study (time frame) relevant?
Economics analysis	What economics analysis did the authors say they used?
	Was this what they really used? If not, what did they use?
	Was the analysis used appropriate?
	Are incremental or marginal costs (outcomes) provided? Are they needed?
Data sources	What type of study was done (randomized controlled trial, naturalistic, other)?
	Was the study prospective, retrospective, or cross-sectional?

Criteria for Evaluating a Pharmacoeconomics or Outcomes Study, cont.

	Was the source of each element of the data provided?
	Was the evidence for the data strong?
	Was discounting needed? Were both costs and outcomes–benefits discounted? What discount rate was used?
	Was sensitivity analysis used and appropriate?
	Was the study robust?
Statistical analysis	Is the power of the study given?
	What is the sample size? Does it provide adequate power for all outcomes?
	What statistical analysis was used? If none, was it needed? If so, were the significance levels appropriate?
	What is the internal validity?
	What are the inclusion and exclusion criteria?
	Was intent-to-treat analysis done? What was included or excluded?
	Is any systematic bias apparent?
Discussion and conclusions	Are the authors' conclusions appropriate based on the results?
	Are the results statistically significant? Are they clinically significant?
	Are the assumptions presented? Are limitations objectively discussed?
	Do the conclusions address the objectives?
	What are the overall strengths and weaknesses of the study?
Application of the study	What is the external validity?
	Can the study be applied to the population in general?
	Is the problem relevant to my practice site? If so, could the study be applied to my practice site?
	How would the costs, consequences. and outcomes differ?
Other study aspects	Do the title and abstract appropriately reflect the content of the study?
	Is the article referenced appropriately and fully?
	Are most of the references primary and current?
	Do the authors have expertise to conduct the study?
	What is the reputation of the journal? Is it peer reviewed?
	Who sponsored the study? Are conflicts of interest disclosed?
	Are any ethical issues apparent?
	Are editorials or letters to the editor related to this study available?

[a]Questions are used to help a reader evaluate a pharmacoeconomics study and determine what information (if any) from the study can be used to answer a pharmacoeconomics question.

Adapted with permission from Chandramouli JC, Tyler LS. How to evaluate an outcomes study. Hosp Pharm 2001;36:131–142.

in this chapter. A basic understanding of these concepts is necessary for critically evaluating a pharmacoeconomics study. The questions listed are used to critique a pharmacoeconomics article and help the pharmacist apply valid information when answering a clinical or pharmacoeconomics question.

The Research Question and General Information

One of the first steps in evaluating a pharmacoeconomics study (or any study) is identifying the research question that the study is attempting to answer and the context in which the question is framed. For pharmacoeconomics studies, the context includes the study perspective and the alternatives that are being compared.

PERSPECTIVE

Pharmacoeconomics is all about **perspectives** (what is important to the decision maker). In general, four perspectives can exist (provider, payer, patient, and society). These perspectives consider the costs and outcomes of healthcare in different ways. Thus the perspective of a study determines which costs and outcomes are considered in the analysis. For example, if a study was conducted from an insurance company's perspective (payer), then only the direct costs of healthcare paid by the insurance company would be included in the analysis. The charges of one perspective may become the cost to another perspective. For example, the amount on a physician's bill is the cost to the insurance company (payer) and the charge from the physician's office (provider). This charge includes the physician's cost plus a profit. The cost to the patient is the amount of the physicians bill paid by the patient (i.e., the copayment and deductible), and the cost to the payer is the amount of the bill not paid by the patient. Table 9-2 demonstrates how the costs included in a pharmacoeconomics study vary by perspective.

Each perspective places its own value on the outcomes. For instance, the provider thinks about health as "absence of disease or symptoms." The patient may not consider "the absence of disease or symptoms" as the ultimate goal. His or her ultimate goal of healthcare may be the ability to maintain a certain level of activity. This idea is consistent with Kaplan's Ziggy Theorem.[6] In one of the *Ziggy* comic strips, the character Ziggy asks the wise man of the mountain the meaning of life. The answer is "doin' stuff," in contrast to death, which is "not doin' stuff."[7] Thus Kaplan proposed that quality of life was the ability to do stuff. The payer, who is often the insurer, and society take these two definitions (absence of disease and ability to be active) and add the concept of health to determine **health capital**. The Human Capital Model was originally described by Grossman in 1972, who described health as "a durable capital stock that yields an output of healthy time."[8] According to this model, health capital is the time available for productivity.

TABLE 9-2	Costs of Interest[a]			
	PERSPECTIVE			
COSTS	PROVIDER	PAYER	PATIENT	SOCIETY
Direct medical	Yes	Yes	Yes	Yes
Direct nonmedical	No	Maybe	Yes	Yes
Indirect	No	Maybe[b]	Maybe	Yes
Intangible	No	No	Yes	Maybe

[a]The types of costs included in a pharmacoeconomics analysis depend on the perspective of the study.

[b]If the payer perspective is that of an indemnity insurance company then indirect costs may not be included. If the payer perspective is that of a self-insured employer group, then indirect costs are included because the payer/employer is interested in productivity issues.

Finally, if the payer perspective is that of an insurance company or HMO that wants to market its services to employees, then indirect costs are included in the analysis.

The perspective of an analysis should be clearly stated in the article, but this is not always the case. Sometimes the reader must determine which costs and outcomes are included in the analysis and infer the perspective from these data. If the perspective of the analysis in an article is different from the perspective of the reader/decision maker, then the article may not be totally useful for addressing the reader's question (this concept is called external validity, discussed later in this chapter). However, if the outcome included in the study is the outcome of interest to the reader, then the fact that the costs included in the analysis are different from the reader's costs may not pose a problem. In essence, if the important outcome is included in the study, then the information from the article may still help the reader answer his or her pharmacoeconomics question.

ALTERNATIVES

Alternatives are the choices from which the decision maker must choose. The clinically relevant alternatives for any particular analysis depends on the question addressed in the study. They may consist of treatment strategies, such as pharmacotherapy, surgery, nonpharmacological therapy, and no treatment. The alternatives could also include preventive measures, such as screenings or investment strategies. In essence, any viable option available to the decision maker could be included as an alternative. However, if the alternative comparators included in an analysis are not clinically relevant to the reader's question, then the article is not as useful for answering his or her pharmacoeconomics question.

TRANSPARENCY

Transparency describes the ease with which the reader can follow the methods and procedures to replicate the analysis. Most pharmacoeconomics analyses require the researcher to make some assumptions about the data used in the analysis. In addition to having a clear and comprehensive description of the methods and procedures for data collection, estimation, and analysis, a transparent study makes all assumptions clear. A major component of transparency in pharmacoeconomics studies is the sources of the data.

 LITERATURE CRITIQUE 9-1

Plains HealthCare is trying to decide if it should cover mammography screenings for women over the age of 65 years. As previously stated, the pharmacoeconomics question of interest is whether mammography screenings for these women are cost effective. Once the literature search has been conducted, it is time to determine if Articles 1 and 2 will help answer the pharmacoeconomics question of interest. Begin by addressing the following questions (Table 9-1):

- Is the reason for conducting the study discussed (what is the problem)?
- Are the study objectives well defined and address the problem?
- Whose perspective is considered?
- What alternatives are compared?
- Are the comparators reasonable?
- Are all the relevant alternatives included?
- Is the do-nothing alternative relevant and included?

ARTICLE 1: BOER ET AL.

The reason Boer et al. conducted their study is clearly explained. A change in Medicare coverage of yearly mammograms for women 65 years and older prompted the study. The objective was to determine whether it would be appropriate to apply a longer screening interval to women > 65 years of age than for those 50–64 years of age. The perspective of this analysis is not explicitly stated, but it can be assumed that it is a payer perspective (i.e., Medicare) because the study is being conducted in response to a change in Medicare coverage.

The authors compare mammogram screening intervals of 1, 2, and 3 years for women > 65 years of age. Given the study objective, the alternatives (the three intervals) seem to be clinically appropriate and over a sufficient range based on the background information presented in the article. The do-nothing alternative is not explicitly included because these screenings are now covered by Medicare. However, the base case is the previous Medicare coverage policy (mammogram screenings every 2 years for women 50–64 years of age).

The article seems to address a research question that is related to Plains HealthCare's pharmacoeconomics question. The alternatives considered in the article are relevant and applicable to the pharmacoeconomics question at hand because at least one of the alternatives in the study includes the decision facing Plains HealthCare.

ARTICLE 2: OSTBYE ET AL.

Ostbye et al. note that the objective of their study is to "determine the frequency of self-reported receipt of screening mammography and Papanicolaou (Pap) tests in older women and investigate important predictors of utilization, based on 2 national longitudinal surveys." Based on the stated purpose, the study is not relevant to Plains HealthCare's pharmacoeconomics question. Therefore this article is dropped from consideration, and the pharmacist focuses on Article 1. ■

Costs and Outcomes

As with all economics, pharmacoeconomics is the study of the use of resources. The ultimate goal is to maximize outcomes at a given cost or to minimize the costs necessary to achieve a given outcome. Techniques are available to analyze resource use and these same methods can be applied to the allocation of healthcare resources. The ideal is to make decisions and to allocate resources based on the application of evidence.

COSTS

A **cost** is a resource consumed in an attempt to produce a positive outcome. Such costs, or inputs, are classified as direct, indirect, or intangible. The inclusion of each type of cost depends on the perspective of the analysis (Table 9-2).

Direct costs are the actual costs of obtaining healthcare. These are often divided into medical and nonmedical costs. Direct costs are expenditures on tangible products or services that contribute to the **gross national product** (the gross national product of the United States is the value of goods and services produced in the country). **Direct medical costs** are used to purchase medical services or supplies directly. These costs include medications, hospitalization, emergency department visits, laboratory tests, and other related goods and services. The cost of salaries, facilities, and other expenses are costs to the provider. **Direct nonmedical costs** are incurred to obtain healthcare but are not supplies or services. Direct nonmedical costs include transportation to the doctor's office and costs incurred by a parent who has to hire a baby-sitter while he or she is in the hospital.

The next type of cost is **indirect cost**. Indirect costs in economics include the cost of morbidity and mortality, which is generally related to productivity costs, such as death, lost workdays, and decreased productivity while at work. Productivity loss is often estimated for individuals not employed outside the home, such as stay-at-home parents and retirees. For example, the productivity of a woman who is a full-time homemaker is measured by determining how much it would cost to hire a baby-sitter to care for the children and a housekeeper to maintain the home. Another type of indirect cost is the **value** of services that are used but are not purchased with cash (e.g., when a relative baby-sits for free).

Indirect costs from an accounting perspective include items such as rent and electricity. These are items that are necessary for conducting business and that can be allocated to all parts of a business. For example, the cost of rent may be proportionally allocated to the dispensing, compounding, and front-end areas of a pharmacy. These indirect costs are included only if an analysis is conducted from the provider perspective. Therefore, in economics, these types of cost become either fixed or variable direct costs.

The final category of costs consists of **intangible costs**. These are often left out of analyses because they are difficult to measure. Intangible costs are the costs of pain, suffering, or lost social time. Intangible costs are based on preferences of patients or society. Many people believe that putting a value on these types of costs is unethical, often because the value applied is different for different people and is often based on their income or potential to earn. Intangible costs are a large part of quality-of-life and cost–utility analyses and should be included in cost–benefit analyses because they are based on patient preferences.

You may also see articles that discuss **opportunity costs**. In economics, opportunity cost is the inability to use a unit of resource for its next best purpose. This becomes a lost opportunity; therefore, these costs are most often considered in relation to indirect costs. For example, if a person sits in the physician's waiting room for 1 hr, he or she cannot use that time to earn money at work. If a hospital uses funds for an immunization clinic, it cannot use that money for a new device for diagnosing cancer. If a new pharmacy graduate completes a 1-year residency that pays $45,000, rather than going to work as a pharmacist for $100,000, the opportunity cost of that decision is $55,000 for that year ($100,000 − $45,000).

 LITERATURE CRITIQUE 9-2

In Literature Critique 9-1, we determined that the perspective and alternatives included in Article 1 are applicable to Plains HealthCare's pharmacoeconomics question. Now it is time to determine if the costs included in the study are also applicable to the question at hand. The following questions guide the next step of evaluation (Table 9-1):

- Are all relevant costs and consequences considered?
- Were the considered costs relevant to the perspective?

The costs were assumed to be $100 per screening with a zero balance of other costs incurred and saved as a result of the screening. The other costs included items such as diagnostics, primary therapy, and prevented palliative care. Specific details about how the costs were determined are not provided. The costs included in the article are consistent with Plains HealthCare's cost of conducting a mammography screening ($110), so the costs included in Article 1 are relevant and applicable to Plains HealthCare's pharmacoeconomics question. ■

OUTCOMES

Kozma et al. divided outcomes into three categories, economic, clinical, and humanistic, and developed the economic, clinical, and humanistic outcomes (ECHO) model.[9] The **ECHO model** shows that many of the outcomes of health are difficult to examine individually. For example, the outcomes from an acute exacerbation of asthma have a component in each of the listed categories. Outcomes are always stated with a direction, such as increased productivity, and decreased emergency department visits.

The measurable positive economic, clinical, and humanistic outcomes that result from the purchase and use of medical products or services are considered direct benefits. Direct economics benefits are measured in dollars and include savings from implementing a new service or adding a new drug to the formulary. Direct clinical benefits are measured in natural or clinical units. Examples of clinical benefits include **life-years** gained, blood pressure reduction measured in millimeters of mercury, symptom-free days, or event avoided (such as myocardial infarction). Direct humanistic outcomes are improvements in satisfaction, quality of life, or **utility**; these outcomes are measured by surveying or interviewing people.

Indirect benefits are benefits derived from avoiding indirect costs. For example, assume an employee who has no sick leave earns $23.75/hr ($190 per 8-hr day). He gets an infection and must take off work for a number of days. If a particular antibiotic will get him back to work 1 day sooner than another antibiotic, then the indirect benefit of the first medication is $190. These outcomes are also measured by surveying or interviewing people, but the *human capital approach* is most often used to value indirect benefits.

Intangible benefits are the benefits derived from avoiding pain and suffering. These benefits are inherently included in cost–utility and cost–benefit analyses because the measurement of **quality-adjusted life-years (QALYs)** (used in cost–utility analyses) and techniques such as willingness to pay (used in cost–benefit analyses) include patient or societal preferences. QALYs and willingness-to-pay estimates are obtained by surveying or interviewing people. Techniques for determining value of outcomes are discussed in more detail later in this chapter.

DISCOUNTING

For interventions or programs that last more than 1 year, a concept called **discounting** is applied to the costs and outcomes. However, the extent to which benefits should be discounted remains controversial.[10] The idea behind discounting future costs and benefits lies in the fact that humans value items in the present (the sure thing or instant gratification) more than they value receiving that item in the future. Spending money in the present costs more than waiting to spend it, a reflection of the opportunity cost. For example, you could spend $100 right now to cover a $100 expense incurred today. However, if you were to defer that $100 expense until 10 years from now, you could invest a smaller amount of money today so you would have the $100 to cover the cost 10 years from now. A formula using a discounting rate to convert future expenditures and gains to the present year's value (the **present value**) is given as equation C in Table 9-3. The discount rate should theoretically be based on society's time preference but is often based on some economic factor that provides a rate of return, such as the rates on government bonds. Discount rates can be obtained from the literature, from government sources, and from other references. Because the discount rate is an estimate, sensitivity analysis (discussed later in this chapter) should be conducted whenever discounting is used.

TABLE 9-3	Common Formulas Used in Pharmacoeconomic Analyses	
FORMULA	**TITLE**	**EQUATION**
A	Net benefit	$\Sigma \text{Benefits} - \Sigma \text{Costs}$
B	Cost–benefit ratio	$\dfrac{\Sigma \text{Costs}}{\Sigma \text{Benefits}}$
C	Net present value	$\Sigma \dfrac{\text{Benefits}_{\text{year}}}{(1 + \text{Rate}_{\text{benefits}})^{\text{year}}} - \Sigma \dfrac{\text{Costs}_{\text{year}}}{(1 + \text{Rate}_{\text{costs}})^{\text{year}}}$
D	Average cost-effectiveness ratio[a]	$\dfrac{\Sigma \text{ Cost}}{\text{Units of outcome}}$
E	Incremental cost-effectiveness ratio[b]	$\dfrac{\text{Cost}_A - \text{Cost}_B}{\text{Unit of outcome}_B - \text{Unit of outcome}_A}$

[a]Each alternative is calculated and then compared.

[b]Marginal cost effectiveness uses essentially the same formula, but the answer is in cost per additional unit.

 LITERATURE CRITIQUE 9-3

Previously, we determined that the study perspective, alternatives, and costs included in Article 1 are applicable to Plains HealthCare's pharmacoeconomics question. Now, it is time to determine if the outcomes included in the study are also applicable to the current concern. The following questions guide the next step of the evaluation (Table 9-1):

- Are the selected outcomes appropriate? Do they make sense relative to the perspective?
- Are the selected outcomes measurable?
- Are intermediate outcomes used appropriately?
- Is the length of the study (time frame) relevant?

The authors included both favorable outcomes—such as deaths prevented and life-years gained—and unfavorable outcomes—such as increased incidence of disease and extra years of life with the disease. These make sense because these are the outcomes of interest for breast cancer. They are relevant to the payer because these outcomes are the major cost drivers. Death avoided and life-years gained are final rather than immediate outcomes.

The time frame covered by the analysis ranged from 17 years in the base case to 29 years in the sensitivity analysis. The study was based on a model, and the authors calculated the expected outcomes based on the life expectancy of women aged 65 years with specific conditions. This is a relevant time frame. The outcomes included in the article are consistent with the clinical situation faced by Plains HealthCare. Therefore the outcomes included in Article 1 are relevant and applicable to Plains HealthCare's pharmacoeconomics question. ■

Types of Pharmacoeconomics Analyses

The analyses used in pharmacoeconomics research can be categorized as partial or complete analyses. Cost analyses and outcomes analyses (such as clinical trials) are considered **partial analyses** because they consider either the costs or the outcomes of an intervention. Another type of partial analysis is the program description that describes the costs and outcomes of a single program or intervention without comparing it to another. Full economics analyses compare at least two alternatives and include both the costs and the benefits in the analysis.[11] Cost–benefit, cost-effectiveness, cost-minimization, and cost–utility analyses are full economics analyses. The question being asked, available data sources, financial resources available to the researcher, and time resources determine if a full or partial analysis is conducted.

COST ANALYSIS

As stated previously, cost analysis is a partial economic analysis because the costs of an intervention or interventions are considered without considering the benefits or outcomes of the intervention(s). Cost analyses can be used by P&T committees to determine the economics effect of adding a new drug to the formulary or for other budget-planning activities.

Cost-of-illness studies are a special form of cost analysis. These studies estimate the economic burden of a disease or condition. They are generally conducted from a societal or payer's perspective and usually include direct and indirect costs. The problem with cost analysis (especially cost of illness) is that the results of the study provide the amount of money spent and the items or services purchased, but the results of the analysis do not indicate if the expenditures were appropriate.

COST–BENEFIT ANALYSIS

Cost–benefit analyses (CBAs) are often used when decision makers are trying to compare two or more options that have entirely different outcomes. A CBA provides a quantitative foundation for decision making because it allows decision makers to determine which program, project, or service should be implemented given the current resource constraints. Because all benefits are converted into dollar amounts, programs with multiple or unrelated outcomes can be compared.[12] An example is a hospital board trying to decide if it should spend money to expand the maternity ward or to build a new cancer treatment center. The types of benefits and the population for whom the benefits accrue are different for these two options. A CBA is grounded in the welfare economics notion of **Pareto efficiency**,[11] also known as **allocative efficiency**. Pareto efficiency is the best possible allocation of resources; no redistribution of resources improves the welfare of one person without reducing the welfare of another.

All costs and benefits (outcomes) are measured in dollars and converted to present value (discounted). This is different from a cost analysis because it includes direct, indirect, and intangible benefits. They are converted to dollars using one of the following techniques: willingness to pay (contingent valuation), the human capital approach, court awards, amount spent on health and life insurance, or expert opinion.[13] The technique chosen affects the strength of the evidence for the analysis. The net benefit is calculated for each alternative by subtracting the costs from the benefits (equation A in Table 9-3). The alternative (intervention or service) with the largest net benefit is selected, followed by the alternative with the next highest positive net benefit until the resources are exhausted.[14]

The basic calculation of net benefit (i.e., costs subtracted from benefits) provides the most information because it allows the actual dollar value to be identified. In contrast, calculating a ratio (either cost–benefit or benefit–cost) allows comparisons of effect but does not reflect the magnitude of the expenditures. Ratios are often given in reports to justify the project. For example, a benefit of $5 for every dollar spent (cost–benefit ratio of 1:5 dollars).

Although cost–benefit analysis grounded in economics theory, several problems prevent its widespread use in healthcare. First is the difficulty of identifying all benefits of a program and converting them to a dollar figure. Second, it is difficult and sometimes unsavory to place a dollar value on human life. Third, there is debate in the economics literature over the best method to use to convert the benefits into dollar amounts: willingness to pay, the human capital approach, court awards, or other approaches.[11,12,14] Finally, any alternative with even a $0.01 benefit would be selected if resources are available. Alternatives with a zero or negative benefit (costs are greater than benefits) would never be selected, which can be extremely unpopular with some groups.

COST-EFFECTIVENESS ANALYSIS

Cost-effectiveness analysis (CEA) is a tool to help decision makers identify which outcomes can be achieved at the least cost or, given a limited budget, which alternative will maximize the overall health **effectiveness**.[15–18] Cost-effectiveness analyses are often used when decision makers are trying to compare drugs or other interventions used to treat a single disease state. An example is a P&T committee trying to decide if a new selective serotonin reuptake inhibitor (SSRI) should replace depression medications currently on the formulary, be added to the formulary in addition to the current drugs that are used to treat depression, or not be added to the formulary.

A cost-effectiveness analysis entails the calculation of a ratio of the costs measured in dollars to a single outcome measure (effectiveness), measured in natural or clinical units.[11,15] Examples of natural units include number of patients responding to a therapy, change in total serum cholesterol levels, increased number of life-years, or number of deaths avoided. Because only one outcome can be used in a cost-effectiveness analysis, the outcomes of the interventions must be common to each alternative in the analysis.[15] This limits the comparisons to programs or interventions with the same outcome. For example, two antihypertension medications could be compared because both alternatives produce the same outcome (decreased blood pressure). The average cost-effectiveness ratio is of interest (equation D in Table 9-3), but the incremental cost-effectiveness ratio is used for determining the most cost-effective alternative. The cost calculations always include direct costs, may include indirect costs, and rarely (if ever) include intangible costs, although the use of intangible costs is not prohibited.

Incremental Cost-Effectiveness Ratios

Although some studies try to determine the most cost-effective alternative by comparing the average cost-effectiveness ratios (the expected cost of an alternative divided by the expected outcome of that alternative), Karlsson and Johannesson claim that using average cost-effectiveness ratios is inappropriate.[18] They demonstrate that even though two different therapies have equal average cost-effectiveness ratios, it is not possible to conclude that they are equally cost effective. The **incremental cost-effectiveness ratio (ICER)**, the cost to achieve one additional unit of outcome, is the only way to determine which alternative is the most cost-effective therapy.[18]

To estimate the ICER, the therapies are ranked in increasing order of effectiveness. Then the incremental cost-effectiveness ratio is calculated by dividing the incremental costs by the incremental outcome for each successively more effective treatment alternative (equation E in Table 9-3); these equations are calculated for two therapies (alternatives) at a time. This ratio shows how much the cost is increased when the next incrementally effective treatment option is chosen.[18]

The standard cost-effectiveness plane reveals the cost-effectiveness decision. The plane is divided into four quadrants with effectiveness of the therapy plotted on the x axis and the cost of the therapy along the y axis. Figure 9-1 is one such plane.[19] A new alternative that falls in quadrant II would never be selected because it is less effective and

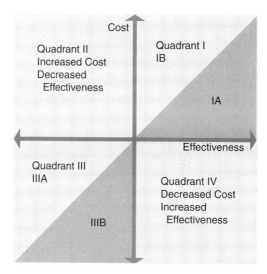

FIGURE 9-1   Cost-Effectiveness Plane. (Adapted with permission from O'Hagan A, Stevens JW, Montmartin J. Inference for the cost-effectiveness acceptability curve and cost-effectiveness ratio. Pharmacoeconomics 2000;17:339–349.)[19]

more expensive than the alternative that is currently being used (it is dominated by the alternative). Likewise, a new alternative that falls into quadrant IV would always be selected because it is more effective and less expensive than the current alternative (it dominates the alternative). Thus quadrant I (or northeast in some reports) and quadrant III (or southwest) are those of interest. The decision of which alternative is more cost effective depends on the slope of the line intersecting the quadrants; alternatives that fall in IA and IIIB (shaded areas in the figure) are selected because they are the most cost-effective alternatives.

Once the ICER is calculated, two decision rules can be used to select the most cost-effective therapy. The first decision rule relies on the budget. The treatment with the lowest incremental cost-effectiveness ratio is implemented first, followed by the next most cost-effective alternative. This continues until the budget is exhausted. Using the budget as the decision rule may result in different treatments within a patient group, which raises ethical issues about distributive justice and equality.

The second decision rule is to set a maximum cost per unit of effectiveness. The decisions involve only alternatives that are either less effective at less cost or more effective at higher cost (IA and IIIB). This maximum cost per unit of effectiveness may include the cost of treating a case, the cost of treating a case plus the cost of a lawsuit, or some other economics value determined within the setting. Using the maximum cost per unit of effectiveness (also known as the willingness-to-pay approach, discussed later), all patients within a treatment group receive the treatment that has an ICER at or below the cutoff point. This approach always leads to the adoption of the same treatment within a patient group.[18] The societal **willingness to pay** has traditionally been determined to be $50,000 per additional unit of effectiveness or, recently, €50,000 per additional unit of effectiveness.

Some authors use the terms *incremental cost-effectiveness analysis* and *marginal cost-effectiveness analysis* interchangeably. Although the fundamental concepts and calculations are similar, their applications are not. **Incremental cost-effectiveness analysis** is used when two or more alternatives are being compared. The **marginal cost-effectiveness analysis** is used when the cost of one more unit of outcome is calculated for using one more sequential application of a given intervention (e.g., one more test or one more counseling session). The classic example (though controversial) of marginal cost-effectiveness is in determining the number of guaiac stool tests needed to cost-effectively detect colon cancer[20].

Cost-Minimization Analysis

A variation of the CEA is the **cost-minimization analysis (CMA)**. The costs included in this analysis are calculated just as they are in the CEA. Similarly, the benefits of the interventions included in the CMA are represented by a single outcome measured in natural units.[12] In addition to having a common outcome for the interventions included in the CMA, the magnitude of the outcome must also be the same. Thus the CEA is reduced to a CMA because the effectiveness of the two interventions is equal. Because both positive and negative (adverse reactions) effectiveness must be essentially equal, CMA can rarely be used. A CMA, as with all economic analyses, must include all costs (labor, supplies and others).

CMAs are used when decision makers are trying to compare drugs or other interventions used to treat a single disease state. An example is a P&T committee trying to decide if a new blood pressure medication should replace a blood pressure medication currently on the formulary. If it turns out that each medication lowers blood pressure to the same degree with the same side effects, then the cheaper alternative is selected.

Cost-Utility Analysis

Cost–utility analysis (CUA) is often considered a subdivision of cost-effectiveness analysis. The advantage is that the unit of measure has been converted into a common unit (similar to cost–benefit in which the unit of measure is the dollar). This allows for comparisons of different outcomes, which is not possible with CEA. The most studied unit is the quality-adjusted life-year, but other units have been developed, such as the **healthy-year equivalent (HYE)**. The most cost-effective alternative is the one with the lowest incremental cost–utility ratio.

Because CUA deals more directly with valuing lives (or the quality of lives) relative to CEA, the maximum cost per QALY is usually much larger than that used for CEA. The cutoff used in CEAs is often $50,000 per additional unit of effect. The cutoff for a CUA may be as high as $100,000 per QALY gained.[21] Thus, any alternative that has a cost per QALY > $100,000 would not be deemed cost-effective, even if it had the lowest ICER. These cutoff values are not set in stone and are controversial.

CUAs are more expensive and complex to conduct than CEAs, so they are reserved for studies where **quality of life (QOL)** is the needed outcome or one of the important outcomes. For example, medications that ameliorate the side effects of chemotherapy do not extend life, but they do improve the patient's quality of life.

The QALY is basically the quality of life (measured as a utility) multiplied by the quantity of life. When examining the results of a CUA, the reader must determine if the result is an increase in quality of life, quantity of life, or both. The most difficult, time-consuming, and controversial aspect of CUA is determining the utility. Basically, a utility is a value applied as satisfaction with a level of health (with health again serving as the indicator of being able to do stuff). Units other than QALYs are usually considered preferences or values rather than utilities. Utilities are determined using the standard gamble or time trade-off methods (discussed later in this chapter).

Utilities range from the worst (death), which equals 0, to full health, which equals 1. The fact that QALYs do not allow any health state to be worse than death and the fact that a QALY for a newborn is the same as a QALY for a 100-year-old are two problems cited for this type of analysis. Utilities that could apply to Plains HealthCare's pharmacoeconomics

TABLE 9-4	Utility Example	
TREATMENT PHASE (HEALTH STATE)	**UNITED KINGDOM UTILITY (STANDARD DEVIATION)[a]**	
Active (start of second-line therapy)	0.64 (0.15)	
Follow-up care (partial or complete response plus stable disease)	0.73 (0.21)[b]	
Supportive care (progressive disease)	0.33 (0.24)	
Terminal care (terminal disease)	0.13 (0.12)	

[a]Values were obtained using the standard gamble technique on a large number of people in the United Kingdom.

[b]Combined category assuming an even split between partial and complete response and stable disease.

Adapted with permission from Martin SC, Gagnon DD, Zhang L, et al. Cost-utility analysis of survival with epoetin-alfa versus placebo in stage IV breast cancer. Pharmacoeconomics 2003;21:1153–1169.

question are given in Table 9-4.[21] In this example, the utilities are derived from subjects participating in a standard gamble study in the United Kingdom and are presented with the standard deviation (SD). The utilities differ by treatment phase, so the subjects rated active treatment (i.e., receiving another phase of chemotherapy) 0.64, which is lower than stable disease (0.73) but higher than progressive (0.33) and terminal (0.13) disease. Utilities obtained in the United Kingdom have been found to be similar to those obtained in the United States This is a good example of where economic analyses can be generalized from one population to another.

LITERATURE CRITIQUE 9-4

So far, we have determined that the study perspective, alternatives, costs, and outcomes included in Article 1 are applicable to Plains HealthCare's pharmacoeconomic question. Now it is time to determine what type of economics analysis was used and if it was done properly. If an analysis is improperly conducted, then the results are not useful. The following questions guide the next phase of the evaluation (Table 9-1):

• What economics analysis did the authors say they used?
• Was this what they really used? If not, what did they use?
• Was the analysis used appropriate?
• Are incremental or marginal costs (outcomes) provided? Are they needed?

In the abstract, the authors claim to use a cost–utility analysis. That is the only place the type of analysis is mentioned. However, because they did not include QALYs or some other utility-based outcome, this is not a cost–utility study. The outcome used in the incremental analysis is life-year gained (the authors calculated the cost per additional life-year gained). This is a natural or clinical unit of measure; therefore, the study used a cost-effectiveness analysis. However, the authors actually conducted a marginal cost-effectiveness analysis because they compared each alternative (screening every 1, 2, or 3 years) to the base case rather than comparing the alternatives to each other based on effectiveness. Incremental costs and benefit analyses are presented.

The authors claim this is a cost–utility analysis, although it is not; however, the results may still be useful for answering the Plains HealthCare's pharmacoeconomics question ■.

Evidence and Data Collection

Many countries require some kind of evidence that a new drug is of benefit economically before the drug can sold in that country. This may be required by the government or an outside reviewer who makes the recommendation to the government. The National Institute for Health and Clinical Excellence (NICE) is the organization in Great Britain (www.nice.org.uk); Canada, Australia, Sweden, and others also have government-backed systems. In the United States, Oregon implements a combined approach: One group performs a systematic review of the effectiveness and safety and a second group calculates cost savings. Other states can purchase these documents.[22]

The strength of the evidence from a pharmacoeconomics study is based on study design and can be evaluated based on the transparency of the methods, whether final outcomes are used, the type of data collection methods and—because economics is a science of uncertainty—the accuracy of the assumptions. Transparency is judged by how many questions the reader has about how the analysis was conducted; the fewer, the better. Final outcomes such as death, myocardial infarctions (MIs), and survival are definitive, but the time to reach these end points is frequently too long for most studies, so other measures are used (intermediate outcomes). The strength of evidence is based on how strong the association is between the intermediate outcome and the final outcome. For example, strong evidence exists that blood pressure (an intermediate outcome) is directly related to the risk of having an MI (a final outcome). The accuracy of assumptions should be tested with sensitivity analysis (discussed later). Data collection methods include primary and secondary data collection or data estimation using modeling techniques.

PRIMARY DATA COLLECTION METHODS

Clinical Trials (Randomized Controlled Trials)

The hierarchy of evidence places the randomized controlled trial (RCT) or meta-analyses of multiple RCTs at the top. Therefore, the best medical evidence is considered to come from well-conducted RCTs. Randomization is used to maximize the possibility of creating a study group that is equivalent to the control group in every aspect except the intervention the study group receives. Usually, these types of studies are attempting to determine the **efficacy** of the study drug (whether the study drug improves the outcome in a controlled situation). However, as discussed in Chapter 8, RCTs have significant limitations. The major limitation is that the study population may not represent the population in society (low external validity).

Pharmacoeconomics analyses can collect data during a RCT that is designed as a clinical study. This so-called piggyback study uses the protocol of the study and collects data on the used resources. The main limitation with this type of economics study is that, to be considered a strong RCT, the study drug is controlled by placebo. This violates the main premise of good economics analyses in that comparison of at least two treatments is needed (this prevents the calculation of opportunity costs because the next best use—standard of care—is not included). Although the do-nothing alternative may be the standard of care, the difference here is that resources are used in the placebo arm. In addition, RCTs are powered for the primary outcomes (clinical) of the study and may not be powered for the economics outcomes.

Another limitation to the piggyback economics study is that the RCT is an artificial situation. The protocol drives the costs and is, of financial necessity, short term. Subjects are required to see physicians, have laboratory tests, and be compliant. Freemantle et al.

state that the outcomes being measured may not be clinically relevant.[25] Finally, a strong RCT has high internal validity and avoids as many factors that could affect the results of the study as possible. This eliminates subjects who are not the same (usually those with multiple disease states or multiple medications). RCTs are designed to control for the potential of bias, but outcomes and pharmacoeconomics studies and analyses are looking at that uncertainty. If an active control (i.e., standard of care) is used in a RCT, then there are at least two alternatives; however, the problem of protocol-driven costs remains.

Naturalistic (Pharmacoeconomics) Trials

Pharmacoeconomics analyses are interested in effectiveness (whether the intervention improves the outcome in a wide range of situations) outcomes achieved in the real world. These studies can be called naturalistic, pragmatic, or practical studies.[25] These studies are considered observational trials and, therefore, have been considered lower on the evidence hierarchy. Few inclusion and exclusion criteria exist (strong external validity); similar to what occurs in actual medical practice. They may be initially randomized or not (quasi-experimental), but are allowed to proceed as the patient would normally proceed with his or her care (i.e., in a natural or real-world way). This includes allowing noncompliance, which may be measured during the study. Blinding is probably undesirable because many outcomes are subtle and can affect whether the patient continues to take treatment. So the strength of the evidence has to be maximized by the data collection and sources.

Measures of Utility, Preferences, and Values

Willingness to Pay and Contingent Valuation

The willingness-to-pay (WTP) technique values an intervention based on preferences of people being interviewed. The preferences are obtained by interview or survey. During the process, a detailed scenario is presented to an interviewee. The scenario contains details about the intervention, current resources available, and the likely positive and negative consequences and outcomes of the intervention. The interviewee is asked to determine what he or she would be willing to pay for the product or intervention being studied (which is carefully described). This may be a specified amount or a bid process. The bid process starts with an amount that has been researched as being a reasonable amount for the product or intervention (or the closest alternative). This is represented by the $100 in the top box of Figure 9-2. The amount is either increased or decreased depending on the answer to the first bid: yes (willing to pay) or no (not willing to pay). The amount is increased to $200 for a yes response and decreased to $25 for a no response in the next level of the figure. If the second bid is accepted, the next bid is larger than the last (but not as large as any previous no bid). This continues for several levels of bid until the interviewee's willingness to pay is determined. The WTP amount from each interviewee is aggregated and the average WTP is determined. This value encompasses indirect and intangible costs and benefits.

Standard Gamble

Standard gamble is a technique by which an interviewer asks the person whose utility is being measured to choose between an outcome that will occur for certain and a gamble. An example is having breast cancer requiring chemotherapy and the associated side effects for the rest of your life (alternative 2 in Figure 9-3) versus having surgery (a mastectomy; alternative 1 in Figure 9-3). There is uncertainty associated with the surgery because this alternative is linked to a probability (p) of obtaining complete health and a

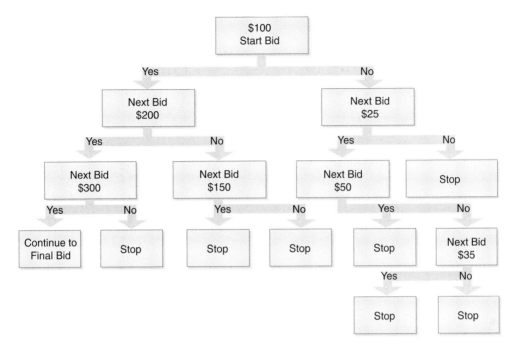

FIGURE 9-2 Willingness to Pay.

probability $(1 - p)$ of death. The choice is usually presented to the respondent as either accepting or rejecting a treatment option. The interviewer varies p from a high value to a low value until the interviewee is ambivalent (undecided) between living with breast cancer and having the surgery. This indifference point is the utility of living with breast cancer.

For example, an interviewer may ask the interviewee if she would have the surgery if there were a 95% chance of obtaining perfect health. Assuming the interviewee says yes, the interviewer would ask if she would have the surgery if there were a 5% chance of obtaining perfect health. If the interviewee says no, then the interviewer would repeat the

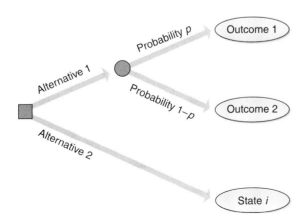

FIGURE 9-3 Standard Gamble. For this example, alternative 1 is surgery; alternative 2 is do nothing beyond standard care; outcome 1 is complete health; outcome 2 is death; and state *i* is having breast cancer for 15 years with its associated treatments, side effects, and complications followed by death.

question using a 90% chance of perfect health. The interviewer would continue present-ing the question, alternating between a high and low probability of perfect health until they reach the probability at which the interviewee does not care if she has the surgery or remains in the breast cancer state.

In this example, assume that when the interviewer asks the interviewee if she would have the surgery if there were a 65% chance of obtaining perfect health (a 35% chance of death), the interviewee cannot decide if she would pick the surgery or live with breast cancer. This is the point of indifference (or ambivalent point). The interviewee is saying that living with breast cancer requiring chemotherapy with the associated side effects has the same value as having an intervention with a 35% chance of death. Therefore, this interviewee's utility for living in the breast cancer state is 0.65. To obtain a utility value for a given state, many people are interviewed and the average (or median) utility value is calculated for the group. The utility values presented in Table 9-4 were obtained in this manner. One of the limitations of the standard gamble technique is that it does not allow a state worse than death.

Time Tradeoff

Time tradeoff is a technique by which an interviewer asks the person whose utility is being measured to determine how much time in a diseased state the person would be will-ing to give up to live for a shorter time in perfect health. An example is presenting a sce-nario to the interviewee in which she would live with breast cancer requiring surgery (as-sume chemotherapy is done for both alternatives) for 15 years followed by death (Fig. 9-4). The interviewer then asks the person how many of the 15 years she would be willing to give up to live in perfect health. To calculate the utility for living 15 years with breast cancer, divide the number of years of living in perfect health by the number of years of liv-ing with breast cancer (x/t). Time (t) is 15 years in this case; if the person is willing to give up 5 years of life living with breast cancer to live 10 years in perfect health, then $x = 10$ ($t = 15$, so $15 - 5 = 10$). Thus the utility of living with breast cancer for 15 years is 0.67 ($10/15 = 0.67$). Time tradeoff is considered by many to be a value rather than a true util-ity because the concept of uncertainty has been removed.

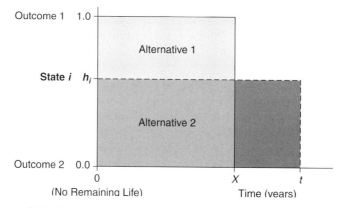

FIGURE 9-4 Time Tradeoff. For this example, alternative 1 is surgery; alternative 2 is do nothing beyond standard care; outcome 1 is complete health; outcome 2 is death; state i is having breast cancer for 15 years with its associated treatments, side effects, and complications followed by death; h_i is the utility of having state i; t is the number of years living with the disease in the current state (15 years); x is the number of years living in perfect health, which is equiva-lent to living t years with the disease in the current state.

Visual Analog Scale

The visual analog scale technique uses a visual scale to assess preference. The interviewer presents the person whose utility is being measured with a line that is anchored on each end by perfect health and death (or the worst possible state). The interviewer then asks the person to rate the desirability for each health state by placing it at some point on the line between the anchors. Respondents are instructed to place the health states on the line so that the intervals between the responses reflect perceived differences. The responses are aggregated across all respondents to obtain the average utility for that health state. The visual analog scale is again not considered a true utility.

Although these techniques have shown strong reliability and validity, one of the areas of debate for all forms of utility, preference, and value data collection is who should be interviewed: healthy individuals, people with the disease of interest, family members, or healthcare providers? Each of these groups has an inherent bias that may affect the data collected.

SECONDARY DATA COLLECTION METHODS

Secondary data collection techniques estimate costs (or outcomes) using data that were collected for some other purpose.

Databases (Clinical and Administrative)

Administrative claims databases are created for accounting and actuarial purposes. However, current uses of claims databases include pharmacoeconomic and epidemiology studies, healthcare resource use patterns, and adherence studies[25,26] The items commonly found on claims in medical claims databases include member identifier, provider identifier, place of service, date of service, procedure code, and financial information. The items commonly found in pharmacy claims databases include member identifier, provider identifier, pharmacy identifier, date of service, prescription number, national drug code (NDC) number, quantity dispensed, days supply, and financial information. In addition to medical and pharmacy claims databases, managed-care organizations usually maintain files containing patient demographic and eligibility information.[26]

Claims databases are a relatively low cost source of data and provide a means of measuring medications and medical services used in the real world.[27] Claims databases contain information on a large number of patients and do not rely on patients to remember which medications or services they received, thus claims databases are free from recall bias.[24] They are useful for descriptive studies of resources used to treat particular diseases (i.e., cost analyses), to conduct regression analyses to predict future costs, for planning and monitoring clinical programs, and for helping decision makers develop clinical and economics targets.[26] Claims databases may have missing data because some medications or services may not be covered, may cost less than the copayment amount, or may lack detailed claims from hospitalizations.[26] In addition, the data may contain a number of errors associated with *International Classification of Disease*, 9th revision, *Clinical Modification* (ICD-9-CM) diagnostic codes, including keystroke errors, improper documentation by the provider, and improper selection of code by coder.[26,28]

Chart Review

Medical chart review is a broad term describing the extraction of data from medical or pharmacy records. This form of data collection is also a relatively low-in-cost source and allows assessment of effectiveness rather than efficacy—that is, how the medication is working in an actual clinical setting versus a clinical trial. Clinical outcome measures are documented in the medical records so the analysis is not restricted to process measures found in claims data. Unfortunately chart reviews are time-consuming, so the number of data points may be fewer than with claims data. This form of data collection is also constrained by the accuracy and completeness of the data in the medical or pharmacy records.[29]

Human Capital Measures

If medical care is seen as an investment in human capital or productivity, then earning potential can be used as an index of value. Data are obtained from wage survey, census reports, market value, or imputed cost calculations. Any improvements or deterioration in productivity, time off work, or social time can be valued based on estimates from these data sources. The largest problem with the human capital measures is that some people are valued lower than others; children, the retired, and the unemployed are valued the lowest. The strength of evidence for human capital measures is the strength of the data source from which the values were obtained.

MODELING

Sometimes the cost and outcomes data cannot be measured directly (using primary data collection techniques) or obtained from secondary data. In these instances, the cost and outcomes data must be estimated using models. The most common forms of models seen in the pharmacoeconomics literature are grounded in decision analysis or statistics.

Decision Analytic Models

Decision analysis was introduced into healthcare in the early 1970s, and its use has increased over the years. Decision analysis is useful when a choice has to be made between two or more alternatives (e.g., treatment interventions or clinical services) and there is uncertainty about which option is more appropriate.[28] It can be considered a roadmap to the decision.

Decision analysis separates a decision into three components: alternatives, probabilities, and outcomes.[30] The viable alternatives differ from one analysis to another and depend on the situation being modeled. The probabilities used in a decision analysis are estimates of the likelihood that a given event will occur; these probabilities can be obtained from a variety of sources, such as randomized controlled trials, observational studies, and clinical databases. The outcomes can be clinical or economic in nature and represent the end point of the decision tree.

The researcher is responsible for defining the characteristics of the decision and the patients being modeled.[30] If the characteristics of the decision and patients included in the model are clear, then it is easier to determine if the results of the analysis can be generalized to the pharmacist's practice setting. For example, rather than stating that a model represents diabetes, the authors should write something like this: The model represents patients with type 2 diabetes mellitus who are currently receiving oral antidiabetic medications.

In addition to specifying the characteristics of the patient population, a decision model should include all key characteristics of the situation or treatment intervention being modeled. However, care should be taken to avoid making the model too complex or cumbersome. An overly complex model has the potential to confuse decision makers without providing any additional information.[31,32]

Although decision analysis is a useful tool, it is not without problems. First of all, it is time-consuming. Novices may underestimate the time and technical expertise required to conduct a proper analysis. Improper model construction will limit the usefulness of the

TABLE 9-5	Steps for Decision Analytic Modeling[a]

1. Conduct a systematic review of the literature, including computerized searches, file-drawer searches, and review of references.

2. If probabilities are found in an applicable meta-analysis, they may be used. Otherwise, the analyst should examine the clinical studies obtained from the search to determine if they are applicable to the current model. Assess the study design, population studied, the study setting, and time frame.

3. Discard nonrelevant studies and studies that are methodologically flawed.

4. If one study is methodologically superior to all the others, then the probabilities obtained in that study may be used. If more than one relevant study exists, average the results of the studies to obtain the probability estimate for the model. A weighted average (weighted by the number of subjects in each study) may be used.

[a]These are the steps involved in deriving the probabilities for a decision analytic model (a decision tree or a Markov model). The process of identifying relevant studies and combining data to estimate probabilities used in such an analysis are similar to the procedures used to combine data when conducting a meta-analysis.

model, which may bias the results.[26] Whether tests of statistical significance should be conducted on decision analysis models—and, if so, how these tests should be conducted—is still to be determined.[30]

The actual probabilities used in any decision analysis are unknown and must be estimated. The estimate can come from a published meta-analysis, a published systematic review, clinical studies, expert opinion, or existing databases.[33] The steps involved in deriving the probabilities for a decision analytic model (a decision tree or a Markov model) are given in Table 9-5. The process of identifying relevant studies and combining data to estimate probabilities (or the percentages) used in a decision tree or Markov model are similar to the procedures used to combine data when conducting a meta-analysis (see Chapter 10).

Decision Trees

The **decision tree** is a common way to operationalize a decision analysis. This is most appropriately used for diseases or conditions that progress in a defined linear manner. Diabetes is a disease that progresses in a linear fashion. Once complications of diabetes appear, such as peripheral neuropathy or heart disease, they usually do not disappear.

The starting point of a decision tree is the decision node or choice node, which is represented by a square.[29,30] This point indicates where the decision maker must choose between several alternatives, which are represented as branches radiating from the decision node. All branches emanating from the same node in a decision tree represent mutually exclusive options (Figure 9-5).

The events that occur in the branches after the decision node are not under the control of the decision maker—that is, the patient may respond favorably to the therapeutic intervention, have an adverse reaction, or die. These events are represented as branches emanating from the chance nodes. Chance nodes are represented as circles, and the branches arising from these nodes should represent all clinically relevant outcomes.[29,30] The probabilities associated with the branches extending from a given chance node must sum to 1. As with the branches emanating from a decision node, the branches from a chance node should represent mutually exclusive events so that a given patient may travel only one path through the decision tree.[29,30] As mentioned previously, decision analysis separates the decision-making process into three components: alternatives, probabilities, and outcome.

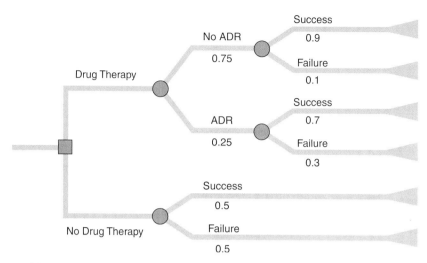

FIGURE 9-5   Decision Tree. *ADR*, adverse drug reaction. See text for details.

A hypothetical situation that can be represented by Figure 9-5 is deciding whether to treat an upper respiratory tract infection with a medication (represented by the drug therapy branch) or to let the infection run its course (represented by the no drug therapy branch). Thus, the two mutually exclusive options are providing drug therapy or not providing therapy. The outcome of interest is resolution of the infection (represented by the success branches). There are several probabilities used in this model. Drug therapy has a 25% chance of causing an adverse drug reaction (ADR). This is indicated by the probability of 0.25 in the figure. If no ADR occurs, then the patient has a 90% chance of being cured (indicated by 0.9). If an ADR does occur, then the patient has a 70% chance of a cure (indicated by the 0.7). In this example, there is a 50% chance of curing the infection if no drug therapy is given.

A dollar value is associated with each branch in the decision tree (this value can be $0). For this example, assume that drug therapy costs $50 and the office visit to obtain the prescription costs $80. Therefore, the cost associated with the drug therapy branch is $130 ($50 + $80 = $130). Further assume that the other branches (no drug therapy, no ADR, and success) have no costs associated with them (e.g., if the infection is cured then the patient will incur no additional treatment costs). Assume there is a $25 cost associated with the ADR branch (on average it costs $25 to treat adverse drug reactions associated with the drug therapy). Assume that if the infection isn't cured initially then the patient has to go to the emergency room for additional treatment, so the cost associated with the failure branch is $1,000.

The expected cost of each alternative (treating the infection with medication or not) is the weighted average cost that is calculated by multiplying the cost associated with a given branch by its probability. This process, known as *rolling back a decision tree*, begins at the right-hand side of the tree (the terminal branches at the end of the tree) and continues until you have calculated the expected cost associated with a given option. In this example, the expected cost associated with the drug therapy alternative is $206.25, which is calculated as follows:

1. The cost of the top success branch is multiplied by the probability of achieving success: $0 × 0.9 = $0.
2. The cost of the top failure branch is multiplied by its probability: $1,000 × 0.1 = $100.

3. The sum of the first two products is added to the cost associated with the no ADR branch and multiplied by the probability associated with that branch: ($0 + $100 + $0) × 0.75 = $75. This the expected cost of the no ADR branch.

This process is continued for the ADR branches

4. The cost the success branch is multiplied by the probability of achieving success: $0 × 0.7 = $0.
5. The cost the failure branch is multiplied by its probability: $1,000 × 0.3 = $300.
6. The sum of the first two products is added to the cost associated with the ADR branch and multiplied by the probability associated with that branch: ($0 + $300 + $25) × 0.25 = $81.25. This the expected cost of the ADR branch.
7. The sums of the expected costs of the no ADR and ADR branches are added to the cost associated with the drug therapy branch: $75 + $81.25 + $50 + $80 = $286.25.

Therefore, the expected cost of treating one person with an upper respiratory tract infection is $206.25. Some people may cost more to treat and some may cost less, but $286.25 is the weighted average treatment cost. The expected cost of the no drug therapy branch is $580. It is calculated as follows: (0.5 × $80) + (0.5 × $1,000) + $80 = $500. The outcome is the number of treatment successes. The expected outcome for the drug therapy alternative is calculated as follows.

1. The probability of achieving success is multiplied by the probability of having no ADR: 0.9 × 0.75 = 0.675.
2. The probability of achieving success is multiplied by the probability of having an ADR: 0.7 × 0.25 = 0.175.
3. The sum of these two products is the expected outcome for the drug therapy alternative: 0.675 + 0.175 = 0.85
4. The expected outcome from the no drug therapy alternative is simply 0.5.

This means that for every 100 patients treated, it will cost $28,625 (100 × $206.25), and 85 patients will be cured with the initial treatment (100 × 0.85). The overall costs of not treating 100 patient is $58,000 (100 × $580), and the infection will resolve itself in 50 patients.

The expected costs and expected outcomes obtained form a decision analytic model such as a decision tree or a Markov model are the estimated costs and outcomes that are plugged into an incremental cost-effectiveness analysis to determine which option is most cost effective.

The time frame encompassed by the model is dictated by the disease state or therapeutic intervention under study. The time frame should be of a duration sufficient to capture key outcomes.[30] For instance, a 1-month time frame would be adequate to model most acute infections such as upper respiratory infection. This time interval would capture the initial office visit and treatment as well as a relapse, if applicable.

Markov Models

Markov models are another common way to operationalize a decision analysis. Markov models are most appropriately used for diseases or conditions that cycle from one state to another and do not progress in a defined linear pathway. The alternatives, probabilities, and outcomes are present in these models as they are in decision tree models. The primary difference is that when you are in a given state there is a probability of remaining in that state or switching to another state.

A Markov model is presented in Figure 9-6.[34] Each line emanating from a given state has a probability associated with it. These probabilities are obtained by the process described in

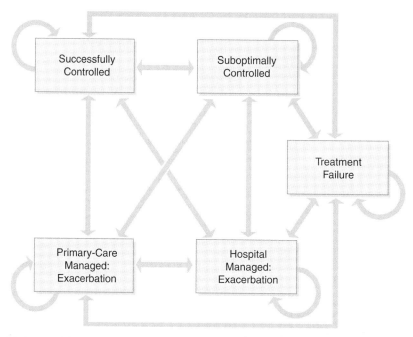

FIGURE 9-6 Markov Model: Asthma. (Adapted with permission from Price MJ, Briggs AH. Development of an economic model to assess the cost effectiveness of asthma management strategies. Pharmacoeconomics 2002;20:183–194.)

the decision analysis section. An example for asthma treatment is presented in the figure. A person who has asthma can transition in and out of different levels of control, each requiring different amounts of resources for treatment. These levels of control are represented by the boxes in Figure 9-6 (successfully controlled, suboptimal control, treatment failure, hospital managed exacerbation, and primary care managed exacerbation). For example, a person who has asthma may be successfully controlled one day, then have an acute exacerbation that is managed in a primary-care clinic, followed by a period of perfect control, and then have an episode that requires admittance to the hospital for treatment.

Again, the probabilities used in a Markov model are obtained the same way probabilities are obtained for a decision tree. In this example, the probability of going from successfully controlled to hospital management could be obtained from the literature (the number of emergency room visits or hospitalizations reported in an asthma study) or from a review of emergency room visits and hospitalizations for acute exacerbations recorded in a claims database.

A decision tree would not be a good option for modeling this condition because each of the different levels of control would have to be included after every branch in the tree, making the model appear like a decision bush. Thus, a Markov model is the most efficient way to model conditions that are cyclical.

Statistical Analysis

The use of statistical models (also called stochastic models) has increased in recent years owing to the development and availability of clinical and administrative databases for outcomes research and because more pharmacoeconomics data are collected during RCTs.

Regression analysis was introduced in Chapter 7. The two uses of regression analysis that are most useful for pharmacoeconomics are developing models to predict responses or costs in patients and describing the relationship between changes in one variable with respect to another variable. For example, regression models can used to determine the difference in total healthcare costs between patients treated with two different medications. In this example, total healthcare costs is the dependent variable and the treatment regimen is the independent variable. Other independent variables could be included in the model to control for confounding factors, such as age, disease severity, and number of other medications the patient is taking. Regression analysis or logistic regression analysis could also be used to identify patients who are good candidates for a new pharmaceutical care intervention. The independent variables in this model may include a measure of disease severity, number of medications, and age of the patient.

Regression models offer an advantage over decision analytic models because they allow patient characteristics to be considered in the analysis.[35] Often, the way in which the data were generated and the nature of the relationship between two variables is unknown, so researchers often make assumptions about the data and use the general linear model (described in Chapter 7) to estimate the relationship between two variables such as the use of a specific medication and total healthcare costs. Regression analysis, an inferential technique, is one of the traditional statistical models used to estimate the relationship between costs (independent variables) and outcomes (dependent variables), allowing predictions to be made.

PERSPECTIVE 9-1

Bayesian analysis is another type of statistical analysis used with increasing frequency in pharmacoeconomic analysis. Bayesian techniques provide a mathematical mechanism to determine the probability that our previous understanding about the relationship between variables was correct given new data or information. This approach differs from linear regression techniques in that it is based on previously determined probabilities and probability distributions associated with the variables of interest. The previous data are the bases of prior probability distributions and new data are the basis of posterior probability distributions. These are manipulated mathematically to clarify the relationship between variables. Thus, Bayesian techniques incorporate old and new information while taking into account uncertainty. Bayesian models can be used when data are missing or highly uncertain. For example, Bayesian analysis can be used to predict outcomes for cancer patients based on cancer cell type as well as characteristics of the patient and disease. Some of the data used in such a Bayesian model must be estimated because they are not known for certain. The statistical functions produced by Bayesian analysis can be used by decision makers to choose an alternative that minimizes loss or maximizes utility.[36]

 ## LITERATURE CRITIQUE 9-5

Earlier, it was determined that the study perspective, alternatives, costs, and outcomes presented in Article 1 are applicable to Plains HealthCare's pharmacoeconomics question and that the analysis was properly conducted. The next set of questions deal with the data collection methods used in Article 1. Again, if the data used in an analysis are not properly collected, then the results may not be useful in answering the pharmacoeconomic question. The following questions guide the next step in the evaluation (Table 9-1):

- What type of study was done (randomized controlled trial, naturalistic, other)?
- Was the study prospective, retrospective, or cross-sectional?
- Was the source of each element of the data provided?
- Was the evidence for the data strong?

The study in Article 1 was a modeling study rather than a randomized controlled study or a naturalistic study. Therefore, the researchers used secondary data to build their model. You could consider this a type of retrospective study. Previous clinical, epidemiology, and observational studies were used as data sources for the Markov model. Thus, the data used to build the model came from appropriate sources. Based on the critique of Article 1 to this point, it appears that the results can be used to help answer Plains HealthCare's pharmacoeconomics question. ◼

SENSITIVITY ANALYSIS: DEALING WITH UNCERTAINTY

Because point estimates of the probabilities, costs, and outcomes are often used to conduct pharmacoeconomic analyses, uncertainty is assessed by a sensitivity analysis.[35] A **sensitivity analysis** is necessary any time cost and outcomes data are estimated. This occurs most frequently when cost and outcomes data are estimated using a decision analytic model. A sensitivity analysis is used to assesses the robustness (ability to change the decision) of the results of a pharmacoeconomic analysis when the value of variables (the costs and probabilities) included in a model are uncertain. The level of uncertainty associated with the costs, probabilities, or outcomes variables used in a model determine which variables will be included in the sensitivity analysis. Those with greater uncertainty will be included in the sensitivity analysis to determine if the model is robust to changes in that variable.

For example, in the decision tree example, the probability of success could have been estimated based on the results of several clinical trials, and the cost of treatment failure could have been estimated by surveying several local emergency rooms. Because these values represent the best guess, it is good to conduct sensitivity analyses on these variables in case our best guess is wrong.

One-way and two-way analyses are most frequently conducted. The decision tree in Figure 9-5 is used to demonstrate a one-way sensitivity analysis. First identify the estimated variables that have the most effect on the model. In this example, the key variables are the cost of treatment failure and the probability associated with a treatment success (or failure). A one-way sensitivity analysis involves changing the value of one key variable at a time to determine if the results of the analysis change. In this example, the cost associated with the failure branch can be increased to $2,000. Then the new expected costs are calculated by rolling back the decision tree again. The incremental cost-effectiveness analysis would be conducted again to determine if the decision changed about which alternative was the most cost effective. These steps are repeated by lowering the cost of the failure branch to $500, then increasing the probability of success by 20%, and then decreasing the probability of success by 20%. The incremental cost-effectiveness analysis is conducted each time to see if any of these changes alter the decision of which alternative is the most cost effective.[29]

If the decision never changes, then the model is **robust**, indicating that the assumptions used to create the model were accurate enough. If the decision changes when one of the variables is altered, then the model is sensitive to that variable. If this is the case, the researcher must make sure the most accurate data were used to build the model and caution readers about the limitations of the estimates produced by the model.

A two-way sensitivity analysis is conducted the same way as a one-way sensitivity analysis, except the values of two variables are altered at the same time. Multiway sensitivity analyses are difficult to interpret, so one-way analyses are seen more frequently in the literature.[37] One type of multiway analysis that is more commonly used is the analysis of the extremes. Two incremental cost-effectiveness computations are compared to the initial cost-effectiveness computation. One incremental cost-effectiveness computation is based on the estimated costs and outcomes obtained from the model that includes the best case values of all variables. The other computation is based on the model that includes the worst case values of all variables.[38]

Because in real life we do not expect only one variable at a time to change or every variable to change in the same direction, several alternative methods have been proposed to assess the variability of the all variables simultaneously. Each variable in a decision analysis is assumed to be fixed at a particular level, the point estimate of that variable. Probabilistic sensitivity analysis takes into account the uncertainty of the probabilities and outcomes used in the decision tree. This type of sensitivity analysis uses an assumed probability density function for each variable and determines the mean and standard deviation of the distribution using algebra.[37,39–41]

 LITERATURE CRITIQUE 9-6

To recap, it has been determined that the study perspective, alternatives, costs, and outcomes given in Article 1 are applicable to Plains HealthCare's pharmacoeconomics question and that data collection and analysis were properly conducted. The next set of questions help assess the level of confidence that can be placed on the results (the believability of the results). The following questions guide the next steps of evaluation (Table 9-1):

- Was discounting needed? Were both costs and outcomes/benefits discounted? What discount rate was used?
- Was sensitivity analysis used and appropriate?
- Was the study robust?
- Were the methods transparent?

It doesn't appear that the costs or outcomes were discounted, even though the model covered a number of years. This is not a fatal flaw that would prevent the use of these results. The costs presented in the results may be overestimated, however.

A sensitivity analysis was conducted using the range of input data obtained from the literature: time frame covered by the analysis (82–94 years) and length of screen-detectable preclinical period. In addition, the data and assumptions used in the model were based on individual distributions of specific variables. The study results did not change during the sensitivity analyses, so the results are robust to these assumptions (or changes). The fact that the results of the study did not change when the values of different variables were altered is a good indication that confidence can be placed in the results.

The methods used in this study are transparent because the source of the data, the Markov model, the assumptions used to create the model, and the variables modified in the sensitivity analyses are clearly stated. The authors explain how they derived the probabilities used in the Markov model, but they do not give the actual probabilities used. This limits the transparency of the model. Nothing presented so far would prevent us from using the results of Article 1 to answer Plains HealthCare's pharmacoeconomic question. ■

External Validity and Application to the Pharmacoeconomics Question

The term **external validity** has been used several times in this chapter. External validity is has to do with applying the results of a study to the population of interest (i.e., the patients with whom you are dealing). If the subjects included in the study are similar to your patient, and if the methods and procedures used in the study are similar to clinical practice in your setting, then it is easy to generalize or apply the results of the study to your setting (i.e., you can use the results of the study to answer your question). If the subjects or procedures differ significantly from your setting, then it is difficult, if not impossible, to use the results of the study to answer your question.

 LITERATURE CRITIQUE 9-7

The final step in critiquing Article 1 is to determine if the results of the article can be generalized to people outside of the group studied, specifically to Plains HealthCare members. The following questions guide this step in the evaluation of Article 1 (Table 9-1):

- What is the external validity?
- Can the study be applied to the population in general?
- Is the problem relevant to my practice site? If so, could the study be applied to my practice site?

The data used to build the model were obtained from women within the correct age range. This increases the external validity of the model and results. Some of the data came from European sources, so if the incidence or characteristics of breast cancer in Europe differ from North America, then this could limit the applicability of the results to a U.S. HMO practice setting. Given the nature of this disease and the variations used in the sensitivity analysis, the use of European data to build the model does not prevent us from using the results to address our question. (Note, however, that a literature search and analysis would be need to be conducted to determine if this assumption is accurate.)

The question facing Plains HealthCare is, Are mammography screenings for women over the age of 65 years cost effective? Article 1 provides evidence for payment for mammograms for women over the age of 65, and that screenings every 3 years is the most cost-effective option. In a real-life situation, additional articles identified during the original literature search would be used to provide additional information for answering this pharmacoeconomics question. ■

Summary

The strength of the evidence from a pharmacoeconomics study is based on the study design and can be evaluated on the transparency of the methods, whether final outcomes are used, the data collection methods, and the accuracy of the assumptions. In this chapter, the basic components of pharmacoeconomic study are explained, including the study perspective, types of costs and outcomes, types of economics analyses, and methods of data collection and modeling. The questions in Table 9-1 can be used as a guide for critiquing articles, and the results can help pharmacists answer pharmacoeconomics questions. This chapter is meant as an introduction to pharmacoeconomics topics; greater details are available in other texts.

STUDY PROBLEMS

1. Obtain a copy of Article 3.[3] Use the questions presented in Table 9-1 to critically evaluate the article. Answer all questions.

2. Based on the article, should Plains HealthCare change their decision to pay for mammograms in women aged 70 and over?

REFERENCES

1. American Community Survey, American Fact Finder [Homepage on the Internet]. Washington, D.C.: U.S. Census Bureau; August 15, 2006. http://factfinder.census.gov/servlet/ADPGeoSearchByListServlet?_lang=en&_ts196861628675. Accessed May9, 2007.
2. Boer R, de Koning HJ, van der Maas PJ. A longer breast carcinoma screening interval for women age older than 65 years? Cancer 1999;86:1506–1510.
3. Ostbye T, Greenberg GN, Taylor DH Jr., Lee AMM. Screening mammography and pap tests among older American women 1996–2000: Results from the Health and Retirement Study (HRS) and Asset and Health Dynamics Among the Oldest Old (AHEAD). Ann Fam Med 2003;1:209–217.
4. Kerlikowske K, Salzmann P, Phillips KA, et al. Continuing screening mammography in women aged 70 to 79 years: Impact on life expectancy and cost-effectiveness. JAMA 1999;282:2156–2163.
5. Chandramouli JC, Tyler LS. How to evaluate an outcomes study. Hosp Pharm 2001;36:131–142.
6. Kaplan RM. The Ziggy theorem: Toward an outcomes-focused health psychology. Health Psychol 1994;13:451–460.
7. By Tom Wilson. Copyright Universal Press Syndicate.
8. Grossman M. The human capital model. In: Newhouse JP, Culyer AJ, eds. Handbook of Health Economics. Vol A. Amsterdam: North-Holland, 2000.
9. Kozma CM, Reeder CE, Schulz RM. Economic, clinical, and humanistic outcomes: A planning model for pharmacoeconomic research. Clin Ther 1993;15:1121–1132.
10. Schulman K, Seils D. Clinical economics. In: Max MB, Lynn J, eds. Sympton Research: Methods and Opportunities [Online Textbook]. Bethesda, MD: National Institutes of Health. Available at: symptomresearch.nih.gov/chapter_12/index.htm. Accessed July 2006.
11. Drummond MF, Sculpher MJ, Torrance GW, et al. Methods for the Economic Evaluation of Health Care Programmes. 3rd ed. Oxford, UK: Oxford University Press, 2005.
12. Bootman JL, Townsend R, McGhan WF, eds. Principles of Pharmacoeconomics. 3rd ed. Cincinnati OH: Whitney, 2004.
13. Pearce DW. Cost-Benefit Analysis. 2nd ed. London: Macmillan, 1983.
14. Bootman JL, McGhan WF, Schondelmeyer SW. Application of cost-benefit and cost-effectiveness analysis to clinical practice. Drug Intell Clin Pharm 1982;16:235–243.
15. Birch S, Gafni A. Cost effectiveness/utility analyses. Do current decision rules lead us to where we want to be? J Health Econ 1992;12:459–467.
16. Weinstein MC, Stason WB. Foundations of cost-effectiveness analysis for health and medical practices. N Engl J Med 1997;296:716–721.
17. Wagstaff A. QALYs and the equity-efficiency trade-off. J Health Econ 1991;10:21–40.
18. Karlsson G, Johannesson M. Decision rules of cost-effectiveness analysis. Pharmacoeconomics 1996;9:113–120.
19. O'Hagan A, Stevens JW, Montmartin J. Inference for the cost-effectiveness acceptability curve and cost-effectiveness ratio. Pharmacoeconomics 2000;17:339–349.
20. Donaldson C, Currie G, Mitton C. Cost effectiveness analysis in health care: contraindications. BMJ 2002;325:891–894.
21. Chapman RH, Berger M, Weinstein MC, et al. When does quality-adjusting life-years matter in cost effectiveness analysis? Health Econ 2004;13:429–436.
22. Martin SC, Gagnon DD, Zhang L, et al. Cost-utility analysis of survival with epoetin-alfa versus placebo in stage IV breast cancer. Pharmacoeconomics 2003;21:1153–1169.
23. National Institute for Health and Clinical Excellence. *National for Health and Clinical Excellence* [Homepage on the Internet]. June 12, 2006. http://www.nice.org.uk/. Accessed June 14, 2006.
24. Helfand M. Incorporating information about cost-effectiveness into evidence-based decision-making: The Evidence-Based Practice Center (EPC) model. Med Care 2005;43:33–42.

25. Freemantle N, Blonde L, Bolinder B, et al. Real-world trials to answer real-world questions. Pharmacoeconomics 2005;23:747–754.
26. Armstrong EP, Manuchehri F. Ambulatory care databases for managed care organizations. Am J Health Sys Pharm 1997;54:1973–1983.
27. Motheral BR, Fairman KA. The use of claims databases for outcomes research: Rationale, challenges and strategies. Clin Ther 1997;19:346–366.
28. Lloyd SS, Rissing JP. Physician and coding errors in patient records. JAMA 1985;254:1330–1336.
29. Weinstein MC, Fineberg HV. Clinical Decision Analysis. Philadelphia: Saunders, 1980.
30. Hagen MD. Decision analysis: a review. Fam Med 1992;24:349–354.
31. Detsky AS, Naglie G, Krahn MD, et al. Primer on medical decision analysis: Part 1—Getting started. Med Decision Making 1997;17:123–125.
32. Moskowitz AJ, Dunn VH, Lau J, Pauker SG. Can "hypersimplified" decision trees be used instead of Markov models? Med Decision Making 1984;4:530.
33. Naglie G, Krahn MD, Naimark D, et al. Primer on medical decision analysis. Part 3—Estimating probabilities and utilities. Med Decision Making 1997;17:136–141.
34. Price MJ, Briggs AH. Development of an economic model to assess the cost effectiveness of asthma management strategies. Pharmacoeconomics 2002;20:183–194.
35. O'Brien BJ, Drummond MF, Labelle RJ, Willan A. In search of power and significance: Issues in the design and analysis of stochastic cost-effectiveness studies in health care. Med Care 1994;32:150–163.
36. Kennedy P. *A Guide to Econometrics*. 3rd ed. Cambridge MA: The MIT Press; 2003.
37. Katz BP, Hui SL. Variance estimation for medical decision analysis. Stat Med 1989;8:229–241.
38. Briggs AH, Sculpher MJ, Buxton M. Uncertainty in the economic evaluation of health care technologies: The role of sensitivity analysis. Health Econ 1994;3:95–104.
39. Willard KE, Critchfield GC. Probabilistic analysis of decision trees using symbolic algebra. Med Decision Making 1986;5:93–100.
40. Critchfield GC, Willard KE. Probabilistic analysis of decision trees using Monte Carlo simulation. Med Decision Making 1986;5:85–92.
41. Doubilet P, Begg CB, Weinstein MC, et al. Probabilistic sensitivity analysis using Monte Carlo simulation, a practical approach. Med Decision Making 1985;5:157–177.

Critical Appraisal of Evidence Derived from Systematic Reviews

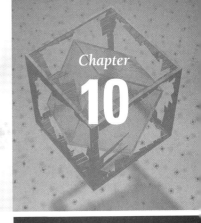

Chapter

10

CHAPTER GOALS

After studying this chapter, the student should be able to:

1. Describe the major types of systematic reviews and indicate their appropriate clinical application.

2. Enumerate the steps in the systematic review process, describing the major purpose of each.

3. Describe the steps in a meta-analysis necessary to identify and evaluate individual research papers.

4. Enumerate the four steps in a statistical analysis and identify them in a published meta-analysis.

To this point, the focus has been on the design and analysis of individual studies. In this chapter, several different approaches to combining individual research studies are described. These approaches are termed systematic reviews. Formally, a **systematic review** is a synthesis or summary of medical literature that uses explicit methods to perform a thorough literature search, evaluate individual studies critically, and synthesize their findings to reach a conclusion. Systematic reviews incorporate strategies to limit bias and random error by assembling and examining critically *all available* high-quality evidence that bears on a specific clinical question.[1-3] Well-executed systematic reviews are transparent in their methods. This means that every step in the process is described in sufficient detail to be replicated by the reader.

It should be noted that a discrepancy exists among clinicians regarding the classification of systematic reviews as primary literature or tertiary literature. The argument for classifying systematic reviews as tertiary literature rests on the fact that the review authors are not performing a new study; they are merely reviewing—either quantitatively or qualitatively—previous research. The argument for classifying systematic reviews as primary literature rests on the fact that the pooled data are evaluated or analyzed in a novel manner.

Regardless of how they are classified—as primary or tertiary literature—systematic reviews are integrative articles that help pharmacists and other healthcare providers obtain in-depth answers to specific, often narrow, clinical questions. Systematic reviews are thus a useful tool in the evidence-based model of clinical practice. They help guide clinical decisions with research evidence, but they don't dictate decisions or obviate the need for sound, compassionate clinical reasoning.

In general, there are two types of systematic reviews: quantitative systematic reviews and qualitative systematic reviews. A **quantitative systematic review** identifies and evaluates individual studies, then integrates and synthesizes the results using inferential statistics to answer a narrow clinical question. In some cases, however, studies are so different in population, research design, execution, or data analysis that a quantitative data synthesis is not possible. An alternative systematic review, a **qualitative systematic review**, is then used. This review process follows a similar methodology but uses descriptive data techniques rather than inferential methods to summarize the data. Conclusions are drawn based on a preponderance of evidence rather than statistical significance.

The goal of this chapter is to describe the general methods used to carry out systematic reviews. Both quantitative and qualitative systematic reviews follow a similar methodology. However, the quantitative method, because it involves a statistical approach, is examined in greater detail. The generalization of the principles to the qualitative systematic review is straightforward and is treated in the final section of the chapter.

Quantitative Systematic Reviews (Meta-Analyses)

A quantitative systematic review is also known as a **meta-analysis.** A meta-analysis combines the outcomes of several independent studies to obtain a statistical estimate of the overall efficacy or safety of a treatment or procedure (Fig. 10-1). Meta-analysis is a way to:

- Explore the consistency among several individual trials and resolve uncertainty when previous trials disagree, are inconclusive, or have small sample sizes.
- Increase power and develop a better estimate of the overall treatment effect.
- Answer new clinical questions not posed in the original trials.

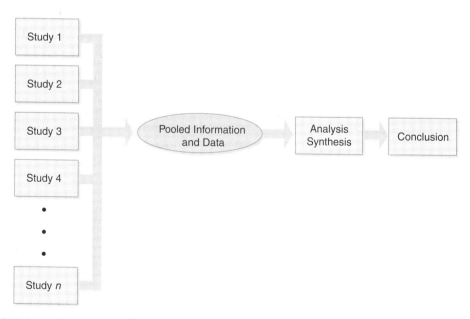

FIGURE 10-1 A Meta-Analysis. Individual research studies (study 1 . . . *n*) are identified, evaluated, and selected for the review. Specific information from those studies is extracted and synthesized using statistical techniques to address a specific question raised by the reviewer.

TABLE 10-1	**Abstract: Quantitative Systematic Review**

BACKGROUND: Albuminuria is an independent risk factor for cardiovascular and renal disease with limited therapeutic options. Data on the effects of statins on albuminuria are conflicting. PURPOSE: To determine whether and to what degree statins affect albuminuria. DATA SOURCES: English-language and non–English-language studies found in PubMed, MEDLINE, EMBASE, BIOSIS, SciSearch, PASCAL, and International Pharmaceutical Abstracts (IPA) databases and the Cochrane Central Register of Controlled Trials that were published between January 1974 and November 2005. STUDY SELECTION: Randomized, placebo-controlled trials of statins reporting baseline and follow-up measurements of albuminuria or proteinuria measured by 24-hour urine collection or the urinary albumin-to-creatinine ratio. DATA EXTRACTION: Two investigators independently abstracted study quality, characteristics, and outcomes. DATA SYNTHESIS: Fifteen studies involving a total of 1384 patients and averaging 24 weeks in duration were included. Meta-analysis of the proportional reduction in proteinuria showed that statins reduced albuminuria (11 studies) and proteinuria (4 studies) in 13 of 15 studies. The reduction in excretion was greater among studies with greater baseline albuminuria or proteinuria: change of 2% (95% CI, −32% to 35%) for those with excretion less than 30 mg/d, −48% (CI, −71% to −25%) for those with excretion of 30 to 300 mg/d, and −47% (CI, −67% to −26%) for those with excretion more than 300 mg/d. Statistical heterogeneity was evident only in the group with excretion greater than 300 mg/d (excretion < 30 mg/d, $I^2 = 23\%$ [$P = 0.27$]; excretion of 30 to 299 mg/d, $I^2 = 0\%$ [$P = 0.64$]; excretion ≥300 mg/d, $I^2 = 63\%$ [$P = 0.020$]). LIMITATIONS: Published studies were not of high quality on average and varied markedly in effect size, as well as in characteristics of the cohorts. Unpublished studies showing no effect could impact these results. CONCLUSION: Statins may have a beneficial effect on pathologic albuminuria. The validity of this finding, and whether this effect translates into reduction of cardiovascular or end-stage renal disease, requires larger studies.

Reprinted with permission from Douglas K, O'Malley PG, Jackson JL. Meta-analysis: The effects of statins on albuminuria. Ann Intern Med 2006;145:117–124.

Meta-analysis is especially useful if definitive trials cannot be conducted or are not yet complete.

Meta-analyses have enjoyed a long history of contributions to social sciences and education as well as to areas of medicine unfamiliar to many pharmacists. However, their application to areas of interest to pharmacists is increasing rapidly. An example of a meta-analysis is the study by Douglas et al.[4] As described in the abstract of the article (Table 10-1), the goal of the study was to determine whether statins reduce the progression to end-stage renal disease as indexed by albuminuria. The authors screened and evaluated 125 papers appearing between January 1974 and November 2005 and identified 15 randomized controlled trials suitable for synthesis. Differences among the 15 studies were quite inconsistent, precluding an overall pooled analysis. Subsequent a priori analyses provided evidence of a role of statins in reducing albuminuria only among those with the highest baseline albuminuria levels (shown in figure 2 of the article). Overall, the included studies proved to be of low quality. These findings, although not definitive, demonstrate the need for larger studies that address the clinical implications of statin-induced albuminuria reductions more adequately.

In general, the approach used to conduct, and therefore to evaluate, quantitative and qualitative systematic reviews involves the following steps:[5]

1. Refine and formulate the research question.
2. Develop inclusion criteria for considering studies for the analysis.
3. Conduct the literature search.
4. Evaluate the studies for acceptability and quality.
5. Perform qualitative and/or quantitative data analysis.
6. Formulate conclusions and interpretations.

Conducting a quantitative systematic review is a complex and time-consuming process. Because of this, meta-analyses are often not yet available to assist pharmacists in answering all clinical queries. However, the number of systematic reviews (including meta-analysis) has increased at least 500-fold in the last decade, and such reports will continue to be useful tools in providing evidence-based care for patients.[6,7] Understanding the complexities associated with conducting a meta-analysis will assist the pharmacist in evaluating this type of systematic review critically. The following sections examine each step of the meta-analytic process in greater detail and highlight specific points of critical evaluation for each.

THE RESEARCH QUESTION

Meta-analysis typically begins with an overview of the literature to characterize the present status of knowledge and to identify issues that require resolution to achieve consensus as a result of the meta-analysis. For example, Morrison et al. used a meta-analysis to resolve the issue of whether patients suffering acute myocardial infarction (AMI) benefited from a thrombolytic agent provided before hospital admission.[8]

As in any research study, it is essential that all major questions and hypotheses be formulated a priori, or before the statistical analysis begins. Findings from post hoc analyses, or those conducted after the primary data analysis, cannot be used to draw firm conclusions in the present analysis, although they may be used to generate hypotheses for subsequent studies.

Morrison et al. state that AMI accounts for a large proportion of cardiovascular disease–related deaths.[8] These deaths can be reduced by thrombolytic therapy, but the therapy's effectiveness decreases with time since the cardiovascular insult. There is some evidence that prehospital administration of thrombolysis is effective in saving lives, but there has not been a critical review of randomized controlled trials. Thus "the primary objective of this meta-analysis was to evaluate all randomized controlled trials of pre-hospital versus in-hospital thrombolysis in AMI patients, using all-cause mortality as the primary outcome variable."[8]

When formulating a research question as part of a meta-analysis, the clinical question must be focused, specific, and answerable using statistical analyses, meaning the research hypotheses must be stated explicitly. The research question must also be clinically relevant and timely. Most often, the clinical question will follow the PICO format (Table 10-2).[9] This format includes a consideration of the major variables that determine the relevance of the meta-analysis to answering a specific clinical question. As part of this determination, the pharmacist should be clear with respect to the research problem addressed and the population studied. Specifically, the research question should fit the need of the pharmacist for information, and the populations examined should be similar to those the pharmacist serves.

Interventions and exposures can be quite difficult to interpret, particularly when studies using different preparations, dosages, and routes of administration are combined. Also important is the inclusion of a control group. Questions concerning the controls are

---

TABLE 10-2	**PICO Format for Asking an Answerable, Specific Clinical Question**

P = People, patients, populations, or problem

I = Intervention or exposure

C = Control group or comparison intervention

O = Outcomes

Adapted with permission from Sackett DL, Straus SE, Richardson WS, et al., eds. Asking answerable clinical questions. In: Evidence-Based Medicine: How to Practice and Teach EBM. 2nd ed. Edinburgh, UK: Churchill Livingstone, 2000: 13–27.

TABLE 10-3	**Framework for Evaluating a Research Question**

- Is the research question clinically needed and timely?
- Is the research question focused and specific?
- Does the research question follow the PICO format?

similar to those involving the study population in general. In addition, however, the pharmacist should be sensitive to changes in the control group that may be the result of a placebo effect. Finally, the pharmacist must evaluate the clinical relevance of the outcomes included in the meta-analysis and consider whether a similar magnitude of effect is to be anticipated in her clinical population. When critically evaluating the research question for a meta-analysis, the pharmacist can use the questions listed in Table 10-3 as a guide.

INCLUSION CRITERIA

To minimize selection bias in systematic reviews such as a meta-analysis, detailed and explicit criteria for the inclusion of studies into the analysis must be developed before the literature search. These inclusion criteria must be consistent with the question focus and should include the details discussed in the following sections.

Types of Study Designs

Are all types of study designs to be included in the meta-analysis? Only randomized trials? What about observational studies? Remember that each type of study design comes with unique strengths and weaknesses. Refer to the Chapter 3 to review the nuances of the various study designs.

Study Subject Characteristics

Are restrictions (per the meta-analysis protocol) in patient characteristics such as gender, age, and national origin important? What are the specific criteria? Are the criteria appropriate for the research question? These types of questions are important in helping the pharmacist decide whether the patients included in the analysis are similar to those seen in his or her clinical practice. In addition, the meta-analysis should seek to include individual studies that involved similar patients.

Published vs. Unpublished Studies

There is little doubt that published studies will be identified, but what about gray and unpublished literature? Gray literature is "any documentary material that is not commercially published and is typically composed of technical reports, working papers, business documents, and conference proceedings."[10] The problems with gray literature are that it is difficult to find (because it may not be indexed extensively by secondary resource databases) and that it is usually unedited. However, gray literature is part of the total literature search strategy.

Are unpublished research results admissible? What kinds of bias will excluding studies introduce into the meta-analysis? For example, studies that show negative findings are less likely to be published than studies that show positive findings. Including studies in the meta-analysis that do not show a treatment effect dilutes the composite effect size of the published studies. Excluding studies that show no effect is tantamount to inflating the effect size of the treatment.[11]

Language Limits

Will only English-language studies be admissible, or will foreign-language studies also be considered for inclusion into the meta-analysis? Often, review authors will consider only English-language articles, especially if it is their language of primary use. But with this restriction, potentially relevant non-English-language studies might be missed.

Treatment vs. Control Groups

What types of treatments will be examined? Are they compatible in terms of duration, safety, and efficacy? Are the treatments similar in terms of time course and biologic activity? Is it legitimate to combine data from drugs in the same class? What comparison groups are used: placebo or active controls? For example, if the meta-analysis seeks to determine if a new angiotensin-converting enzyme (ACE) inhibitor is better than a standard ACE inhibitor for reducing albuminuria, inclusion criteria should be created to allow only studies that compared equipotent doses of the ACE inhibitors.

Time Frame

What is the time frame for the included studies? For example, will the analysis include studies published only in the last 10 years? Will the analysis include studies that are only a year or more in duration? The pharmacist must evaluate if the time parameters used are appropriate and think about if any potentially relevant evidence will be excluded from the analysis because of the time frame imposed by the analysis protocol.

The answers to these and other questions go a long way to contributing to an unbiased, systematic literature search. However, even though specific inclusion criteria are met, significant differences can still exist between both patient populations and methods to reduce bias for each individual study included in the meta-analysis. Such discrepancies can lead to an interesting debate about the value and risks of pooling different studies, a topic discussed later in this chapter. When critically evaluating a meta-analysis then, the clinician must assess the inclusion criteria. The major points are summarized in Table 10-4.

TABLE 10-4	**Framework for Critically Evaluating the Inclusion and Exclusion Criteria in a Meta-Analysis**

- Did the authors provide explicit detail on how studies were eligible for the analysis?
- Was their rationale provided and reasonable?
- Do the inclusion criteria fit the research question?
- Did authors specify the type of study designs to be eligible for inclusion and whether unpublished studies were eligible?
- Did the authors specify study subject characteristics?
- Did the authors specify the time frame or study duration for the included trials?
- Did the authors specify language limits?
- Did the authors specify drug therapies or treatments to be included? Is it reasonable to group the included treatments?

THE LITERATURE SEARCH

The next step in conducting a meta-analysis is to find all the literature that is relevant to the research issue under examination. Ideally, authors must make every effort to search the world's literature—published, gray, and unpublished. Multiple secondary sources such as MEDLINE, EMBASE, and International Pharmaceutical Abstracts (IPA) should be used to find published studies. In addition, review authors can search the Cochrane Central Register of Controlled Trials (CCTR), a database that includes reports published in conference proceedings and in many other sources not currently listed in MEDLINE or other bibliographic databases. Another technique is a manual search of journals and other sources likely to contain studies of interest. Finally, the reference sections of the identified papers can be examined.

Authors should also expend reasonable effort to find unpublished literature by contacting pharmaceutical companies or consulting experts in the field who may know of unpublished studies. Despite even the best efforts though, there is no guarantee that all relevant studies will be identified.

In conducting the literature search, several critical issues arise. The most important of these is whether all of the relevant research articles have been identified by the search. As mentioned previously, a corollary issue is whether unpublished results should be included. In the current scientific environment, data that do not evidence statistically significant differences in efficacy or safety are oftentimes considered not to merit publication. (The only exception that the we are aware of is the negative findings of a randomized placebo controlled trial.) This phenomenon is known as **publication bias.** Excluding studies with negative results, however, may lead to an overestimation of the effect size. On the other hand, it may be that statistically significant results were not obtained because the study was poorly designed or conducted and therefore the findings suffer from excess measurement error, which obscures the treatment effect.

An associated problem is **file-drawer phenomenon**, the tendency of researchers not to submit papers for publication or to otherwise promulgate findings that do not show statistically significant effects but to keep them in a file drawer. Once again, the general consensus is that meta-analyses including only published research reports probably overestimate the true treatment effect.

Returning Morrison et al.'s AMI meta-analysis,[8] to identify all relevant research efforts, The Cochrane search strategy, a highly regarded comprehensive and systematic method of finding and reviewing literature, was used. This strategy includes the following:

- Electronic bibliographic databases search
- Inspection of reference sections of primary research articles and narrative review articles
- Review of conference proceedings
- Search of research registries
- Inquiries to researchers and manufacturers
- Search of the Internet

Contrast this with the literature search method of Douglas et al. (Table 10-1). In their statins and albuminuria paper;[4] the authors restricted their analysis to published reports in any language between January 1974 and November 2005 that had appeared in the most popular abstracting and indexing databases.

When critically evaluating a meta-analysis then, the clinician must assess whether the search strategy was thorough and appropriate. Table 10-5 provides some guidelines. Confidence in the results of a meta-analysis is increased when the pharmacist can be certain that no relevant and high-quality studies—published or unpublished—were overlooked.[12]

TABLE 10-5	Framework for Critically Evaluating the Search Strategy of a Meta-Analysis

- Is it likely that important, relevant studies were missed?
- Were search strategies explicit?
- Were multiple secondary databases used to find primary literature?
- Were both published and unpublished research reports included?

Adapted with permission from Hunt DL. McKibbon KA. Locating and appraising systematic reviews. Ann Intern Med 1997;126:532–538.

SELECTING AND APPRAISING THE STUDIES FOR INCLUSION

Once the review authors have established criteria for study inclusion and have thoroughly searched the world's literature to find all relevant articles, the next step is to select the specific studies to be included in the analysis. To minimize bias, authors typically follow an inclusion protocol and are blinded to the reports' authors and affiliations and to the results and other telling features of each study. The thought here is that if review authors are blinded, they are not as apt to include only studies that demonstrate positive findings or studies that were performed by colleagues. Instead, each study is judged only with respect to how well it meets the predefined inclusion criteria.

An index to the quality of a systematic review is the methodology involved in evaluating the suitability of studies for analysis. In higher-quality reviews two or more experts first rate each paper independently and then resolve discrepancies, as in the Morrison et al. meta-analysis.[8]

Once the relevant research papers have been selected for inclusion to the meta-analysis, the next steps are to categorize the major outcome variables and findings in each paper in such a way that the different studies can be compared on these metrics and to provide an index of the relative quality of the studies included in the meta-analysis. Evaluating the included studies with respect to major variables is termed data extraction or **coding**. Coding research papers involves categorizing various characteristics of the methods so that similar features can be combined. This process essentially overlooks small differences in methods and procedures so that variables can be compared across studies.

Coding is best done with the reviewers blinded to the report authors, authors' affiliations, journal, and other information that might bias the evaluation. Also, coding should be carried out independently by at least two experts, and the extent of their agreement should be determined by calculating a kappa (κ) statistic or an interclass correlation coefficient.

The κ statistic indicates the level of agreement between authors of the review beyond that expected by chance.[13] κ ranges from 0 to 1; the closer the value is to 1, the greater the level of agreement between review authors. Guidelines for the interpretation of κ statistic are presented in Table 10-6. In the Morrison et al. study, the extent of agreement between the raters based on an evaluation of article content was 0.86. This indicates a very high level of agreement between the authors of this meta-analysis.

While coding procedures do not capture the nuances of the different study methodologies, some loss of detail is inevitable if the results of individual studies, each using a different methodology, are to be compared. In the Morrison et al. study, for example, the authors claim that differences in pharmaceutical interventions were small and not sufficient to prevent the combining of the study results. Morrison et al. sent the extracted data to the primary author of the individual study to verify the outcome.

The next step in the evaluation process is the rating of the research reports for quality. The quality criteria used by Morrison et al. in their AMI analysis are the Detsky Criteria (Table 10-7).[14] Note that some of the responses to the Detsky Criteria require a judgment

TABLE 10-6	Interpretation of the Kappa (κ) Index of Interobserver Agreement
κ VALUE	DEGREE OF AGREEMENT BEYOND CHANCE
0	None
0–0.2	Slight
0.2–0.4	Fair
0.4–0.6	Moderate
0.6–0.8	Substantial
0.8–1.0	Almost perfect

Reprinted with permission from McGinn T, Wyer PC, Newman TB, et al. Tips for learners of evidence-based medicine: 3. Measures of observer variability (kappa). Can Med Assoc J 2004;171:1369–1373.

by the raters. Quality ratings for papers included in Morrison et al.'s analysis ranged from 0.43 to 0.93 on a scale in which 1.0 is the highest score possible. An interclass correlation coefficient of 0.86 suggested excellent agreement among the review authors rating the quality of the studies contained in the AMI analysis.

At this point, the characteristics of the studies to be included in the meta-analysis are typically presented. This consists of a listing of the articles used for the meta-analysis. Such a summary allows the reader to judge whether the studies selected are sufficiently similar in key characteristics to merit a quantitative synthesis. Such characteristics include subjects, methods, data analytic techniques, and quality.

TABLE 10-7	Detsky Criteria Used to Assess the Quality of Individual Studies Included a Meta-Analysis

- Were the patients assigned to treatments randomly? ☐ yes ☐ no
- Describe the randomization. ☐ adequate ☐ partial ☐ inadequate
- Do you believe there could have been bias in the treatment assignment (e.g., if clinicians weren't blind to treatment assignment before enrolling patients into the trials)? ☐ yes ☐ no
- Was there a description of the criteria for measuring outcomes? ☐ yes ☐ no
- Were the criteria objective? ☐ yes ☐ no
- Were the outcome assessors blind to the treatment received? ☐ yes ☐ no
- Were the inclusion and exclusion criteria clearly defined? ☐ yes ☐ partial ☐ no
- Do you know how many patients were excluded from the trial (not enrolled for logistical reasons, refused consent, not eligible)? ☐ yes ☐ partial ☐ no
- Was the therapeutic regimen fully described for the treatment group? ☐ yes ☐ partial ☐ no
- Was the therapeutic regimen fully described for the control group? ☐ yes ☐ partial ☐ no
- Is there a statistical analysis and is the test stated? ☐ yes ☐ no
- Is the p value stated? ☐ yes ☐ no
- Is the statistical analysis appropriate? ☐ yes ☐ partial ☐ no
- If the trial is negative, were confidence intervals or post-hoc power calculations performed? ☐ yes ☐ no ☐ not applicable
- Was there a sample size justification before the study? ☐ yes ☐ no

Adapted with permission from Detsky AS, Naylor CD, O'Rourke K, et al. Incorporating variations in the quality of individual randomized trials into meta-analysis. J Clin Epidemiol 1992;45:255–265.

TABLE 10-8 Trial Characteristics for Studies Included in a Meta-Analysis

STUDY (YEAR)[a]	PROVIDER	THROMBOLYTIC AGENT	QUALITY SCORE	TIME FROM SYMPTOM ONSET TO THROMBOLYSIS (SE) [MEDIAN]			ALL-CAUSE HOSPITAL MORTALITY		
				MEAN MINUTES		INTERVAL DIFFERENCE (MIN) AND/OR P VALUE	PREHOSPITAL (NO./TOTAL)	IN HOSPITAL (NO./TOTAL)	OR (95% CI)
				PREHOSPITAL	IN HOSPITAL				
MITI trial (1993)	Paramedics	rt-PA	0.91	92 (58) [77]	120 (49) [110]	$p < 0.001$; 33 (18)	10/175	15/175	0.69 (0.30–1.57)
EMIP group (1993)	MICU	Anistreplase	0.85	[130]	[190]	[55]	251/2750	284/2719	0.86 (0.72–1.03)
GREAT study (1992)	GPs	Anistreplase	0.78	101 [25–360]	240 [80–540]	130 [40–370]	11/163	17/148	0.56 (0.25–1.23)
Roth et al. (1990)	MICU	rt-PA	0.65	94 (36)	137 (45)	$p < 0.001$	4/72	3/44	0.80 (0.17–3.77)
Schofer et al. (1990)	MICU	Urokinase	0.63	85 (51)	137 (50)	$p < 0.001$	1/40	2/38	0.46 (0.14–5.31)
Castaigne et al. (1989)	MICU	Anistreplase	0.48	[131]	[180]	60	3/57	3/43	0.74 (0.14–3.86)

[a]See Morrison et al. for references.

CI, confidence interval; EMIP, European Myocardial Infarction Project; GPs, general practitioners; GREAT, Grampian Region Early Anistreplase Trial; MICI, mobile intensive care unit; MITI, Myocardial Infarction Triage and Intervention; OR, odds ratio; rt-PA, recombinant tissue-type plasminogen activator.

Adapted with permission from Morrison LJ, Verbeek PR, McDonald AC, et al. Mortality and pre-hospital thrombolysis for acute myocardial infarction. A meta-analysis. JAMA 2000;283 2686–2692.

TABLE 10-9	Studies Excluded from a Meta-Analysis
EXCLUDED STUDY (YEAR)[a]	**REASON FOR EXCLUSION**
Castalgne et al. (1987)	Mortality numbers unclear
Barbash et al. (1990)	All mortality at 60 days and 2 years only
Bolssel (1995)	Same data set as the European Myocardial Infarction Project trial
Gotsman et al. (1996)	Same study as Rozenman et al.
McAleer et al. (1992)	Open allocation, not a randomized controlled trial, only vascular mortality cited
McNeill et al. (1989)	Cardiac mortality cited (not all mortality), trial question unclear, suspect this to be a trial of recombinant tissue-type plasminogen activator
Risenfors et al. (1991)	Randomization by convenience, additional concurrent control group, not intent-to-treat analysis
Rozenman et al. (1995)	Not a randomized controlled trial, consecutive patients

[a]See Morrison et al. for references.

Adapted with permission from Morrison LJ, Verbeek PR, McDonald AC, et al. Mortality and pre-hospital thrombolysis for acute myocardial infarction. A meta-analysis. JAMA 2000;283 2686–2692.

In addition, review authors should also provide a list of studies excluded from the meta-analysis so that readers may decide whether such exclusions were justified. Not only did Morrison et al. tabulate the key characteristics of the papers included in the meta-analysis but they also presented the papers that were excluded and provided explanations of the reasons for their exclusion (Tables 10-8 and 10-9).

In summary, when selecting and appraising included studies, review authors have four main objectives (Table 10-10):

- To ensure that all relevant studies are considered for the analysis
- To understand the validity of the included studies

TABLE 10-10	Framework for Critically Evaluating the Study Selection and Appraisal Process in a Meta-Analysis

- Was the validity of included studies assessed?
  - Quality of study designs included?
  - Study methodologies sound?
  - Did included studies have similar inclusion and exclusion criteria and similar patients?
- Were the assessments of included studies reproducible?
  - Any problems with reviewers' judgments?
  - Bias apparent?
  - Conflict of interest seen?
  - Kappa statistic or correlation coefficient calculated and show good agreement?
- Were the results similar from study to study?
  - Did each study use the same drug and/or measure the same outcomes?

Adapted with permission from Hunt DL. McKibbon KA. Locating and appraising systematic reviews. Ann Intern Med 1997;126:532–538.

- To uncover reasons for differences among study results other than chance
- To provide readers with sufficient information with which to judge the applicability of the meta-analysis to their particular clinical practice.

THE STATISTICAL ANALYSIS

There are two different methods of examining a meta-analysis. One involves constructing a composite data set by combining data files from the original studies and then analyzing the composite data set using standard statistical procedures, such as those described in earlier chapters. For example, two studies showed that linezolid and vancomycin have equivalent outcomes in their ability to successfully treat methicillin-resistant *Staphylococcus aureus* (MRSA).[15,16] Based on the results of an analysis indicating that a difference in survival might be related to the acute physiology and chronic health evaluation (APACHE) II scores of the participants, the data from the two individual studies were combined into one data set and reanalyzed.[17] The results of the combined analysis indicated that "patients in the MRSA subset had better survival (80.0% vs. 63.5%, $p = 0.03$) and clinical cure rates (59.0% vs. 35.5%, $p < 0.01$) if they were treated with linezolid rather than with vancomycin."[17]. Thus, by combining the data sets, the statistical power of the data analysis was increased to the point to which a statistically significant difference between the two conditions could be detected.

A more common approach to statistical analysis within the meta-analysis framework is examination of the statistical results of individual research reports in lieu of the raw data. This process involves four steps. First, treatment effects from individual studies are converted to a common metric, like effect size, and then synthesized into an overall expression of the treatment effect. In addition, the data are examined to explore variation in the results from individual studies and to assess the presence of publication bias. Finally, a sensitivity analysis is conducted to determine whether the findings of the meta-analysis are influenced by other variables.

Although it is desirable to use the original measurement scale from each of the individual studies in the meta-analysis, this is not always possible. For example, studies of changes in blood pressure after the introduction of a new treatment may be reported in mmHg, percent change, or risk reduction. To compare the results of these studies, the various effects must be converted to a common measurement scale, or metric.

The type of metric used depends on the scale of measurement of the data. For continuous measurements such as blood pressure, the effect is calculated in terms of standard deviation units, like effect size. Nominal data, like frequencies, in contrast, are converted to odds or risk ratios. Survival data are best expressed in terms of hazards. In each case, the power of the synthesized statistic is greatly increased, enabling the detection of differences that might not be found in individual research efforts.

In the Morrison et al. meta-analysis involving prehospital thrombolysis, odds ratios (ORs) were used as the metric to compare treatment effects among individual studies and were presented as a **forest plot**. On the left side of Figure 10-2, each individual study is identified with the number of participants and quality score. To the right is the corresponding OR and 95% confidence interval (CI) for each study. The right side of the figure also contains a scale indicating that ORs < 1 suggest that prehospital thrombolysis is preferred and ORs > 1 suggest that in-hospital thrombolysis is more effective. The vertical line indicates the point of no difference between the groups, or an equal level of risk for both procedures. The results of each study are interpreted as indicating a statistically significant effect if the confidence interval surrounding the OR does not intersect the vertical line. As the forest plot depicts, none of the individual studies support the preference of one thrombolytic method over the other.

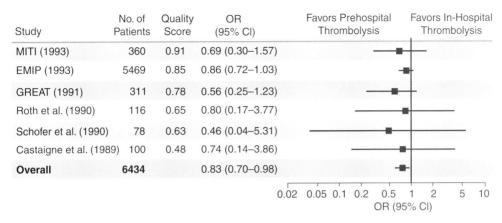

Study	No. of Patients	Quality Score	OR (95% CI)	Favors Prehospital Thrombolysis Favors In-Hospital Thrombolysis
MITI (1993)	360	0.91	0.69 (0.30–1.57)	
EMIP (1993)	5469	0.85	0.86 (0.72–1.03)	
GREAT (1991)	311	0.78	0.56 (0.25–1.23)	
Roth et al. (1990)	116	0.65	0.80 (0.17–3.77)	
Schofer et al. (1990)	78	0.63	0.46 (0.04–5.31)	
Castaigne et al. (1989)	100	0.48	0.74 (0.14–3.86)	
Overall	**6434**		0.83 (0.70–0.98)	

0.02 0.05 0.1 0.2   0.5   1   2   5   10
OR (95% CI)

FIGURE 10-2   A Forest Plot. The *filled squares* indicate the odds ratio for each study, the *horizontal line* that bisects each square indicates the 95% confidence interval (*CI*), and the *vertical line* indicates the point of no difference at which neither prehospital nor in-hospital thrombolysis is favored. Thus, according to this forest plot, each individual study found no statistically significant difference in mortality between prehospital and in-hospital thrombolysis (because the 95% CI crosses 1 for each study). However, the overall effect found by combining the data from the studies does show a statistically significant difference favoring prehospital thrombolysis (because the 95% CI does not cross 1). *EMIP*, The European Myocardial Infarction Project, *GREAT*, Grampian Region Early Anistreplase Trial; *MITI*, Mycardial Infarction Triage and Intervention; see Morrison et al. for references. (Adapted with permission from Morrison LJ, Verbeek PR, McDonald AC, et al. Mortality and pre-hospital thrombolysis for acute myocardial infarction. A meta-analysis. JAMA 2000;283:2686–2692.)

The horizontal line labeled "Overall" presents the overall statistical result of the meta-analysis. Using one of several techniques,[18] the authors synthesized the statistical results of the individual trials into a composite estimate of the treatment effect, which is tested for statistical significance. In the Morrison et al. study, the composite OR equals 0.83 with a 95% CI ranging from 0.70 to 0.98. Because this confidence interval did not include 1.0, the overall results indicate a statistically significant reduction in mortality as a result of prehospital administration of thrombolytic agents.[8]

The second step in the statistical analysis is to check for heterogeneity. **Heterogeneity** refers to the variation between studies owing to factors related to differences in experiments rather than to chance. For example, the results of two studies might differ as a result of differences in protocol regarding drug type or dose regimen. Because better estimates of the composite treatment effect are obtained with studies whose methods are consistent, several measures of heterogeneity have been developed.

Heterogeneity in studies may be assessed by computing statistical indices and by visually examining a graphical display of the data.[19] Traditionally, the most common statistical index is Cochrane's Q, which is distributed as chi squared (χ^2). A statistically significant Q suggests that the individual study results should not be combined. The I^2 statistic is related to Q but expresses the amount of homogeneity among studies as a percent.[20] This index was used in the Douglas et al. meta-analysis of statins and albuminuria (described earlier), and there it indicated that the data should not be pooled.[4]

Heterogeneity in a meta-analysis can also be evaluated graphically. One method is to construct a **L'Abbe diagram** or plot. A L'Abbe plot was used in the Morrison et al. study to compare prehospital and in-hospital mortality rates for each study (Fig. 10-3).[8] If there were no treatment effect, the mortality rates for the groups in each study would be similar, and their intersection would lie on a line of identity. In Figure 10-3, however, each study displays a lower mortality rate for prehospital thrombolysis than for in-hospital

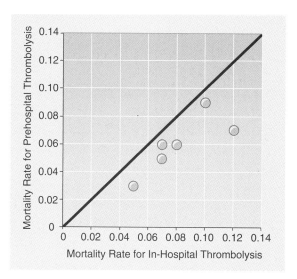

FIGURE 10-3   L'Abbe Diagram. The point estimates of mortality rates for in-hospital thrombolytic treatment are plotted against the mortality rates for prehospital treatment. All data points are consistently below the diagonal line, indicating that the studies are homogenous (or are not heterogeneous). (Adapted with permission from Morrison LJ, Verbeek PR, McDonald AC, et al. Mortality and pre-hospital thrombolysis for acute myocardial infarction. A meta-analysis. JAMA 2000;283:2686–2692.)

thrombolysis. This indicates a consistent pattern in which prehospital treatment mortality rates are lower than in-hospital treatment mortality rates. The finding of such consistency suggests that the study results are homogeneous, and supports the main overall effect found by the meta-analysis.

Heterogeneity may be controlled by adopting a random effects model for the statistical analysis. A *random effects model* assumes that the studies in the meta-analysis represent a random sample of all possible studies and can control the effects of heterogeneity statistically. An alternative model, the *fixed effects model,* is appropriate when the data are homogeneous. Under conditions in which heterogeneity is minimal, both models provide similar estimates of effect size. When heterogeneity exists, the random effects model is less likely to exhibit a statistically significant treatment effect and to provide a wider CI. It is said to be more conservative than the fixed effect model.

The recommendation, however, is to explore potential sources of heterogeneity using subgroups analyses. This method is exemplified by the statins and albuminuria meta-analysis: After finding significant sources of heterogeneity, the investigators sought to determine whether the variability between studies was the result of baseline urinary excretion and loss to follow-up. Results indicate that differences in baseline urinary excretion rate contributed to heterogeneity. Subgroup analyses, however, have the potential to inflate the α, or type I, error rate, leading to the rejection of true null hypotheses.

A third step of the data analysis involves a study of whether publication bias affected the results. This possibility is usually explored with a **funnel plot** and is not typically presented as part of the data reporting in a meta-analysis. A funnel plot is simply a scatter plot of the variability among individual study treatment effects against an index of sample size or effect size (Fig. 10-4). The variability among study results, and therefore the extent of the variability in study results, should be greatest at the base of the graph (where for example the sample size is small) and become less variable as the sample size increases and the effect size estimates become more stable.

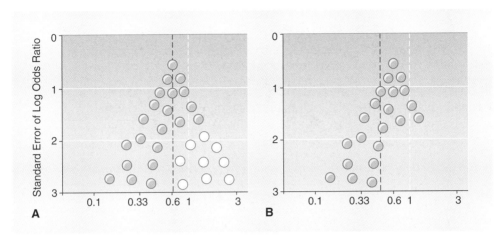

FIGURE 10-4 Funnel Plots: Relationship between Effect Size (x) and standard error (y). **A.** No publication bias. **B.** Publication bias indicated by a lack of studies in the lower right area of the funnel. (Adapted with permission from Sterne JA, Egger M, Smith GD. Investigating and dealing with publication and other biases in meta-analysis. Br Med J 2001;323:101–105.)

The ideal funnel plot resembles an inverted, symmetrical funnel (Fig. 10-4A). Deviations from symmetry indicate a systematic exclusion of studies that should have been included in the analysis, and suggested a biased effect size estimate (Fig. 10-4B).

The final step of analyzing the data in a meta-analysis is to perform a **sensitivity analysis**. Because there are different approaches to conducting a meta-analysis, it is important to ask how sensitive the results are to assumptions that were made when coding the data or to changes in the way the analysis was carried out. Sensitivity analyses provide an approach to testing how robust the overall results are relative to key decisions and assumptions that were made in the process of conducting the analysis. Types of decisions and assumptions that may be examined by sensitivity analysis include the following:[21]

- Changing the inclusion criteria
- Including or excluding studies in which there was some ambiguity as to whether the study met the inclusion criteria
- Excluding unpublished studies
- Excluding studies of lower methodologic quality
- Reanalyzing the data using different statistical approaches, imputing reasonable ranges of values to missing data or resolving uncertainty about study results exists

Morrison et al. carried out two sensitivity analyses of their AMI meta-analysis. The first examined the effect of the quality rating scale in the data by examining changes in the composite OR owing to the inclusion of poorer-quality studies. However, selectively removing these trials from the data synthesis did not affect the results, suggesting that the findings were not affected by trial quality. The forest plot of this sensitivity analysis is presented in Figure 10-5.

A second sensitivity analysis was conducted to examine whether the outcome changed as a function of the person administering the thrombolytic drug. No differences, however, were found when results obtained from physician providers were compared to those from non-physician providers. This suggests that the staff of emergency response vehicles is competent to administer the drug to the patient. The forest plot of this sensitivity analysis is presented in Figure 10-6.

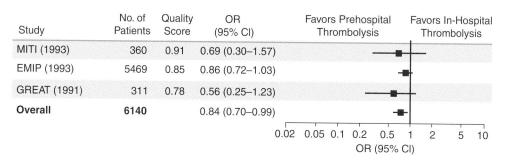

Study	No. of Patients	Quality Score	OR (95% CI)	Favors Prehospital Thrombolysis / Favors In-Hospital Thrombolysis
MITI (1993)	360	0.91	0.69 (0.30–1.57)	
EMIP (1993)	5469	0.85	0.86 (0.72–1.03)	
GREAT (1991)	311	0.78	0.56 (0.25–1.23)	
Overall	**6140**		0.84 (0.70–0.99)	

FIGURE 10-5   Forest Plot. Note that when the data from only the highest-quality studies are pooled, the overall odds ratio (*OR*) and 95% confidence interval (*CI*) are similar to the pooled results of all the studies included in Figure 10-2. Thus study quality did not affect the overall mortality rate. *EMIP*, European Myocardial Infarction Project; *GREAT*, Grampian Region Early Anistreplase Trial; *MITI*, Myocardial Infarction Triage and Intervention; see Morrison et al. for references. (Adapted with permission from Morrison LJ, Verbeek PR, McDonald AC, et al. Mortality and pre-hospital thrombolysis for acute myocardial infarction. A meta-analysis. JAMA 2000;283:2686–2692.)

In summary, the Morrison et al. AMI meta-analysis[8] showed that prehospital administration of thrombolytics favored survival after acute myocardial infarction independent of the administrator of the thrombolytic agent or the quality of the study. The results suggested that one life could be saved for every 62 patients who received prehospital thrombolysis. Table 10-11 summarizes the steps used when evaluating the statistical methods reported in a meta-analysis.

CONCLUSIONS AND INTERPRETATIONS

The final step for meta-analysis authors involves drawing conclusions and making recommendations from the synthesized evidence. Care must be taken to not make recommendations beyond scope of the meta-analysis findings.

In addition, check that the authors' interpretations and recommendations were commensurate with the strength of evidence displayed in the meta-analysis. Table 10-12 provides an example scheme for determining levels of evidence in a systematic review

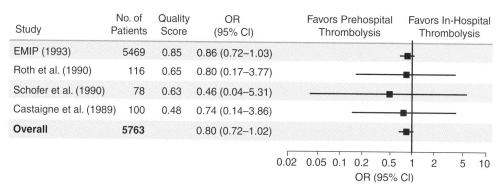

Study	No. of Patients	Quality Score	OR (95% CI)	Favors Prehospital Thrombolysis / Favors In-Hospital Thrombolysis
EMIP (1993)	5469	0.85	0.86 (0.72–1.03)	
Roth et al. (1990)	116	0.65	0.80 (0.17–3.77)	
Schofer et al. (1990)	78	0.63	0.46 (0.04–5.31)	
Castaigne et al. (1989)	100	0.48	0.74 (0.14–3.86)	
Overall	**5763**		0.80 (0.72–1.02)	

FIGURE 10-6   Results of a Sensitivity Analysis. This forest plot shows that when data are pooled from only studies using non-physician-administration of thrombolysis, the overall odds ratio (*OR*) and 95% confidence interval (*CI*) are similar to the overall pooled results of all the studies included in Figure 10-2. Thus the overall mortality outcome did not change as a function of the person administering the thrombolytic drug. *EMIP*, European Myocardial Infarction Project; see Morrison et al. for references. (Adapted with permission from Morrison LJ, Verbeek PR, McDonald AC, et al. Mortality and pre-hospital thrombolysis for acute myocardial infarction. A meta-analysis. JAMA 2000;283:2686–2692.)

| **TABLE 10-11** | **Framework for Evaluating the Statistical Analysis of a Meta-Analysis** |

- Were statistics used to determine the homogeneity (or heterogeneity) of included studies?
- Were appropriate statistics used to evaluate the pooled data?
  - ◆ Sensible statistical model used (i.e., random vs. fixed effects)?
  - ◆ Descriptive statistics (i.e., measures of central tendency and dispersion) employed correctly?
- What were the overall results and how precise were they?
- Was a sensitivity analysis performed?

Adapted with permission from Hunt DL. McKibbon KA. Locating and appraising systematic reviews. Ann Intern Med 1997;126:532–538.

such as a meta-analysis. Next, the reader must assess the authors' recommendations and then must decide to agree or disagree with the report's authors. Finally, the clinician must consider how the results of the meta-analysis will apply to his or her patient group. Table 10-13 provides a checklist for evaluating the conclusions of a meta-analysis.

How to Evaluate a Meta-Analysis

The steps for conducting a meta-analysis have been detailed in this chapter. In addition, points of critical evaluation for each step have been elucidated. Here, additional practice is offered. The evaluation of a meta-analysis is illustrated using a report by Simpson et al. (see Appendix C for a reprint).[22] Reading the meta-analysis before proceeding with the text will aid your understanding.

Simpson et al. begin their paper with an introduction that presents an overview the clinical problem—namely, noncompliance with prescription drug therapy remains a

| **TABLE 10-12** | **Example Scheme for Strength of Evidence for Different Study Designs.** |

LEVEL	EVIDENCE
1a	SR with homogeneity of RCTs
1b	Individual RCT with narrow CI
1c	All or none: met when all patients died before the treatment became available but some now survive on it, or when some patients died before the treatment became available but none now dies on it.
2a	SR with homogeneity of cohort studies
2b	Individual cohort study (including low-quality RCT [(e.g., < 80%] follow-up)
2c	Outcomes research; ecological studies
3a	SR with homogeneity of case-control studies
3b	Individual case-control study
4	Case-series (and poor-quality cohort and case-control studies)
5	Expert opinion

CI, confidence interval; *RCT*, randomized controlled trial; *SR*, systematic review.

Adapted with permission from Phillips B, Ball C, Sackett D et al. Levels of Evidence and Grades of Recommendation. Centre for Evidence-Based Medicine, Oxford, UK. Available at www.cebm.net/levels_of_evidence.asp#levels. Accessed Feb 2007.

TABLE 10-13	**Framework for Evaluating the Conclusions and Interpretations of a Meta-Analysis**

- Did authors derive conclusions beyond what the meta-analysis can support?
- Can the results be easily applied to patients in the clinical practice?
- Did the included studies measure all clinically important outcomes?
- Are the overall benefits worth the overall risks or costs?

leading challenge to healthcare providers. It is estimated that as many as 25% of patients taking prescription medications do not adhere well to their regimen.[22] Several studies have attempted to identify potential risk factors for noncompliance and have attempted to link good medication adherence (including placebo adherence) to good health outcomes, including a benefit on mortality. Although most clinicians believe that placebos do not affect health outcomes, the possible association of good health to good placebo adherence drove Simpson et al. to determine if adherence acts as an identifiable surrogate marker for overall healthy behavior—the so called healthy adherer effect. The research question addressed by this meta-analysis is whether there is a relationship between adherence to a prescription drug or placebo therapy and mortality.[22] Table 10-3 presents a framework for critically evaluating the research question of a meta-analysis.

 LITERATURE CRITIQUE 10-1

As Simpson et al. describe in the introductory section of the paper, patient nonadherence to drug therapy remains a critical problem. Most pharmacists would also surmise that nonadherence to medications could lead to poorer health outcomes among noncompliant patients. It is interesting that good adherence to placebo, which should not render a therapeutic effect, has also been associated with good health outcomes, creating the idea of a healthy adherer effect, meaning, patients who take a more conscientious approach to using their medications most likely expand that approach to their overall health and well-being (e.g., following a healthy diet and exercise program).

However, Simpson et al. lack focus and specificity in formulating their research question. They did not clearly define who the subjects were—adults, children, elderly, patients who are very ill, patients with symptomatic diseases, patients with asymptomatic conditions, and so on. For example, medication compliance issues and mortality may greatly differ in subjects who are HIV positive versus subjects who are taking medication to treat hypertension. Antiretroviral regimens tend to be more cumbersome, more difficult to take, and more apt to cause side effects, which could affect compliance. Better defining the patient population within the meta-analysis objective or research hypothesis would aid the reader in deciding up front whether the meta-analysis applies to his or her clinical practice. In sum, to be clinically useful, a more focused research question is desired.

Overall, this meta-analysis was conceived to provide a broad-ranging systematic review on compliance and its relationship to mortality. Medication compliance and its effects is a clinically relevant question—particularly to the pharmacist. Although evidence is currently lacking in this area, the meta-analysis would be more useful if it were more focused on a particular patient population. ■

The methods section of the adherence meta-analysis describes study eligibility—namely, to be included in the analysis, studies could be randomized controlled trials (RCTs), retrospective analyses from RCTs, or observational designs. No language limits were applied. Each study had to evaluate the association between medication adherence and mortality. Medication adherence, including the method used to measure it and a clear definition of what constituted good versus poor adherence, had to be detailed in each study. Subjects in each study had to be stratified into good and poor adherence groups for comparison. Table 10-4 provides a framework for critically evaluating the inclusion criteria of a meta-analysis.

 LITERATURE CRITIQUE 10-2

Although Simpson et al. provided some detail on study eligibility in an attempt to minimize selection bias, much detail is lacking. The information that was provided by the inclusion criteria does allow the reader to understand precisely what individual original research designs were included. In this case, both randomized and observational studies were allowed. It is important for the reader to remember the potential pitfalls associated with each of these designs.

In addition, the inclusion criteria allowed for various study languages, which is a good method to minimize study selection bias. The inclusion criteria also delineated some of the attributes each study must have displayed (e.g., mortality measured as an outcome, precise definitions of compliance supplied, and subjects stratified into good and poor adherence groups). Although these seem reasonable and fit the research question, the rationale for these was not explicitly explained by the review authors. This hinders the reader's ability to fully grasp and evaluate the authors' intentions for the inclusion criteria.

Despite the aforementioned positive points, the inclusion criteria were limited in that Simpson et al. failed to provide criteria for study subject characteristics or for study duration. This allows selection bias to enter the analysis. As previously discussed, this makes it difficult for the reader to decide whether the meta-analysis applies to his or her clinical practice or if only certain subjects were sought for inclusion. In addition, because the authors did not define the subject characteristics, problems may arise when pooling the data if subjects in the included studies were not similar. It's difficult to compare apples to oranges.

Furthermore, lack of inclusion criteria to define study duration creates a problem for the reader. For example, does the analysis include only studies < 1 year in duration? Within this time frame, compliance issues may not have emerged in the individual studies. Additionally measuring mortality within only 1 year may not supply an accurate long-term assessment of this outcome; thus the data pooled in the meta-analysis may be skewed.

Overall, this meta-analysis is weakened by a lack of detail regarding how studies were included. Recall that the overarching concept for a systematic review such as a meta-analysis is to provide explicit details on how the analysis was carried out so the reader can fully evaluate each step to ensure the systematic nature of the review and have confidence in its validity. Providing enough detail so the reader could assess the presence and extent of selection bias would have strengthened the analysis. The literature search may also be affected by the lack of explicit inclusion criteria. ■

The literature search was performed by a librarian who used multiple secondary databases, including MEDLINE and EMBASE, to find pertinent literature. Reference listings in textbooks and review articles on adherence were also searched. The search of secondary databases included a time frame of the database inception date to June 20, 2005. Synonyms for *adherence* and *mortality* were searched as keywords and subject headings in each database. Table 10-5 provides a framework for critically evaluating the search strategy of a meta-analysis.

LITERATURE CRITIQUE 10-3

Although use of multiple secondary databases and review of reference lists in tertiary resources is a strength, the lack of additional search details raises concern. For example, it is difficult for the reader to determine the appropriateness of the search without knowing the exact search terms used. What synonyms for *mortality* and *adherence* were used? Were all synonyms searched? What combinations of search terms were used? It also appears that Simpson et al. did not expend reasonable effort locating unpublished research on the subject, which could bias the pooled results. The shortcomings of the adherence meta-analysis search strategy are highlighted when comparing it to the search strategy employed by the AMI meta-analysis by Morrison et al.[8] Confidence in the findings of the current meta-analysis is weakened because the reader cannot be certain that a thorough search was performed; thus relevant studies might have been missed. ■

Two authors independently screened citation titles and abstracts of items generated from the literature search. If either author thought the article was potentially pertinent, it was retained. Tertiary literature was excluded. Each article was then evaluated further to determine if it indeed met the meta-analysis inclusion criteria. If the two raters disagreed, a third review author weighed in and broke the tie. Inter-reviewer agreement was measured via a qualitative scale developed by Landis and Koch on both on the initial citation and abstract screening (agreement level was 0.68, which was deemed "substantial") and on the full article evaluation (agreement level was 0.97, which was deemed "almost perfect").[24] Figure 1 in the Simpson et al. article reveals the literature selection process. The authors also provide a listing and characteristics of the included studies as Table 1 of their article.

Relevant data from each research paper were extracted using a standardized form. Data extracted included disease state, drug therapy group, adherence measurement method, definition of good adherence, and mortality. The investigators compared their standardized forms to ensure accuracy of the data collection. When mortality information was lacking or insufficient, the review authors either calculated the outcome from available information or contacted the study's corresponding author to obtain the data. Table 10-10 provides a framework for critically evaluating the study selection and appraisal process of a meta-analysis.

LITERATURE CRITIQUE 10-4

This meta-analysis is strengthened by using more than one investigator to determine study inclusion and by assessing their level of agreement. The level of agreement was deemed high. However, none of the investigators were blinded to the results of each individual study, which could lead to selection bias—the reader cannot dismiss the possibility that review authors chose to include only studies that demonstrated positive associations between good compliance and mortality or studies that support the healthy adherer effect hypothesis. A listing of excluded studies might assist the reader in evaluating the presence of selection bias. A list of the 58 excluded studies was not provided. Given that the amount of journal space to carry this out is excessive, the authors should have offered to provide the citations upon request.

The use of standard forms to extract data is a strength of the meta-analysis. These forms were compared to determine agreement of the data collection between reviewers. However, the data were extracted from studies that differed widely in terms of their design, patient population, drugs used, and definitions of adherence. These differences contribute to heterogeneity among the studies and might preclude the synthesis of a composite effect size estimate.

Another concern includes the lack of a validity assessment of each individual study included in the meta-analysis. From Table 1 of the Simpson et al. paper, it appears that cohort studies and RCTs were included. Per the inclusion criteria, the authors allowed retrospective analyses of RCTs. The table lacks detail as to whether data extracted from the RCTs were in fact retrospective analyses. This information is buried within the text of the paper (in the results section). As previously discussed in this chapter, it is important for the reader to remember the potential strengths and weaknesses of each study design. A lack of study validity assessment from the review authors severely compromises the validity of the pooled data. Compare the literature selection and appraisal process of this meta-analysis to those of Morrison et al. to further appreciate the shortcomings of the adherence meta-analysis. ▪

The statistical analysis employed in the adherence meta-analysis is described next. Separate statistical analyses were carried out for drug adherence and placebo adherence groups. Each used ORs and 95% CIs to characterize the synthesized treatment effect. Heterogeneity was assessed with Cochrane's Q and I^2. Preplanned subgroup analyses searched for sources of heterogeneity.

The investigators reported better survival among good adherers than among poor adherers for both prescribed drugs (OR 0.56; 95% CI 0.50–0.63) and placebo (OR 0.56; 95% CI 0.43–0.74). A forest plot of the individual and pooled OR and 95% CIs for the placebo adherence analysis and for the drug adherence analysis are presented in the article.

Statistically significant heterogeneity was apparent only in the placebo adherence analysis (Q statistic: $p = 0.05$; $I^2 = 51.2\%$), and could be attributed in large part to the mortality experience of studies treating myocardial infarction patients. Another heterogeneity analysis comparing subgroups of patients receiving beneficial drug therapy indicated that a statistically significant vector of homogeneity was associated with the method of measuring adherence. Table 10-11 provides a framework for critically evaluating the statistical analysis of a meta-analysis.

 LITERATURE CRITIQUE 10-5

Recall that there are four steps in the statistical analysis of a meta-analysis.

1. Synthesis of the overall treatment effect
2. Test for and explore heterogeneity
3. Examine publication bias
4. Use a sensitivity analysis to test assumptions.

A quite remarkable finding is that the benefit of survival is similar in both the drug-adherent and the placebo-adherent groups: Both ORs are 0.56, and the 95% CIs are quite similar. This suggests that mortality reductions may be the result of characteristics that promote adherence rather than any pharmacologic effect of the drug. However, the meta-analysis was not structured to compare drug to placebo with regard to mortality reduction; it was designed to compare good compliance to poor compliance. Nonetheless, this interesting finding of similar mortality benefits between drug and placebo might prompt further research.

Analysis of heterogeneity in the data was appropriate. The reader should note that Cochrane's Q is used in the calculation of I^2, so that the two measures are not independent. Further, Q has low power. That studies of myocardial infarction constituted a source of heterogeneity is perhaps not surprising considering that such studies made up almost 40% (8/21) of the studies in the analysis. Explorations of heterogeneity associated with beneficial drug adherence seem more like the findings of a sensitivity analysis (presented in Table 2 of the article). It is unclear why a similar analysis was not carried out with the placebo adherent data.

Publication bias was not addressed. In the next section of the paper, Simpson et al. contend that "important studies relevant to the research question may have been missed during the literature search, although this was unlikely." Sensitivity analyses were not reported. At a minimum, authors should check whether the treatment effect is influenced by sample size and by quality rating. ▪

The authors concluded that good adherence resulted in an approximate 50% reduction in risk of death compared to subjects who were noncompliant. These data supported the hypothesis of the healthy adherer effect, because the analysis showed that good compliance with placebo resulted in lower mortality rates. The authors suggested that good compliance is a surrogate marker for good overall healthy behaviors. Table 10-13 provides a framework for critically evaluating the conclusions of a meta-analysis.

LITERATURE CRITIQUE 10-6

The authors did a fairly good job of not drawing conclusions beyond the scope of their analysis; for example, the authors state that good compliance is associated with positive health outcomes. They are correct not to conclude a cause-and-effect relationship because many of their included studies were cohorts that cannot be used to determine such a relationship. Furthermore, a meta-analysis is an observational study, even when it is applied to RCTs.

However, the results of this meta-analysis cannot be applied easily to clinical practice. It appears from the original research question and lack of inclusion criteria specifying subject characteristics that the authors were making a broad analysis of compliance and its association with mortality. However, the authors ended up including only studies in which certain disease states and drugs were examined. The included studies mainly related to cardiovascular disease and HIV infection. Thus, results cannot be easily extrapolated to other patients with disease states.

In addition, although the authors accepted the healthy adherer effect hypothesis, they did not fully consider other confounders that may affect healthy behavior, such as socioeconomic status. For example, poorer, less-educated patients may have fewer healthy behaviors because they cannot afford quality healthcare or healthy lifestyle practices, or perhaps they don't possess the knowledge of these behaviors and practices. Compliance is not the only determinant of healthy behavior.

It is also important to keep in mind that subjects included in studies are more highly motivated than the general population. Recall the Hawthorne effect (discussed in Chapter 8). Subjects tend to receive better care as a result of their participation and thus may exhibit better compliance and outcomes than the general population. This point was not addressed in the authors' discussion or conclusions.

The absence of data on publication bias and sensitivity represent real shortcomings to this systematic review. Overall, given the limitations discussed in this chapter's Literature Critique sections, the reader cannot be confident that the results of the Simpson et al. meta-analysis impart a valid representation of the association between compliance and mortality. ▓

The ability to combine the results of several similar, independent studies using the techniques of meta-analysis has special advantages. It can increase statistical power, reduce bias, and increase the precision of the data. However, the results of a meta-analysis are quite sensitive to the studies that are analyzed, which is why there are tests for heterogeneity and publication bias. Furthermore, assumptions made during the meta-analysis to extract data may have a profound effect on the results, and should be examined with sensitivity analyses.

Meta-analyses are not panaceas, however. These reviews are subject to the same pitfalls as are all publications (e.g., bias, error) and may not coincide with the findings of large, well-executed RCTs. In addition, the quality of the meta-analysis depends on the quality of the individual trials included in the analysis, which can vary widely. A meta-analysis is an observational study, even if it analyzes RCTs, and is susceptible to the same shortcomings as an individual observational study. Another criticism of meta-analyses is that the process of extraction of data masks the most important information regarding subject and methodologic characteristics that modulate the effect under study. Finally, remember that the principles, applications, methods, and conclusions of meta-analysis are by no means agreed to by all investigators. The methods of meta-analysis itself are evolving.

Qualitative Systematic Reviews

Qualitative systematic reviews are also often termed overviews. These reports follow a similar methodology as meta-analyses with respect to identifying and examining individual research reports. The analysis of the data, however, is based on similarity of findings rather than on a statistical synthesis. A qualitative systematic review was published by Mehra et al.[25] The abstract for this review is reprinted in Table 10-14.

It is important to note here that systematic reviews differ from narrative reviews. A narrative review is a qualitative article that deals with a broad range of issues related to a given topic rather than addressing a particular issue in depth. A narrative review article often

TABLE 10-14	Abstract: Qualitative Systematic Review

BACKGROUND: The association between marijuana smoking and lung cancer is unclear, and a systematic appraisal of this relationship has yet to be performed. Our objective was to assess the impact of marijuana smoking on the development of premalignant lung changes and lung cancer. METHODS: Studies assessing the impact of marijuana smoking on lung premalignant findings and lung cancer were selected from MEDLINE, PSYCHLIT, and EMBASE databases according to the following predefined criteria: English-language studies of persons 18 years or older identified from 1966 to the second week of October 2005 were included if they were research studies (ie, not letters, reviews, editorials, or limited case studies), involved persons who smoked marijuana, and examined premalignant or cancerous changes in the lung. RESULTS: Nineteen studies met selection criteria. Studies that examined lung cancer risk factors or premalignant changes in the lung found an association of marijuana smoking with increased tar exposure, alveolar macrophage tumoricidal dysfunction, increased oxidative stress, and bronchial mucosal histopathologic abnormalities compared with tobacco smokers or nonsmoking controls. Observational studies of subjects with marijuana exposure failed to demonstrate significant associations between marijuana smoking and lung cancer after adjusting for tobacco use. The primary methodologic deficiencies noted include selection bias, small sample size, limited generalizability, overall young participant age precluding sufficient lag time for lung cancer outcome identification, and lack of adjustment for tobacco smoking. CONCLUSION: Given the prevalence of marijuana smoking and studies predominantly supporting biological plausibility of an association of marijuana smoking with lung cancer on the basis of molecular, cellular, and histopathologic findings, physicians should advise patients regarding potential adverse health outcomes until further rigorous studies are performed that permit definitive conclusions.

attempts to integrate information from a variety of research areas to provide a state-of-the-art vision of the research or clinical area. Clinically oriented narrative reviews are often much like a chapter from a medical textbook. They provide a comprehensive description of a disease or condition, including epidemiology, pathophysiology, and treatment approaches. Narrative reviews often reflect the personal views of the senior author.

Narrative reviews are not systematic in nature and do not always analyze and synthesize evidence from all relevant primary literature. Authors of narrative reviews typically do not provide explicit descriptions of methods used to include research papers in their review. Narrative reviews are particularly subject to publication bias. Thus, while useful for obtaining a broad perspective on a topic, narrative reviews are less useful than systematic reviews for providing specific answers to specific clinical questions.

One narrative review was written by Huang et al.[26] Because this article does not contain an explicit abstract, the introductory paragraph, which describes the review, is presented in Table 10-15. This narrative review discusses data and evidence from the primary literature, but lacks a systematic approach to identifying, selecting, and evaluating the studies. The review is classified as a narrative rather than a systematic review because of this lack of systematic methodology.

Evaluating a qualitative systematic review is accomplished using the same criteria outlined for meta-analysis, disregarding the data analysis—that is, the research question should be well defined and specific. The parameters of the literature search, the selection of research papers, and the extraction of data from those studies should be explicitly stated. The synthesis of the research papers is qualitative in that the authors describe in detail similarities among studies and attempt to resolve discrepancies. Based on this information, a conclusion pertinent to the original question is proposed. Evaluating a qualitative systematic review is patterned after the assessment criteria used for meta-analysis and is left as an exercise for the student.

TABLE 10-15	**Narrative Review (Opening Paragraph)**[a]

Antiretroviral therapy has increased the life expectancy of patients who are infected with the human immun-odeficiency virus (HIV) and has reduced the incidence of illnesses associated with the acquired immunodeficiency syndrome (AIDS). However, the frequency of pulmonary, cardiac, gastrointestinal, and renal diseases that are often not directly related to underlying HIV disease has increased. Although the guiding principles of management in the intensive care unit (ICU) pertain to critically ill patients with HIV infection, antiretroviral therapy and unresolved questions regarding its use in the ICU add an additional level of complexity to already complicated cases. This review focuses on some of the important clinical problems related to the use of anti-retroviral therapy in critically ill patients with HIV infection and on the challenging issues associated with the intensive care of such patients, including legal statutes concerning HIV testing and disclosure, the administration of antiretroviral medications, important potential drug interactions with medications commonly used in the ICU, and controversies surrounding the use of antiretroviral therapy in the ICU.

[a]Reference citations have been deleted.

Reprinted with permission from Huang L, Quartin A, Jones D, et al. Intensive care of patients with HIV infection. N Engl J Med 2006;355:173–181. Copyright © 2007 Massachusetts Medical Society.

Summary

Systematic reviews are successful in making the whole greater than the sum of the parts. Systematic reviews can integrate findings from individual studies into a unitary index of a treatment effect. Well-executed meta-analyses can identify significant effects that are undetectable in individual studies, explore consistencies among individual trials, resolve uncertainties and discrepancies among studies, and address clinical questions not raised in the original trials. Systematic reviews are useful if definitive trials cannot be conducted or are not yet complete.

However, systematic reviews are susceptible to the same sources of error, confounding, and bias as are individual studies. Furthermore, details of patients or treatments, which may be important in specific clinical settings, are often neglected in the systematic review to make data extraction possible. With an understanding of both the advantages and the disadvantages of meta-analysis, however, pharmacists can integrate this information source with others and, using sound clinical judgment and reasoning, arrive at a treatment decision in the best interest of their patients.

STUDY PROBLEMS

1. Describe how meta-analyses are useful while practicing in the evidence-based model of medicine.

2. You are caring for a 63-year-old man who has painful osteoarthritis in both knees and no other major medical conditions. Although he can still carry out his normal daily activities, he has limited mobility and reports pain at rest. You are now reviewing his history and current care with him. You had previously recommended acetaminophen 1000 mg four times daily, which provided minimal pain relief. The patient is eager to try a different medication. You mention that nonsteroidal anti-inflammatory drugs (NSAIDs) are generally not associated with improved analgesia compared to acetaminophen, but the patient still wants to try something else. You agree to offer him short-term NSAID therapy but are not sure which agent has the lowest rate of serious gastrointestinal complications such as

hemorrhage. Critically evaluate the meta-analysis by Henry et al.[27] using the framework discussed in this chapter to provide a recommendation for this patient.

3. Why might a meta-analysis be the approach of choice to answer the drug information question detailed in study problem 2 instead of an RCT or other primary literature designs?

4. Search the Internet for a description of the Cochrane search strategy. Apply this strategy to a clinical question raised in a pharmacy course. Establish criteria that you would use to identify and evaluate relevant literature. Share your ideas with other members of your student group and resolve discrepancies.

5. Select three primary research articles that address an area of interest to you. Rate them for quality using the Detsky criteria. Compare your findings with another student's, perhaps computing a statistical index of agreement, like kappa.

6. Select a qualitative systematic review from the literature and critique it using the criteria provided for a meta-analysis. Check your critique with those of other students and resolve discrepancies. Discuss as a group the clinical issue addressed in the review, the adequacy of the information identification and synthesis process, and the authors' discussion of the findings. Do the results of the review provide you with actionable information with respect to patients you might encounter?

REFERENCES

1. Cook CJ, Sackett DL, Spitzer WO. Methodologic guidelines for systematic reviews of randomized control trials in health care from the Potsdam Consultation on Meta-Analysis. J Clin Epidemiol 1995;48:167–171.
2. Mulrow CD. The medical review article: State of science. Ann Intern Med 1987;106:485–488.
3. Mulrow CD, Cook DJ, Davidoff F. Systematic reviews: Critical links in the great chain of evidence. Ann Intern Med 1997;126:389–391.
4. Douglas K, O'Malley PG, Jackson JL. Meta-analysis: The effects of statins on albuminuria. Ann Intern Med 2006;145:117–124.
5. Egger M, Smith GD, Phillips AN. Meta-analysis: Principles and procedures. Br Med J 1997;315: 1533–1537.
6. Chalmers TC, Lau J. Meta-analysis stimulus for changes in clinical trials. Stat Meth Med Res 1993;2:161–172.
7. Chalmers I, Haynes RB. Reporting, updating, and correcting systematic review of the effects of health care. In: Chalmers I, Altman DG, eds. Systematic Reviews. London: British Medical Journal, 1995.
8. Morrison LJ, Verbeek PR, McDonald AC, et al. Mortality and pre-hospital thrombolysis for acute myocardial infarction. A meta-analysis. JAMA 2000;283:2686–2692.
9. Sackett DL, Straus SE, Richardson WS, et al., eds. Asking answerable clinical questions. In: Evidence-Based Medicine: How to Practice and Teach EBM. 2nd ed. Edinburgh, UK: Churchill Livingstone, 2000;13–27.
10. Matthews BS, Gray literature: Resources for locating unpublished research. Coll Res Library News [Online] 2004;65. Available at: www.ala.org/ala/acrl/acrlpubs/crlnews/backissues2004/march04/graylit.htm. Accessed July 2006.
11. Gould, SJ. Cordelia's dilemma. Natural Hist 1993;102:10–18.
12. Hunt DL. McKibbon KA. Locating and appraising systematic reviews. Ann Intern Med 1997;126:532–538.
13. McGinn T, Wyer PC, Newman TB, et al. Tips for learners of evidence-based medicine: 3. Measures of observer variability (kappa). Can Med Assoc J 2004;171:1369–1373.
14. Detsky AS, Naylor CD, O'Rourke K, et al. Incorporating variations in the quality of individual randomized trials into meta-analysis. J Clin Epidemiol 1992;45:255–265.
15. Vincent JL, Bihari DJ, Suter PM, et al. The prevalence of nosocomial infection in intensive care units in Europe: Results of the European Prevalence of Infection in Intensive Care (EPIC) Study; EPIC International Advisory Committee. JAMA 1995;274:639–644.

16. Rubinstein E, Cammarata SK, Oliphant T, et al. Linezolid (PNU-100766) versus vancomycin in the treatment of hospitalized patients with nosocomial pneumonia: a randomized, double-blind, multicenter study. Clin Infect Dis 2001;32:402–412.

17. Wunderink RG, Rello J, Cammarata SK, et al. Linezolid vs. vancomycin. Analysis of two double-blind studies of patients with methicillin-resistant *Staphylococcus aureus* nosocomial pneumonia. Chest 2003;124:1789–1797.

18. Berlin JA, Laird NM, Sacks HS, et al. A comparison of statistical methods for combining event rates from clinical trials. Stat Med 1989;8:141–151.

19. Shakiba B. Heterogeneity. Systematic Review [Online]. Available at: ssrc.tums.ac.ir/SystematicReview/Heterogeneity.asp#. Accessed August 2006.

20. Higgins JP, Thompson SG, Deeks JJ, Altman DG. Measuring heterogeneity in meta-analyses. Br Med J 2003;327:557–560.

21. Oxman AD. Systematic reviews: Checklists for review articles. Br Med J 1994;309:648–651.

22. Simpson SH, Eurich DT, Majumdar SR, et al. A meta-analysis of the association between adherence to drug therapy and mortality. Br Med J 2006;333:15.

23. DiMatteo MR. Variations in patients' adherence to medical recommendations: A quantitative review of 50 years of research. Med Care 2004;42:200–209.

24. Landis JR, Koch GG. The measurement of observer agreement for categorical data. Biometrics 1977;33:159–174.

25. Mehra R, Moore BA, Crothers K, et al. The association between marijuana smoking and lung cancer: A systematic review. Arch Intern Med 2006;166:1359–1367.

26. Huang L, Quartin A, Jones D, et al. Intensive care of patients with HIV infection. N Engl J Med 2006;355:173–181.

27. Henry D, Lim LL, Garcia Rodriguez LA, et al. Variability in risk of gastrointestinal complications with individual non-steroidal anti-inflammatory drugs: Results of a collaborative meta-analysis Br Med J 1996;312:1563–1566.

Clinical Decision Making Using Contemporary Healthcare Information

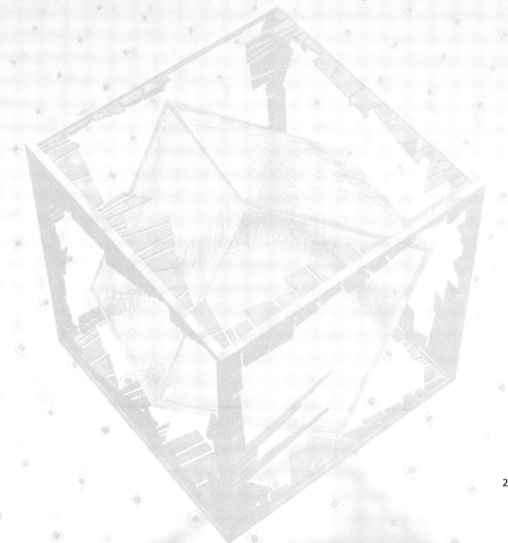

11

Evaluating and Implementing Practice Guidelines

CHAPTER GOALS

After studying this chapter, the student should be able to:

1. Explain the rationale for clinical practice guideline development.

2. Discuss the potential limitations of implementing clinical practice guidelines.

3. Differentiate between the various developmental methods for clinical practice guidelines.

4. Evaluate clinical practice guidelines.

5. Describe a pharmacist's role in implementing clinical practice guidelines.

6. Make clinical decisions when guidelines differ.

7. Integrate new evidence from primary literature along with practice guidelines to make clinical decisions.

As defined by the Institute of Medicine, **clinical practice guidelines** are systematically developed statements created to assist practitioner and patient decisions about healthcare for specific circumstances.[1] Guidelines are developed by various organizations, such as government agencies, managed-care organizations, and professional associations. Properly developed practice guidelines provide a concise summary of current best evidence on what works and what does not work in consideration of specific healthcare interventions. Although guidelines should not dictate every clinical decision, quality guidelines can provide the practitioner with current best evidence summaries to inform the decision-making process.

Why the need for clinical practice guidelines? Simply put, guidelines can help:

- Improve healthcare quality
- Improve patient outcomes
- Improve frequency of appropriate care
- Reduce unnecessary or inappropriate care and thus reduce healthcare costs
- Enhance communication and continuity of care between various healthcare providers and patients

The National Healthcare Quality Report (NHQR), developed by the Agency for Healthcare Research and Quality (AHRQ) on behalf of the U.S. Department of Health and Human Services, tracks the current state of healthcare quality for the United States on an annual basis. The 2005 NHQR, the third report of its kind, provides evidence that healthcare quality is improving in the United States but that major improvements can still be made in specific areas.[2] Four key themes emerged from this report: (1) quality is improving at a modest pace across most measures of quality; (2) quality improvement is variable, with notable areas of high performance and notable areas of poor performance; (3) further improvement in healthcare is needed to achieve optimal quality; and (4) sustained rates of quality improvement are possible.

Clinical practice guidelines can play a key role in improving the quality of care in the United States by calling attention to under-recognized health problems, clinical services, and preventive interventions and to neglected patient populations and high-risk patient groups. Furthermore, practice guidelines help promote distributive justice, advocating better delivery of healthcare services to those in need. And, finally, practice guidelines can improve the efficiency of healthcare to free up resources needed for other healthcare services.

In today's age of spiraling healthcare costs, inappropriate use of diagnostic and laboratory tests, surgical procedures, and medications can inflate healthcare expenditures. Clinical practice guidelines can help deter unnecessary medical expenses in several ways. First, guidelines influence clinical decisions to improve patient and population healthcare. Second, guidelines provide the best current practices for disease prevention, screening, diagnosis, treatment, or palliation. Finally, guidelines help minimize the geographic variations in patient care and thus provide a consistent level of healthcare for all citizens, whether they are located in rural or metropolitan areas or in the east, midwest or west.[3] Table 11-1 summarizes the rationale for guideline development.

PERSPECTIVE 11-1

With the growing emphasis on the practice of evidence-based medicine, guidelines play an important role in the provision of evidence-based pharmaceutical care. But is there evidence to support the use of guidelines as a means to improve healthcare? Do guidelines do what they purport to do?

The answer is yes. The MAHLER survey (Medical Management of Chronic Heart Failure in Europe and Its Related Costs) showed that when physicians adhered to treatment guidelines, rates of heart failure (HF) and cardiovascular-related hospitalizations decreased significantly.[4] A study by Shibata et al. evaluated the implications of treatment guidelines on reducing costs of HF related hospitalizations.[5] The study demonstrated that a mere 10% increase in the use of angiotensin-converting enzyme (ACE) inhibitors, β-blockers, spironolactone, and digoxin as recommended by practice guidelines, would result in a $6.6 million savings as a result of avoided hospital admissions.

Evidence also supports the use of antibacterial therapy, per practice guideline recommendations, to reduce the length of stay, costs, and mortality associated with community-acquired

TABLE 11-1   Rationale for Guideline Development

- Influence clinician decisions
- Improve patient and population healthcare
- Deter rising healthcare costs
- Minimize geographic variations in clinical practice

pneumonia.[6,7] *In another study, Manuel et al. demonstrated improved patient outcomes—namely, avoidance of death from coronary heart disease over a 5-year period—when national practice guidelines were followed for the screening and treatment of hyperlipidemia.*[8]

Evidence also suggests that compliance with the American Heart Association's (AHA) practice guideline for acute stroke and transient ischemic attack improves stroke outcomes. A study by Micieli et al. demonstrated that the relative risk of death was doubled in patients who did not adhere to guideline recommendations compared to those who did adhere.[9] *After 6 months, patients who had good adherence to the AHA's guideline recommendations benefited from a 15% (95% CI 9.1–17.5) decrease in mortality rate.*

A wealth of evidence exists to show that many guidelines actually meet their goals: improving patient care and outcomes along with decreasing costs. However, it is important to recognize that this evidence does not exist for all available practice guidelines. When deciding whether to use a guideline, it may be prudent for the pharmacist to search the medical literature to see if evidence exists to support the guideline.

Limitations of Implementing Clinical Practice Guidelines

Despite the positives of clinical practice guidelines, potential limitations and harms to implementing practice guidelines do exist and should be considered from the perspective of the clinician, the patient, and the healthcare system. For example, consider the clinician. Flawed practice guidelines can compromise the quality of care; encouraging ineffective, harmful, or wasteful interventions that are not in the best interest of the patient.[10]

Practice guidelines can be inconvenient and time consuming to use. Some clinicians believe that guidelines are cookbook medicine, precluding the application of the art of medicine. Guidelines often do not change clinician practice behavior. Studies show that dissemination of practice guidelines through common passive measures, such as continuing education programs or publication in medical journals, is an ineffective means of changing clinician practice behavior.[11]

Auditors, managers, and third-party payers may unfairly judge the quality of care provided by a clinician based on criteria from potentially flawed or invalid guidelines, because guidelines often do not account for the complexities of clinical decision making. And finally, guidelines may even offer citable evidence for potential malpractice litigation, meaning law suits could be filed for instances in which the clinician did not follow guideline recommendations.[12]

PERSPECTIVE 11-2

It is interesting that malpractice suits could be filed in instances in which the clinician did follow guideline recommendations. One such case involved a resident physician who followed national practice guidelines from the American Academy of Family Physicians, the American Urological Association, and the American Cancer Society in regard to screening for prostate cancer.

The physician followed the approach recommended by each guideline: Discuss the risks and benefits of screening with the patient, provide thorough informed consent, and come to a shared decision regarding screening. The patient and physician came to a shared decision not to screen for prostate cancer.

However, a few years later the patient saw another physician who did not discuss the risks versus benefits of prostate cancer screening with the patient and instead ordered the prostate-specific antigen (PSA) screening test. Unfortunately, the patient was found to have an advanced form of prostate cancer.

Although the literature does not support that early detection would have changed the patient's clinical outcome, the patient filed a malpractice suit against the resident physician and the physician's residency program. The physician was exonerated, but the residency program was found liable for $1 million.[13]

From the patient's perspective, practice guidelines may reduce individualized care, especially for patients with special needs. Guidelines do not always account for specific patient attributes or situations, and thus individualized care may be lacking. For example, consider a 75-year-old female with diabetes who recently suffered a hip fracture. The American Diabetes Association's (ADA) Standards of Medical Care for Diabetes[14] recommends a goal hemoglobin A_{1c} (HbA1$_c$) of $< 7\%$ for adults with diabetes. This patient's current HbA1$_c$ is 7.6%. Should her diabetes pharmacotherapy be augmented to lower the HbA1$_c$ level to meet guideline recommendations? Considering that her life expectancy may be substantially decreased as a result of the hip fracture, lowering her HbA1$_c$ to $< 7\%$ may or may not be the best course of action. If the ADA's guidelines were followed precisely, the patient may not receive the best individualized care. Thus guideline recommendations that reduce complex clinical decisions to simplistic algorithms should be tempered with consideration for the individual patient.

Another consideration on behalf of the patients' concerns lay versions of guidelines. Guidelines for professional healthcare workers are written in precise language targeted to an audience that is trained in that communication medium. Explanations written for the general public are necessarily less technical and thus are less precisely written. Furthermore, the information is interpreted by a group of patients with a wide range of experiences and conditions. As such, lay versions of guidelines may actually confuse and mislead some patients and disrupt the patient–healthcare provider relationship.

From the healthcare system's perspective, the system may feel a strain if implementing and promulgating practice guidelines escalates medical benefit use, compromises operating efficiency, or wastes limited resources.[12] Guidelines can adversely affect policy for societal or public healthcare if they increase costs of care or divert resources away from more effective healthcare interventions.[15] Thus, although clinical practice guidelines are an increasingly familiar part of clinical practice and can help improve healthcare, pharmacists must also be mindful of their potential pitfalls.

Methods for Clinical Practice Guideline Development

Several methods for developing clinical practice guidelines exist and are used commonly. Whatever the method employed, development strategies should generally aim to meet the following objectives:

- Produce guidelines that are accurate
- Provide recommendations that are accountable, enabling the clinician to review the data and reasoning behind each recommendation made
- Allow for anticipation of health and financial consequences of applying the guideline to individual patients and populations
- Facilitate resolution of conflicts with other guidelines
- Facilitate application of policy

In this section, three methods of developing clinical practice guidelines are summarized: the informal consensus method, the formal consensus method, and the evidence-based method.

INFORMAL CONSENSUS METHOD

The **informal consensus method** is a development strategy in which a group of experts makes recommendations based on a subjective assessment of the evidence, with little description of the specific evidence or process used to derive the recommendations. Because this method is quick, simple, and economical compared to other development methods, the informal consensus method is used commonly. Recommendations are typically generated after a meeting of an expert panel. Panel members publicly express their views, the aggregate of which may be summarized by the panel's leader and considered the final decision. Recommendations contained in the guideline are reached not through a structured process but through open discussion and consensus of members on the expert panel.

Although this approach is often used, it is not without limitations. The resulting guideline document itself frequently lacks details about the panel's process for deriving its recommendations. Because a systematic approach is not used to gather and evaluate evidence, recommendations can be easily influenced by special interests of panel members, group dynamics, dominant personalities, and organizational and specialty politics.[16] Evidence is often cited within the guideline, but usually little information is provided on the quality of the cited evidence or the methods used to minimize bias.

Generally, in guidelines developed by the informal consensus method, little background information is provided on how evidence was sought, obtained, evaluated, and applied to support the recommendations. This lack of explicit, documented methodology raises questions concerning how consensus was achieved or whether relevant evidence was overlooked. For example, if the panel recommends a certain drug or surgical procedure as first-line care, and that drug or surgical procedure generates income for panel members, questions about potential conflicts of interest may be raised when methods and rationale are not well documented.[16] As a result, a clinician evaluating the guideline is not sure whether the panel's recommendations were founded on solid evidence or justified only by the panel's clinical opinion and special interests.

The informal consensus method was developed by the American College of Chest Physicians (ACCP) to develop guidelines for managing community-acquired pneumonia.[17]

FORMAL CONSENSUS METHOD

The **formal consensus method** was introduced in the mid-1970s and is frequently used by the National Institutes of Health (NIH). This method provides more structure to the analytic process than the informal consensus method in that much advanced planning and preparation is carried out to provide expert panel members with the most current reviews of the evidence.

Using the formal consensus method, a guideline is developed after a planning session and open discussion among subject experts. Guidelines are produced using a structured 2.5-day conference, and recommendations are typically presented to a professional audience and/or members of the press and public on the third day.

Structuring the interaction within the panel is accomplished using different techniques. One approach is the **nominal group technique**. After participants record views independently and privately, the panel facilitator collects one view from each individual and creates a list. After an open discussion of the listed topics, individual panel members privately record their judgments and vote for the options. Further discussion and voting may take place. The individual judgments are aggregated statistically to come up with a group judgment.[18]

Another technique of structured interaction is the **consensus development method**. A selected group of ~ 10 experts is brought together to reach consensus about an issue in an open meeting. Evidence is presented by various groups and experts (who are not part of the decision-making panel), and the panel retreats to consider the issue and evidence.[18]

Despite the added structure, the formal consensus method also lacks explicit criteria with respect to finding, analyzing, and applying evidence to support recommendations. As with the informal consensus method, the formal consensus method may add to confusion regarding the application of its recommendations.

A guideline developed via the formal consensus method is the NIH's recommendations for celiac disease.[19]

EVIDENCE-BASED METHOD

The **evidence-based method** for developing clinical practice guidelines by far provides more scientific rigor than either the informal and the formal consensus methods. The evidence-based method involves a systematic search for evidence along with extensive documentation, evaluation, and communication of the evidence used to support recommendations.

The evidence-based process involves defining specific clinical questions to be answered, establishing criteria for inclusion of potential evidence, and specifying a systematic process for locating and evaluating relevant evidence. Recommendations made are anchored directly to the scientific evidence; they explicitly reflect the weight of the accumulated evidence. Developing a guideline via the evidence-based method can take a year or more, but this method produces science-based, pilot-tested, peer-reviewed recommendations.

The downside to the evidence-based development method is obvious. It generally is a time-consuming, technically demanding, and expensive means ($350,000–$1 million) of developing a practice guideline. An additional limitation to this method is that recommendations are difficult to develop when evidence is scanty. When evidence is lacking, guideline writers are often forced to make relatively neutral recommendations, which are not particularly useful to practicing clinicians.

In fact, if the evidence-based method for guideline development were strictly adhered to, then the vast majority of medicine would be excluded from consideration because clinical studies are lacking to support much of clinical practice.[16] Thus a modified evidence-based approach is often performed, which allows for expert consensus or opinion when evidence is lacking for a recommendation. The key, though, is for guideline writers to specify clearly which recommendations are supported by evidence and which are expert opinion.

Despite the time, energy, and money spent developing a practice guideline using the evidence-based method, the quality of individual guidelines is inconsistent. In a recent systematic review of 279 practice guidelines, only 43% adhered to established methodologic standards for guideline development.[20] Similarly, of practice guidelines developed by specialty societies (e.g., the American College of Cardiology [ACC] and the American Association of Clinical Endocrinologists [AACE]), 82% did not apply explicit criteria to grade scientific evidence that supported recommendations, and 87% did not report whether a systematic literature search was used to find evidence for the guidelines.[21]

In April 2002, the Conference on Guideline Standardization (COGS) was convened to create standards and a more uniform methodology for the development and reporting of evidence-based guidelines in an effort to promote the quality and implementation of practice guidelines.[22] The COGS panel consisted of representatives from various medical specialty societies, government agencies, and private groups, along with representatives from groups that disseminate and implement guidelines. To allow for evaluation of the validity and usability of guidelines, the COGS panel proposed a checklist of essential elements that such a guide should contain (Table 11-2).

TABLE 11-2   The COGS Checklist for Reporting Clinical Practice Guidelines

TOPIC	DESCRIPTION
1. Overview material	Provide a structured abstract that includes the guideline's release date, status (original, revised, updated), and print and electronic sources
2. Focus	Describe the primary disease or condition and intervention, service, or technology that the guideline addresses; indicate any alternative preventive, diagnostic, or therapeutic interventions that were considered during development
3. Goal	Describe the goal that following the guideline is expected to achieve, including the rationale for development of a guideline on this topic
4. Users and setting	Describe the intended users of the guideline (e.g., provider types, patients) and the settings in which the guideline is intended to be used
5. Target population	Describe the patient population eligible for guideline recommendations and list any exclusion criteria
6. Developer	Identify the organization(s) responsible for guideline development and the names, credentials, potential conflicts of interest of individuals involved in the guideline's development
7. Funding source and sponsor	Identify the funding source or sponsor and describe its role in developing and/or reporting the guideline; disclose potential conflict of interest
8. Evidence collection	Describe the methods used to search the scientific literature, including the range of dates and databases searched and criteria applied to filter the retrieved evidence
9. Recommendation grading criteria	Describe the criteria used to rate the quality of evidence that supports the recommendations and the system for describing the strength of the recommendations; recommendation strength communicates the importance of adherence to a recommendation and is based on both the quality of the evidence and the magnitude of anticipated benefits or harms
10. Method for synthesizing evidence	Describe how evidence was used to create recommendations (e.g., evidence tables, meta-analysis, decision analysis)
11. Prerelease review	Describe how the guideline developer reviewed and/or tested the guidelines before release
12. Update plan	State whether or not there is a plan to update the guideline and, if applicable, an expiration date for this version of the guideline
13. Definitions	Define unfamiliar terms and those critical to correct application of the guideline that might be subject to misinterpretation

TABLE 11-2	The COGS Checklist for Reporting Clinical Practice Guidelines, cont.
TOPIC	**DESCRIPTION**
14. Recommendations and rationale	State the recommended action precisely and the specific circumstances under which to perform it; justify each recommendation by describing the linkage between the recommendation and its supporting evidence; indicate the quality of evidence and the recommendation strength, based on the criteria described in 9
15. Potential benefits and harms	Describe anticipated benefits and potential risks associated with implementation of guideline recommendations
16. Patient preferences	Describe the role of patient preference when a recommendation involves a substantial element of personal choice or values
17. Algorithm	Provide, if appropriate, a graphical description of the stages and decisions in clinical care described by the guideline
18. Implementation considerations	Describe anticipated barriers to application of the recommendations; provide reference to any auxiliary documents for providers or patients that are intended to facilitate implementation; suggest review criteria for measuring changes in care when the guideline is implemented

COGS, Conference on Guideline Standardization.

Reprinted with permission from Shiffman RN, Shekelle P, Overhage JM, et al. Standardized reporting of clinical practice guidelines: A proposal from the conference on guideline standardization. Ann Intern Med 2003;139:493–498.

A guideline developed via the evidence-based method was created by the ACC and the AHA for treating heart failure.[23] This guideline is evaluated in detail in the next section.

Evaluating Clinical Practice Guidelines

To determine if guideline recommendations should be integrated into clinical practice, the pharmacist must make a critical assessment of the guideline. In general, there are three main questions:[24,25]

- Are the recommendations valid?
- What are the recommendations?
- Will the recommendations help me in caring for my patients?

Consider this clinical scenario: A pharmacist working in an interdisciplinary heart failure clinic and has been asked to consult on a 69-year-old white male who is diagnosed with New York Heart Association (NYHA) stage III heart failure and who is currently prescribed captopril 100 mg twice daily, digoxin 0.125 mg daily, furosemide 60 mg twice daily, and metoprolol XL 50 mg daily. The patient is currently experiencing increased shortness of breath and increased edema in his lower extremities. His current serum creatinine is 1.9 mg/dL, and his serum potassium is 4.3 mEq/L. Based on the ACC/AHA heart failure guideline,[23] the team is considering the addition of spironolactone, an aldosterone antagonist, to the patient's regimen.

The pharmacist must evaluate the validity, importance, and applicability of the ACC/AHA guideline.

ARE THE RECOMMENDATIONS VALID?

It is obvious that guideline recommendations that are not valid should not be used in clinical practice. When assessing the validity of guideline recommendations, the clinician can use the framework given in Table 11-3.

TABLE 11-3	**Are the Recommendations Valid?**

- What method was used to develop the guideline?
- Who were the guideline developers and do potential conflicts of interest exist?
- Was a transparent and rational process used to search for, select, and combine evidence?
- Was an explicit and rational process used to consider the relative value of different outcomes?
- What is the scheduled review of the guideline? Are recent developments accounted for?
- Has the guideline been subject to peer review and/or testing?

Adapted with permission from Hayward RSA, Wilson MC, Tunis SR, et al. User's guides to the medical literature: How to use clinical practice guidelines. Are the recommendations valid? JAMA 1995;274:570–574.

 LITERATURE CRITIQUE 11-1

Using the framework presented in Table 11-3 to assess the ACC/AHA heart failure guide-line,[23] one can conclude that the recommendations possess strong validity. The guideline developers used an evidence-based methodology. The guideline was developed by a medical society (ACC) and a professional association (AHA) in collaboration with the ACCP and the International Society for Heart and Lung Transplantation. Guideline writers are all physicians and most are fellows of either or both the AHA or ACC; and their financial disclosures, conflicts of interest, and roles in the guideline development are fully disclosed. The guideline was funded by the ACC and AHA.

Guideline developers used a systematic approach to collect and select evidence, including hand searches of published literature and use of MEDLINE and EMBASE to identify pertinent English-language articles. Although details such as specific search terms are not provided, the pharmacist deems that guideline developers employed a reasonable search strategy for compiling evidence. Perusal of the reference list at the end of the guideline statement indicates that almost 200 references are cited, suggesting a comprehensive search and review of currently available literature. ■

It is important to keep in mind that guideline developers must bring together all relevant evidence and synthesize that evidence in an appropriate manner that avoids bias and distortion. The best guidelines explicitly define how the developers determined eligibility of evidence and report how evidence was selected and synthesized to support the recommendations. Making key data available in the guideline is also a positive.[24]

Practice guidelines pertain to decisions, and decisions involve choices and consequences. Thus, to appreciate why a particular intervention or practice is recommended, the pharmacist should make sure that guideline developers have thoughtfully considered all reasonable practice options and all important potential outcomes such as morbidity, mortality, and quality of life—outcomes patients would care about.[24]

In addition, the pharmacist should always look for information about who specifically was involved in assigning value to outcomes. Because expert panels and consensus groups are often used to develop guideline recommendations, the pharmacist needs to bear in mind that panels dominated by members of specialty groups may be subject to intellectual, territorial, and financial biases. Panels that include a well-balanced mix of practicing generalists and specialists along with research methodologists and public representatives are more likely to have considered diverse views and values in their deliberations.[24]

LITERATURE CRITIQUE 11-2

Major outcomes considered in the ACC/AHA heart failure guideline include the following:

• Sensitivity and specificity of diagnostic instruments
• Morbidity and mortality owing to heart failure
• Symptoms of heart failure
• Cardiovascular events
• Risk of heart failure
• Risk of death and hospitalization
• Survival rates
• Quality of life and sense of well-being
• Cost analysis

ACC/AHA heart failure guideline developers explicitly state that review of data on efficacy and clinical outcomes constituted the primary basis for preparing recommendations in the guidelines. However, patient-specific modifiers, comorbidities, and issues of patient preference that might influence the choice of particular tests or therapies were also considered. Other considerations are frequency of follow-up and cost effectiveness. This seems like a rational approach to weighing the relative value of the listed outcomes; however, the guideline panel consisted mainly of cardiologists and thus may suffer from lack of diverse viewpoints in assigning value to outcomes. ■

To be useful and valid, practice guidelines need to be up to date. One group of researchers assessed the current validity of 17 clinical practice guidelines published by the AHRQ and found that only 3 of the 17 guidelines in circulation at the time of the review were still current and valid. Another 7 guidelines warranted major revision in light of currently available evidence. The researchers recommended that, in general, practice guidelines need to be reassessed for validity and currency every 3 years.[26]

 LITERATURE CRITIQUE 11-3

The ACC/AHA heart failure guideline was originally released in November 1995, was first updated in 2001, and was most recently updated in August 2005. The guideline developers state that the ACC/AHA Task Force on Practice Guidelines regularly reviews existing guidelines to determine when an update or full revision is needed.[23]

Because the word *regularly* is not explicitly defined by the guideline developers, the pharmacist must always consider new therapy options or new evidence that may not be included in the latest version of this or any guideline. ■

Scanning the bibliography of the guideline helps give an impression of how current the guideline is. Find the publication date of the most recent study considered in the guideline and look for the date on which final recommendations were made to help determine currency. In addition, the pharmacist should perform a literature search because any new evidence must always be considered along with guideline recommendations when making clinical decisions about patient care. (The integration of new evidence with current guidelines is discussed later in this chapter.)

Finally, confidence in the validity of the guideline increases if it has been subjected to external review and if that review has determined the guideline to be reasonable and applicable to clinical practice.

 LITERATURE CRITIQUE 11-4

The ACC/AHA heart failure guideline was subjected to both internal and external peer review. The guideline was evaluated by official reviewers nominated by a variety of organizations, such as the ACC, AHA, American Academy of Family Physicians, ACCP, American College of Physicians (ACP), Heart Failure Society of America, and International Society for Heart and Lung Transplantation. Furthermore, a numbers of committees reviewed the document, including a committee representing the European Society of Cardiology and a quality-care committee. ■

Returning to the clinical scenario of the 69-year-old white male who has heart failure, the pharmacist can be reasonably sure that the ACC/AHA heart failure guideline does provide valid recommendations.

WHAT ARE THE RECOMMENDATIONS?

Once the pharmacist is reasonably sure that the guideline recommendations are valid, the recommendations themselves need to be considered. Practical, unambiguous recommendations are desirable. To be important clinically, the guideline should convince the pharmacist that the benefits of following the recommendations outweigh the expected risks or costs. The questions listed in Table 11-4 can help in this process.

The ACC/AHA heart failure guideline provides recommendations on the diagnosis, evaluation, management, prevention, risk assessment, and treatment of heart failure in adult patients. The question of whether to add spironolactone to the treatment of a heart failure patient is addressed by the guideline; the recommendation and specific evidence to support it are given in Table 11-5.

TABLE 11-4   What are the Recommendations?

- Are the recommendations practical, clinically important, and relevant?
- How strong are the recommendations?
- What is the effect of uncertainty associated with the evidence and values used in the guidelines?

Adapted with permission from Hayward RSA, Wilson MC, Tunis SR, et al. User's guides to the medical literature: How to use clinical practice guidelines. Are the recommendations valid? JAMA 1995;274:570–574; and Wilson MC, Hayward RSA, Tunis SR, et al. User's guides to the medical literature: How to use clinical practice guidelines. What are the recommendations and will they help you in caring for your patients? JAMA 1995;274:1630–1632.

TABLE 11-5   Recommendation from the ACC/AHA Heart Failure Guideline[a]

RECOMMENDATION

Addition of an aldosterone antagonist is reasonable in selected patients with moderately severe to severe symptoms of HF and reduced LVEF who can be carefully monitored for preserved renal function and normal potassium concentration. Creatinine should be less than or equal to 2.5 mg/dL in men or less than 2.0 mg/dL in women and potassium should be less than 5.0 mEq/L. (Under circumstances where monitoring for

TABLE 11-5	**Recommendation from the ACC/AHA Heart Failure Guideline[a], Cont.**

hyperkalemia or renal dysfunction is not anticipated to be feasible, the risks may outweigh the benefits of aldosterone antagonists.) [Class of Recommendation: I; Level of Evidence: B]

EVIDENCE PROVIDED

In a large-scale, long-term trial, low doses of spironolactone (starting at 12.5 mg daily) were added to ACEI therapy for patients with class IV HF symptoms or class II symptoms and recent hospitalization. The risk of death was reduced from 46% to 35% (30% relative risk reduction) over 2 years, with 35% reduction in HF hospitalization and an improvement in functional class.

[a]Reference citations have been deleted.

ACC, American College of Cardiology; *ACEI*, angiotensin-converting enzyme inhibitor; *AHA*, American Heart Association; *HF*, heart failure; *LVEF*, left ventricular ejection fraction;

Adapted with permission from Hunt SA, Abraham WT, Chin MH, et al. ACC/AHA 2005 guideline update for the diagnosis and management of chronic heart failure in the adult. A report of the American College of Cardiology/American Heart Association Task Force on Practice Guidelines. Circulation 2005;112:e154–e235. © 2005, American Heart Association, Inc.

 LITERATURE CRITIQUE 11-5

Using the framework for assessing the recommendations, the addition of spironolactone is important (a decreased risk of death) and practical if careful monitoring of potassium and renal function is feasible. The guideline also provides a grade or strength for its recommendation to help the pharmacist assess the relative amount of certainty of the advice. The rating scheme for the strength of recommendations used by the ACC/AHA heart failure guideline is outlined in Table 11-6. Based on this rating scheme, the pharmacist can clearly see that the recommendation for addition of spironolactone is the strongest level of recommendation; the developers generally agreed that the addition of spironolactone is beneficial, useful, and effective.

In addition, the ACC/AHA heart failure guideline provides a rating scheme for the strength of evidence used to support the recommendations (Table 11-7). Based on this scheme, the pharmacist can understand clearly the amount and quality of evidence used to support the recommendations. For the use of spironolactone, the supporting evidence is derived from the Randomized Aldactone Evaluation Study (RALES) trial, a landmark, large randomized controlled study.[27] ■

TABLE 11-6	**Rating Scheme for Strength of Recommendations Made in the ACC/AHA Heart Failure Guidelines**

CLASS	DESCRIPTION
I	Conditions for which there is evidence and/or general agreement that a given procedure or treatment is beneficial, useful, and effective
II	Conditions for which there is conflicting evidence and/or a divergence of opinion about the usefulness or efficacy of a procedure or treatment
IIa	Weight of evidence or opinion is in favor of usefulness or efficacy
IIb	Usefulness or efficacy is less well established by evidence or opinion
III	Conditions for which there is evidence and/or general agreement that a procedure or treatment is not useful or effective and in some cases may be harmful

ACC, American College of Cardiology; *AHA*, American Heart Association.

Adapted with permission from Hunt SA, Abraham WT, Chin MH, et al. ACC/AHA 2005 guideline update for the diagnosis and management of chronic heart failure in the adult. A report of the American College of Cardiology/American Heart Association Task Force on Practice Guidelines. Circulation 2005;112:e154–e235. © 2005, American Heart Association, Inc.

TABLE 11-7	Rating Scheme for Levels of Evidence in the ACC/AHA Heart Failure Guidelines.
LEVEL OF EVIDENCE	**DESCRIPTION**
A	Data derived from multiple randomized clinical trials or meta-analysis
B	Data derived from a single randomized trial or nonrandomized studies
C	Only consensus opinion of experts, case studies, or standard of care

Adapted with permission from Hunt SA, Abraham WT, Chin MH, et al. ACC/AHA 2005 guideline update for the diagnosis and management of chronic heart failure in the adult. A report of the American College of Cardiology/American Heart Association Task Force on Practice Guidelines. Circulation 2005;112:e154–e235. © 2005, American Heart Association, Inc.

The strength, grade, level, confidence, or force of a recommendation should be formed by many factors and considerations, including the following:

- Quality of the studies that provide evidence for the recommendations
- Magnitude and consistency of positive outcomes relative to negative outcomes (e.g., costs, adverse drug reactions)
- Relative value placed on different outcomes

Other rating schemes are available from, for example, the Centre for Evidence-Based Medicine, the American Board of Family Practice, and the Infectious Disease Society of America. These three rating schemes are provided in Tables 11-8 to 11-10.[28–30]

It is important to note that many guidelines will not provide a rating scheme for recommendations and level of evidence, especially those developed by consensus methods. This makes it difficult for the pharmacist to determine the validity and strength of the recommendations.

TABLE 11-8	Rating Scheme for Levels of Evidence and Grade of Recommendations from the CEBM
GRADE	**LEVEL OF EVIDENCE**
A	1a: SR of homogeneous RCTs
	1b: Individual RCT
B	2a: SR of homogeneous cohort studies
	2b: Individual cohort study or low-quality RCT
	2c: Outcomes research
	3a: SR of homogeneous case-control studies
	3b: Individual case-control study
C	4: Case series or poor-quality cohort or case-control studies
D	5: Expert opinion without explicit critical appraisal or based on physiology or bench research

CEBM, Centre for Evidence-Based Medicine; *RCT*, randomized controlled trial; *SR*, systematic review.

Adapted with permission from Phillips B, Ball C, Sackett D et al. Levels of Evidence and Grades of Recommendation. Centre for Evidence-Based Medicine, Oxford, UK. Available at www.cebm.net/levels_of_evidence.asp#levels. Accessed Feb 2007.

TABLE 11-9 **American Board of Family Practice Strength of Recommendation Taxonomy**

STRENGTH OF RECOMMENDATION[a]	DEFINITION
A	Recommendation based on consistent and good-quality patient-oriented evidence[b]
B	Recommendation based on inconsistent and limited-quality patient-oriented evidence
C	Recommendation based on consensus; usual practice; opinion; disease-oriented evidence;[c] and case series for studies of diagnosis, treatment, prevention, or screening

STUDY QUALITY	TYPE OF STUDY[d]		
	DIAGNOSIS	TREATMENT, PREVENTION, SCREENING	PROGNOSIS
Level 1 (see A above)	• Validated clinical decision rule • SR or meta-analysis of high-quality studies • High-quality diagnostic cohort study[e]	• SR or meta-analysis of RCTs with consistent finding • High-quality individual RCT[f] • All-or-none study[g]	• SR or meta-analysis of good-quality cohort studies • Prospective cohort study with good follow-up
Level 2 (see B above)	• Unvalidated clinical decision rule • SR or meta-analysis of lower-quality studies or with inconsistent findings • Lower-quality diagnostic cohort or diagnostic case-control study	• SR or meta-analysis of lower-quality clinical trials or of studies with inconsistent findings • Lower-quality clinical trial • Cohort study • Case-control study	• SR or meta-analysis of lower-quality cohort studies or with inconsistent results • Retrospective cohort study or prospective cohort study with poor follow-up • Case-control study • Case series
Level 3 (see C above)	Consensus guidelines; extrapolations from bench research; usual practice; opinion; disease-oriented evidence; and case series for studies of diagnosis, treatment, prevention, or screening		

(continued)

American Board of Family Practice Strength of Recommendation Taxonomy, cont.

TYPE	CONSISTENCY ACROSS STUDIES
Consistent	• Most studies found similar or at least coherent[h] conclusions or • If high-quality and up-to-date SRs or meta analyses exist, they support the recommendation
Inconsistent	• Considerable variation among study findings and lack of coherence or • If high-quality and up-to-date SRs or meta analyses exist, they do not find consistent evidence in favor of the recommendation

[a]In general, only key recommendations for readers require a grade of the "strength of recommendation"; recommendations should be based on the highest quality evidence available. *Example:* Vitamin E was found in some cohort studies (level 2) to have a benefit for cardiovascular protection; but good-quality randomized trials (level 1) have not confirmed this effect. Thus it is preferable to base clinical recommendations on level 1 studies.

[b]Measures outcomes that matter to patients (morbidity, mortality, symptoms, costs, quality of life).

[c]Measures intermediate, physiologic, or surrogate end points that may or may not reflect improvements in patient outcomes (blood pressure, blood chemistry, physiologic function, pathologic findings)

[d]Use this table to determine whether a study measuring patient-oriented outcomes is of good or limited quality and whether the results are consistent among studies.

[e]Rated on design, size, spectrum of patients, blinding, and reference standard.

[f]Rated on allocation concealed, blinding (if possible), intention-to-treat analysis, statistical power, and follow-up.

[g]The treatment causes a dramatic change in outcomes, such as antibiotics for meningitis and surgery for appendicitis; precludes study in a controlled trial.

[h]Meaning, differences are explainable.

RCT, randomized controlled study; *SR,* systematic review.

Reprinted with permission from Ebell MH, Siwek J, Weiss BD, et al. Strength of Recommendation Taxonomy (SORT): A patient-centered approach to grading evidence in the medical literature. J Am Board Fam Pract 2004;17:59–67 by the American Board of Family Medicine.

TABLE 11-10	Infectious Disease Society of America and U.S. Public Health Service Grading System for Ranking Recommendations in Clinical Guidelines.	
CATEGORY, GRADE	**DEFINITION**	
STRENGTH OF RECOMMENDATION		
A	Good evidence to support a recommendation for use	
B	Moderate evidence to support a recommendation for use	
C	Poor evidence to support a recommendation	
D	Moderate evidence to support a recommendation against use	
E	Good evidence to support a recommendation against use	
QUALITY OF EVIDENCE		
I	Evidence from > 1 properly executed randomized controlled trial	
II	Evidence from > 1 well-designed clinical trial (no randomization), cohort or case-control analytic study (preferably multicenter), or multiple time series; or dramatic results from uncontrolled experiments	
III	Evidence from opinions of respected authorities, based on clinical experience, descriptive studies, or reports of expert committees	

Adapted with permission from Kish MA. Guide to development of practice guidelines. Clin Infect Dis 2001;32:851–854.

WILL THE RECOMMENDATIONS HELP YOU IN CARING FOR YOUR PATIENTS?

As noted, guidelines are not meant to dictate every clinical decision, but high-quality guidelines can be an invaluable tool in providing evidence-based care. To be really useful, the guideline needs to describe the management of the patient well enough to be duplicated exactly. The pharmacist must determine if his or her patient and practice are the intended target of the guideline. The framework found in Table 11-11 can help in this endeavor.

The ACC/AHA guideline developers state their intent is to assist healthcare providers in making clinical decisions by describing a range of clinically appropriate prevention, diagnosis, and management strategies for adults with chronic heart failure and normal or lower left ventricular ejection fraction. The target population of this guideline is adult men and women, high-risk ethnic minority groups, elderly patients, and those adults who may be at high risk for developing heart failure. Intended users of the guideline are physicians and other healthcare providers.[23]

TABLE 11-11	Will the Recommendations Help You in Caring for Your Patients?

- Is the main objective of the practice guideline consistent with your objective?
- How applicable are the recommendations to your specific patients?
- Can the recommendations be easily duplicated?

Adapted with permission from Hayward RSA, Wilson MC, Tunis SR, et al. User's guides to the medical literature: How to use clinical practice guidelines. Are the recommendations valid? JAMA 1995;274:570–574; and Wilson MC, Hayward RSA, Tunis SR, et al. User's guides to the medical literature: How to use clinical practice guidelines. What are the recommendations and will they help you in caring for your patients? JAMA 1995;274:1630–1632.

LITERATURE CRITIQUE 11-6

The ACC/AHA guideline is aimed at helping patients that seem to be similar to the 69-year-old male patient under consideration. The guideline provides explicit instructions for initiating and monitoring spironolactone:

> Spironolactone should be initiated at a dose of 12.5 to 25 mg daily, or occasionally on alternate days. Potassium supplementation is generally stopped after the initiation of aldosterone antagonists, and patients should be counseled to avoid high potassium-containing foods.. . . Potassium levels and renal function should be rechecked within 3 days and again at 1 week after initiation of an aldosterone antagonist. Subsequent monitoring should be dictated by the general clinical stability of renal function and fluid status but should occur at least monthly for the first 3 months and every 3 months thereafter.[*]

The pharmacist and interdisciplinary team should be able to confidently and precisely duplicate the guideline's instructions knowing that the recommendations for spironolactone are valid and applicable to the patient. ◼

The Pharmacist's Role in Implementing Guidelines

From reading this chapter, it should be fairly easy to infer that, in general, the evidence-based method provides the most valid guidelines for clinical practice. However, how does the pharmacist implement guidelines that were developed by the informal or formal consensus method? Should guidelines that are developed by consensus be implemented into clinical practice? The question is not an easy one and answering it requires careful evaluation of the validity and credibility of the consensus guideline, using the frameworks provided in this chapter.

The pharmacist should seek to implement guidelines that were developed via the evidence-based method. However, it is important to realize that for some diseases there is not enough available evidence for developing a practice guideline using this method. In addition, the disease might be so rare that it may not be feasible to invest time and money into developing an evidence-based guideline. In these instances, clinicians must rely on guidelines that were developed via consensus.

However, it is important to always keep in mind that guidelines, no matter what method was used to develop them, are meant to *guide* healthcare decisions and not *dictate* them. Recall that the evidence-based approach to medicine involves not only the use of evidence but also the use of sound clinical reasoning and consideration of patient values.

Despite even the highest-quality practice guideline, many potential barriers exist that preclude healthcare practitioners from implementing such recommendations into their practice. Some these barriers are:

- Lack of familiarity or awareness that a specific guideline exists
- Disagreement with the guideline recommendations

---

[*]Reprinted with permission from Hunt SA, Abraham WT, Chin MH, et al. ACC/AHA 2005 guideline update for the diagnosis and management of chronic heart failure in the adult. A report of the American College of Cardiology/American Heart Association Task Force on Practice Guidelines. Circulation 2005;112:e154–e235. ACC/AHA 2005 Guideline Update for the Diagnosis and Management of Chronic Heart Failure in the Adult. © 2005, American Heart Association, Inc.

- Fear of cookbook medicine and loss of autonomy
- Time constraints or lack of personnel to implement the guidelines effectively

To overcome the first barrier—a lack of familiarity and awareness—the pharmacist must make an effort to be familiar with the available practice guidelines and know how to locate them. Various sources of guidelines exist, but the most widely available is the National Guideline Clearinghouse (NGC), at www.guideline.gov. This government-sponsored, publicly available Web site is a comprehensive database for clinical practice guidelines and related documents. The NGC's mission is to offer healthcare providers an accessible mechanism for obtaining objective, detailed information on clinical practice guidelines and to further the dissemination, implementation, and use of guidelines.

Many practice guidelines are published in peer-reviewed biomedical journals and thus are searchable through secondary sources, such as MEDLINE or EMBASE. MEDLINE has a search function in which the pharmacist can choose to limit the search to guidelines only. In additionally, the pharmacist can conduct a search using "practice guidelines" as a medical subject heading (MeSH) in conjunction with the disease or therapy of interest to find guidelines.

A number of medical societies and professional organizations, such as the ACC and AACE provide links to practice guidelines on their Web sites.[31,32] Do not forget to try one of the more popular search engines, such as Google or Yahoo! to locate practice guidelines. Use search terms such as "practice guidelines." Because practice guidelines are widely available online, pharmacists should find it easy to become aware of, locate, and use them. Since many guidelines relate to the provision of pharmacotherapy, it stands to reason that pharmacists should know which guidelines exist and be intimately involved with not only evaluating them but also implementing them in the practice setting.

Research has indicated that even practitioners who are aware of practice guidelines are sometimes reluctant to implement them into their practice. In a cross-sectional survey, Tunis et al. measured physician attitude toward clinical practice guidelines among > 1500 internal medicine physicians.[33] The survey showed that only 11% of respondents were familiar with the ACP guideline on exercise treadmill testing, and only 59% of respondents were aware of the National Cholesterol Education Program (NCEP) guidelines.

Confidence in using practice guidelines was increased when the guideline was developed by the ACP or by the physician's medical subspecialty professional organization. Only 6% of respondents had confidence in practice guidelines generated by a managed-care organization. Approximately 70% of respondents thought that guidelines would improve the quality of healthcare, and 43% thought guideline implementation would result in higher healthcare costs. It is interesting that 34% of physicians thought that implementation of guidelines would make their clinical practice less satisfying.[33]

Pharmacists can play a key role in overcoming these barriers by encouraging use and implementation of high-quality guidelines into clinical practice. Implementation strategies include recognition of potential barriers and efforts to overcome them. For example, if physicians in a particular practice setting are not aware that certain practice guidelines exist, the pharmacist could employ implementation strategies such as academic detailing (a process by which the pharmacist visits a physician to provide a 10- to 15-min educational intervention on a specific topic) or in-service offerings to help increase awareness of the guideline. Important algorithms outlining specific treatment approaches for particular diseases could be posted where physicians could easily consult them during patient care.

If the physician disagrees with a guideline recommendation, the pharmacist could find, evaluate, and share the evidence that supports the guideline recommendation. Academic detailing or in-services might be useful in this regard as well. In addition, the pharmacist could look for evidence to validate the guideline recommendations—for example, that the recommendations improve patient care and outcomes or lowers cost.

Using Practice Guidelines to Make Clinical Decisions

In many cases, incorporating the guideline recommendations into patient care is fairly straightforward; but sometimes it may not be as easy. For example, what does the pharmacist do when guideline recommendations differ? What about new evidence that becomes available but has not yet been incorporated into the current version of the guideline?

For example, the ADA and AACE both provide practice guidelines for the treatment of diabetes. As noted, the ADA recommends a HbA1$_c$ goal of $< 7\%$ in adults who have diabetes.[14] But the AACE recommends a HbA1$_c$ goal of $< 6.5\%$.[34] Which guideline should be followed? The answer is that it depends. It depends on the pharmacist's evaluation of the validity and applicability of each guideline. Of course, the pharmacist would want to implement the guideline that he or she deems most valid and applicable to the situation at hand. However, if validity and applicability are deemed equal, then the decision on which guideline to implement depends on the patient and the clinical situation. Unfortunately, there is no easy formula to follow and no right or wrong answer in a situation such as this. Again, this is where clinical judgment comes into play. Does the patient need the more stringent HbA1$_c$ goal as recommended by the AACE? Or, for example, is the patient a frail and elderly person who might suffer from hypoglycemia if diabetes medications were intensified to meet the lower HbA1$_c$ goal? (See this chapter's study questions for practice making these types of clinical decisions.)

As discussed earlier in this chapter, the pharmacist must also be aware of the currency of the guideline and then check if newer evidence is available that might affect guideline recommendations. Pharmacists may need to integrate newly available evidence with existing guidelines when making a clinical decision. For example, a report of the NCEP's Adult Treatment Panel III (ATP III) provided an update to the treatment guidelines for high blood cholesterol in adults.[35] This update evaluated the implications of several recent studies to propose a new optional goal of < 70 mg/dL for low-density lipoprotein (LDL) cholesterol in high-risk patients (those with coronary heart disease). This update did not include the later published Treating New Targets (TNT) trial, which showed that using high-intensity statin therapy to attain a lower LDL goal (mean LDL cholesterol of 77 mg/dL in the study) provided significant clinical benefit in patients with stable coronary heart disease.[36]

To recommend appropriate therapy and treatment goals for a patient, the pharmacist is compelled to evaluate and consider any new evidence that may not have been available at the time of guideline publication. It would be necessary then to use the new evidence alongside the guideline to make recommendations. Further practice with this is provided in the study problems at the end of this chapter.

Summary

Although not perfect, practice guidelines often provide evidence-based recommendations regarding the treatment of different maladies. Proper selection and application of the guidelines, requires an understanding of their purpose, rationale, development methods, critical evaluation, and potential implementation strategies. Principles and examples of the use of practice guidelines in clinical decision making are illustrated in the chapter.

While guidelines are created to assist both practitioner and patient in making decisions about healthcare for specific circumstances, it is imperative to remember the overarching paradigm of evidence-based clinical decision making: the compilation of using the best evidence along with clinical expertise and patient values. Practice guidelines, particularly those that are high quality, constitute a key component in this practice model.

However, practice guidelines are meant to be guides; they are not meant to dictate every clinical decision. The pharmacist's expertise and judgment must be used along with consideration of the patient's specific attributes and values. The pharmacist must be aware of the available guidelines, be able to critically evaluate these guidelines for validity, and be able to implement the guidelines appropriately and effectively in clinical practice.

STUDY PROBLEMS

1. Compare and contrast the informal and formal consensus methods with the evidence-based method of practice guideline development. Make an argument to support the evidence-based method as producing more valid guidelines. Under what conditions might the consensus methods provide more valuable information? (For example, what about orphan diseases and those with highly variable sequelae?)

2. Interview a clinical pharmacist and ask how he or she has attempted to overcome common barriers to implementing practice guidelines.

3. Use the National Guideline Clearinghouse Web site (www.guideline.gov) to locate the ADA clinical practice recommendations and the AACE's guidelines for diabetes. Use the framework provided in the chapter to critically evaluate these practice guidelines.

4. Consider the following patient cases:

Case 1

CG is a 46-year-old black male. He is active (exercises regularly), has two kids, and is an engineer. CG states that he is feeling well—no hypoglycemia or hyperglycemia symptoms and no problems with tolerating medications. CG states that he is compliant with his medications.

Past Medical History:
  Diabetes type 2 (diagnosed 2 years ago)
  Hypertension (diagnosed 5 years ago)
  Hyperlipidemia (diagnosed 1 year ago)
Current Medications:
  Metformin 1000 mg b.i.d.
  Atenolol 50 mg daily
  Hydrochlorothiazide 25 mg daily
  Lisinopril 20 mg daily
  Simvastatin 20 mg h.s.
  Aspirin 325 mg daily
Diet: Follows a strict 1800- to 2000-calorie per day ADA-compatible diet
Physical Examination: height = 6'2"; weight = 190 lb; blood pressure = 122/68 mmHg; pulse = 72 bpm.
Current Laboratory Values:
  HbA1$_c$ 6.9% (reflects current treatment)
  Home blood glucose readings: A.M. (fasting) = 85–100; P.M. (preprandial) = 95–135 mg/dL
  Urine microalbumin/Cr 50 mg/dL (increased from 9 mg/dL measured 1 year ago)
  Low-density lipoprotein 85 mg/dL

Case 2

LT is a 76-year-old somewhat feeble white female. She has no acute complaints except for hypoglycemic symptoms occurring approximately three times weekly in the early evening (reports blood sugar level is in the 60s when symptoms occur).

Past Medical History:
   Diabetes type 2 (diagnosed 12 years ago)
   Hypertension (diagnosed 15 years ago)
   Hyperlipidemia (diagnosed 8 years ago)
   Breast cancer (right breast mastectomy 2 years ago)
   Osteoporosis (hip fracture 1 year ago)
Current medications:
   Metformin 1000 mg b.i.d.
   Humulin 70/30 22 U q A.M., 14 U q P.M.
   Atorvastatin 10 mg daily
   Hydrochlorothiazide 12.5 mg daily
   Quinapril 10 mg daily
   Aspirin 325 mg daily
   Tamoxifen 10 mg daily
   Fosamax 70 mg weekly
Diet: Eats regularly 3 meals daily; watches sugar and carbohydrate consumption; follows a low-fat, low-cholesterol diet
Exercise: Ambulatory now but minimal physical activity; does take physical therapy owing to previous hip fracture
Physical Examination: height = 5′5″; weight = 130 lb; blood pressure = 134/76 mmHg
Laboratory values:
     $HbA1_c$ 7.2% (reflects of current treatment)
     Low-density lipoproteins 105 mg/dL
     Home blood glucose readings: A.M. = 90–140; P.M. = 59–90 mg/dl

Which practice guideline recommendation in regard to goal HbA1c would you follow for each of these patients—ADA or AACE? Support and justify your decision.

5. The updated NCEP ATP III recommendations for high blood cholesterol in adults are available.[35] The revision evaluated the implications of several recent studies that propose a new optional goal of < 70 mg/dL for low-density lipoprotein cholesterol for high-risk patients. The update did not include the TNT trial.[36] Read and evaluate the TNT trial and answer the following question: Should the NCEP ATP III update change its recommendations about a < 70 mg/dL LDL goal in high-risk patients from "optional" to "absolutely recommended" based on the evidence from the TNT trial?

REFERENCES

1. Institute of Medicine. Clinical practice guidelines: Directions for a new program. Washington, DC: National Academy Press, 1990.
2. U.S. Department of Health and Human Services. Agency for Healthcare Research and Quality. National healthcare quality report 2005. Available at: www.ahrq.gov/qual/nhqr05/nhqr05.pdf. Accessed Mar 2006.
3. Chassin MR, Kosecoff J, Park RE et al. Does inappropriate use explain geographic variations in the use of health care services? A study of three procedures. JAMA 1987; 258:2533–2537.
4. Komajda M, Lapuerta P, Hermans N, et al. Adherence to guidelines is a predictor of outcome in chronic heart failure: The MAHLER survey. Eur Heart J 2005;26:1653–1659.

5. Shibata MC, Nilsson C, Hervas-Malo M, et al. Economic implications of treatment guidelines for congestive heart failure. Can J Cardiol 2005;21:1301–1306.

6. Brown PD. Adherence to guidelines for community-acquired pneumonia: Does it decrease cost of care? Pharmacoeconomics 2004;22:413–420.

7. Nathwani D, Rubinstein E, Barlow G, et al. Do guidelines for community-acquired pneumonia improve the cost-effectiveness of hospital care? Clin Infect Dis 2001;32:728–741.

8. Manuel DG, Kwong K, Tanuseputro P, et al. Effectiveness and efficiency of different guidelines on statin treatment for preventing deaths from coronary heart disease: Modeling study. Br Med J 2006;332:1419.

9. Micieli G, Cavallini A, Quaglini S, et al. Guideline compliance improves stroke outcome: A preliminary study in 4 districts in the Italian region of Lombardia. Stroke 2002;33:1341–1347.

10. Woolf SH. Do clinical practice guidelines define good medical care? The need for good science and the disclosure of uncertainty when defining "best practices." Chest 1998;113:166S–171S.

11. Davis DA, Thomson MA, Oxman AD, et al. Evidence for the effectiveness of CME: A review of 50 randomized controlled trials. JAMA 1992;268:1111–1117.

12. Woolf SH, Grol R, Hutchinson A, et al. Clinical guidelines: Potential benefits, limitations and harm of clinical guidelines. Br Med J 1999;318:527–530.

13. Merenstein D. A piece of my mind: Winners and losers. JAMA 2004;291:15–16.

14. American Diabetes Association. Standards of Medical Care in Diabetes. Diabetes Care 2006;29(suppl 1):s4–s42.

15. Woolf SH. Evidence-based medicine and practice guidelines: An overview. Cancer Control 2000;7:362–367.

16. American College of Rheumatology. Guidelines for the development of practice guidelines. Available at: www.rheumatology.org/publications/guidelines/guidesonguides.asp?aud = mem. Accessed Feb 2006.

17. Ramsdell J, Narsavage GL, Fink JB, et al. Management of community-acquired pneumonia in the home: An American College of Chest Physicians Clinical position statement. Chest 2005;127:1752–1763.

18. National Guideline Clearing House. Methods used to formulate the recommendations. Available at: www.guideline.gov/about/classification.aspx#methodformulate. Accessed Feb 2006.

19. National Institutes of Health Consensus Development Panel on Celiac Disease. Celiac Disease. Bethesda, MD: U.S. Department of Health and Human Services, 2004.

20. Shaneyfelt TM, Mayo-Smith MF, Rothwangl J. Are guidelines following guidelines? The methodological quality of clinical practice guidelines in the peer reviewed medical literature. JAMA 1999;281:1900–1905.

21. Grilli R, Magrini N, Penna A, et al. Practice guidelines developed by specialty societies: The need for a critical appraisal. Lancet 2000;355:103–106.

22. Shiffman RN, Shekelle P, Overhage JM, et al. Standardized reporting of clinical practice guidelines: A proposal from the conference on guideline standardization. Ann Intern Med 2003;139:493–498.

23. Hunt SA, Abraham WT, Chin MH, et al. ACC/AHA 2005 guideline update for the diagnosis and management of chronic heart failure in the adult. A report of the American College of Cardiology/American Heart Association Task Force on Practice Guidelines. Circulation 2005;112:e154–e235. [Also available at: circ.ahajournals.org/cgi/content/full/112/12/1853. Accessed Feb 2007.]

24. Hayward RSA, Wilson MC, Tunis SR, et al. User's guides to the medical literature: How to use clinical practice guidelines. Are the recommendations valid? JAMA 1995;274:570–574.

25. Wilson MC, Hayward RSA, Tunis SR, et al. User's guides to the medical literature: How to use clinical practice guidelines. What are the recommendations and will they help you in caring for your patients? JAMA 1995;274:1630–1632.

26. Shekelle PG, Ortiz E, Rhodes S, et al. Validity of the agency for healthcare research and quality clinical practice guidelines. How quickly do guidelines become outdated? JAMA 2001;286:1461–1467.

27. Pitt B, Zannad F, Remme WJ, et al. The effect of spironolactone on morbidity and mortality in patients with severe heart failure. Randomized Aldactone Evaluation Study investigators. N Engl J Med 1999;341:709–717.

28. Phillips B, Ball C, Sackett D et al. Levels of Evidence and Grades of Recommendation. Centre for Evidence-Based Medicine, Oxford, UK. Available at www.cebm.net/levels_of_evidence.asp#levels. Accessed Feb 2007.

29. Ebell MH, Siwek J, Weiss BD, et al. Strength of Recommendation Taxonomy (SORT): A patient-centered approach to grading evidence in the medical literature. J Am Board Fam Pract 2004;17:59–67.

30. Kish MA. Guide to development of practice guidelines. Clin Infect Dis 2001;32:851–854.

31. American College of Cardiology. Clinical statements/guidelines. Available at: www.acc.org/qualityandscience/clinical/statements.htm. Accessed Sept 2006.

32. American Association of Clinical Endocrinologist. AACE guidelines. Available at: www.aace.com/pub/guidelines/. Accessed Sept 2006.

33. Tunis SR, Hayward RSA, Wilson MC, et al. Internist' attitudes about clinical practice guidelines. Ann Intern Med 1994;120:956–963.

34. Field S. American Association of Clinical Endocrinologists medical guidelines for the management of diabetes mellitus: The AACE system of intensive diabetes self management—2002 update. Endocr Pract 2002;8(suppl 1):41–82.

35. Grundy SM, Cleeman JI, Bairey-Merz CN, et al. Implications of recent trials for the National Cholesterol Education Program Adult Treatment Panel III guidelines. Circulation 2004;110:227–239.

36. LaRosa JC, Grundy SM, Waters DD, et al. Intensive lipid lowering with atorvastatin in patients with stable coronary disease. N Engl J Med 2005;352:1425–1435.

Keeping Current with the Medical Literature—Becoming an Information Master

Chapter

12

CHAPTER GOALS

After studying this chapter, the student should be able to:

1. Explain the importance of keeping current with the medical literature.

2. Develop and employ strategies to manage information efficiently and effectively.

3. Differentiate between patient-oriented and disease-oriented evidence.

4. Use foraging and hunting tools to become an information master.

5. Explain the importance of maintaining literature evaluation skills.

It's time to come full circle. Throughout this text, evidence-based medicine has been the overarching paradigm for providing drug information; the pharmacist not only accesses and evaluates tertiary sources of information efficiently and effectively but also searches for and critically evaluates primary sources of literature, generally considered the most current evidence available. Besides the procedures for evaluating various types of primary literature, we have discussed biostatistical applications to help the pharmacist draw appropriate inferences and apply those inferences to the clinical decision-making process. But now what? How does the pharmacist put all of this into practice? How does he or she keep up with the medical literature to maintain professional competency and provide evidence-based recommendations in a clinical practice setting? The answers to these questions are not easy ones. The goal of this chapter is to provide the pharmacist with one approach to keeping current with the medical literature.

Keeping current with the medical literature is of paramount importance—pharmacists take an oath and have a fiduciary responsibility to provide the best care to their patients (see Chapter 1). To provide the best care, pharmacists must maintain professional competency, which is in part accomplished by keeping current with medical literature. As discussed in Chapter 1, pharmacists must become information masters.

However, knowledge in medicine and pharmacy is growing at a phenomenal rate. MEDLINE alone contains more than 16 million citations from almost 5,000 biomedical journals from the United States and 70 other countries; approximately 500,000 new citations are added each year. With the vast amount of new information available, it is becoming increasingly difficult for clinicians to keep up. Faced with this deluge of information, how can the pharmacist maintain a current information base?

Clinicians rely on many sources of medical information, including scientific studies, biomedical journal articles and reviews, throw-away journals (generally not peer reviewed and laden with advertisements), textbooks and compendia, electronic databases, colleagues, continuing-education forums, and pharmaceutical company representatives.[1] Each source has advantages and limitations. For example, getting an opinion from a colleague may be a fast-and-easy means of obtaining information, but the colleague may not be any better informed on the subject than the questioner. The colleague, in fact, may feel pressured to offer some sort of information even if that information is not the most current or accurate. Expert medical opinion is far from infallible.

Continuing education symposia are an efficient way to keep current, but many symposia are funded by pharmaceutical companies. As such, the information provided is often at risk of being slanted or biased. In addition, continuing education programs are not an effective means for changing clinician practice behavior.[2]

Textbooks, although great for providing an overview or background on a subject, are often outdated with respect to the most recent evidence. Furthermore, buying textbooks year after year is an expensive and impractical means of keeping current.

To overcome these shortcomings, some authors have suggested that clinicians must read and critically assess information for themselves.[3] Indeed, a major goal of this text has been to provide frameworks for evaluating the most commonly published types of research studies. But with thousands of studies being published every year, how can pharmacists manage this wealth of information in a practical and efficient manner? The ever-increasing constraints of a busy clinical practice all too often preclude keeping up with the vast amount of current information. A clinician who wished to keep ahead of the flood of information by reading everything of possible importance to medicine would have to read 6000 articles each day![4] Clinicians must recognize the need for adapting a systematic approach to keeping current with the medical literature.

A Patient-Centered Strategy for Distilling Clinically Relevant Information

One approach to keeping current is to use a patient-centered strategy. That is, pharmacists should consider their clinical practice and the patients they routinely encounter as a way of focusing their efforts to find new medical literature that is most pertinent to their own situation.

Generally, clinicians gather information for four basic reasons:[1]

- To keep up to date with new developments in medicine
- To answer a patient- or population-specific clinical question
- To review and/or reinforce previously learned information
- To keep up with a specific area of interest or for fun

The ultimate goal of gathering information for these reasons is to find the best information using the least amount of time and effort. To be useful, information must possess three traits:[5]

- It must be relevant to everyday practice.
- It must be accurate (valid).
- It must require minimal work to obtain and be readily available.

These attributes can be conceptualized by the equation in Table 12-1. Notice that the usefulness of information gained is a positive function of relevance and validity but is

TABLE 12-1	**Usefulness of Medical Information Equation**

$$\text{Usefulness of medical information} = \frac{(\text{Relevance} \times \text{Validity})}{\text{Work}}$$

Reprinted with permission from Slawson DC, Shaughnessy AF, Bennett JH. Becoming a medical information master: Feeling good about not knowing everything. J Fam Pract 1994;38:505–513.

diminished by the effort required to obtain the information. This is an important equation for pharmacists, because it is a key component to managing the vast amounts of available medical literature. The goal of this strategy is to find articles that are most useful to patient care. The preeminent articles are the ones that are highly relevant and valid yet take minimal time to acquire. Unfortunately, such articles are often rare. Consequently, the pharmacist must often settle for a tradeoff between these components. For example, the pharmacist may need to sacrifice time to find an article that is highly relevant and highly valid.

RELEVANCE

Looking in greater detail at each component of the usefulness equation, the relevance aspect refers to applicability to clinical practice. Is the subject matter of the article germane to the clinician's particular practice? For example, a pediatrician would most likely not find studies performed in adult subjects very relevant to his or her clinical practice.

In addition, the clinician needs to consider how often the disease or problem under study is encountered in his or her practice. A primary-care physician may see 15 patients per day who have hypertension but only 1 person per year with a rare genetic condition such as Huntington disease. Thus finding studies that pertain to hypertension would be more relevant than finding articles pertaining to Huntington disease.

Finally, the clinician needs to evaluate what is being studied—drug pharmacokinetics, the pathophysiologic aspects of a disease, the causes of a disease, disease markers—and think about what outcomes would matter most to patients. The primary goals of the clinician should be to improve the patient's quality of life, ease pain and suffering, and prolong life without significant complications. Studies that measure these outcomes would be highly relevant to the clinician's practice. In this regard, further discernment of study outcomes is needed. In general, study outcomes can be categorized into **disease-oriented evidence (DOE)** or **patient-oriented evidence (POE)**.

What is the difference between DOE and POE? Disease-oriented evidence involves the measurement of an intermediate outcome in a study, such as a surrogate marker or end point. DOE outcomes are aimed at increasing understanding of a disease and its incidence and prevalence, diagnosis and treatment, and prognosis. Disease-oriented evidence is important because clinicians need to first understand the physiologic derangements and pathologic sequelae of a malady before they can provide effective diagnosis and treatment.[1]

Patient-oriented evidence concerns outcomes that patients care most about—morbidity, mortality, and quality of life. For example, a study that measures the number of hospitalizations from heart failure exacerbations or the risk of stroke secondary to atrial fibrillation is categorized as POE, because hospitalizations and stroke are examples of morbidity parameters. A study that measures risk of fatal acute myocardial infarctions is another example of POE. Quality of life might be measured by questionnaires to capture the personal and social context of patients and their disease. Measuring quality of life ensures that evaluations and treatments focus on the patient rather than on the disease only. Table 12-2 lists the characteristics DOE and POE.

TABLE 12-2	**Disease-oriented Evidence vs. Patient-oriented Evidence**[a]
DOE OUTCOMES	POE OUTCOMES
Intermediate outcomes	Mortality/death
Surrogate markers	Morbidity
Disease markers	Quality of life
Outcomes that are important in understanding a disease but are not considered POE	Outcomes that patients are most concerned about; patients want to live longer and/or better

[a]If the study does not measure items listed under POE Outcomes, it is considered DOE.

Often, DOE precedes publication of POE. For example, DOE would derive from a study examining the use of fasting blood glucose as a diabetes screening tool. Although measuring fasting blood glucose is an effective screening method for detecting the presence of diabetes, it does not provide evidence as to whether identifying patients with diabetes early on will result in a positive patient-oriented outcome such as a decrease in mortality risk. Of course, it can be *assumed* that early detection of diabetes would lead to better patient-oriented outcomes, but it is not *proven* explicitly by a DOE study. To *know* that use of fasting blood glucose for diabetes screening reduces mortality risk, a trial evaluating the mortality effects of this screening practice would need to be performed.

Another example of differences between DOE and POE is provided by the effects of bisphosphonate treatment. Bisphosphonates are used commonly to treat osteoporosis. Although increasing bone mineral density (BMD) is a goal of osteoporosis treatment, BMD is considered DOE or a **surrogate outcome**, defined as a laboratory measurement or a physical sign used as a substitute for a clinically meaningful end point.[6] That is, BMD is used as a substitute for a clinically meaningful POE end point, such as increased resistance of long bones to fracture. The latter outcome has a direct effect on how the patient feels, functions, or survives. In contrast, the patient is unaware of changes in BMD.

PERSPECTIVE 12-1

As stated previously, surrogate outcomes are laboratory measurements or physical signs used as a substitute for clinically meaningful end points that measure directly how the patient feels, functions, or survives.[6] The pharmacist should consider the pros and cons of surrogate outcomes.

On the positive side, DOE outcomes may provide preliminary evidence of the efficacy and safety of a treatment before POE outcomes emerge. For example, it takes only 3 months to lower hemoglobin $A1_c$ (HbA1c) levels, a common laboratory index of glycemic control. In contrast, the POE benefits, in terms of reductions in nephropathy or neuropathy, may not be evident for several years.

On the other hand, reliance on DOE outcomes may lead to inaccurate conclusions about the POE clinical end point of interest. For example, consider the statin drug class. There are currently six available statins, including rosuvastatin. Although other statins in the class—such as pravastatin, lovastatin, and simvastatin—have evidence-based support for their ability to lower cholesterol and reduce morbidity and mortality,[7–9] the morbidity and mortality benefit should not be automatically extrapolated to rosuvastatin, because studies measuring POE outcomes with rosuvastatin have yet to be published at the writing of this book.

Some studies do provide evidence that rosuvastatin reduces cholesterol levels (DOE);[10,11] but the benefits in terms of reduced morbidity and mortality are less clear. This is because the decreased risk of morbidity and mortality may be the result of an effect of the statin drug that is unrelated to its cholesterol-lowering properties, a so-called pleiotropic effect.[12] Thus it might be premature to conclude that just because rosuvastatin reduces cholesterol, it also reduces the more patient-oriented outcomes of morbidity and death. Trials that measure clinically relevant, patient-oriented outcomes should generally be performed before new interventions are widely accepted.[13]

Furthermore, there are cases in which a surrogate outcome was not related to a patient-oriented outcome. The Heart and Estrogen/Progestin Replacement Study (HERS) trial[14] was a multicenter randomized controlled trial (RCT) conducted in > 2700 postmenopausal women with coronary heart disease (CHD). The study was performed to evaluate whether conjugated estrogen plus medroxyprogesterone would decrease the recurrence of coronary events. Previous epidemiologic research had associated estrogen use with low-density lipoprotein (LDL) cholesterol reduction and high-density lipoprotein (HDL) cholesterol increase. It was hypothesized that estrogen's effect on these surrogate cholesterol end points would be associated with a reduction in coronary events. The results of the HERS trial did not support this hypothesis, however. Although women receiving estrogen plus medroxyprogesterone experienced an 11% decrease in LDL cholesterol and a 10% increase in HDL cholesterol during the trial, the risk of death owing to myocardial infarction or CHD was similar to that of women who received placebo (hazards ratio [HR] = 0.99, 95% confidence interval [CI] = 0.80–01.22).

It's important to keep in mind that patient-oriented evidence is not always available, leaving the clinician to rely on surrogate markers (or DOE). How does the pharmacist judge the utility of a surrogate outcome? Utility of the surrogate outcome is increased if there is a causal connection between changes in both the surrogate and the patient-oriented outcome. The surrogate outcome must be in the causal pathway of the disease process, and an intervention's entire effect on the patient-oriented outcome should be fully captured by a change in the surrogate outcome.[15] Returning to the bisphosphonate and BMD example, do you think that BMD is a reliable surrogate outcome to measure in a study?

As stated earlier, studies that include POE are typically carried out after disease-oriented studies have been performed. Whereas DOE studies examine intermediate outcomes, POE studies look at final outcomes—outcomes of greatest clinical interest and importance to patients. Actually, POE can be taken one step further—for what patients and clinicians are truly seeking is **Patient-Oriented Evidence That Matters (POEM)**.[1] POEM, if valid, requires the clinician to change his or her clinical practice.[1]

To be considered POEM, the study should meet all three of the following criteria:[16]

- The study focuses on outcomes that patients care most about (i.e. POE).
- The issue under study is common to clinical practice, and the intervention is feasible.
- If the information is valid, a change in clinical practice is required.

POEM studies mainly differ from POE studies in that the former require clinicians to change their practice. For example, a study measures the effect of a new antibiotic compared to a standard antibiotic for reducing hospitalizations secondary to community-acquired pneumonia (CAP). However, the study was performed in a small patient sample, and the novel antibiotic did not show statistically or clinically meaningful reductions in hospitalizations. Although the study would be classified as POE, because it measured a patient-oriented outcome (i.e. hospitalizations), the findings of the study do not prompt the clinician to modify his or her practice.

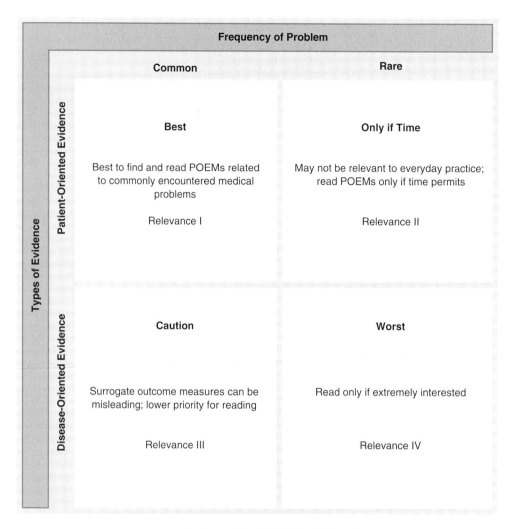

Relevance Scale I (High) to IV (Low)

FIGURE 12-1 Relationship of the Types of Evidence and Frequency of the Clinical Problem to the Relevance of the Information. The clinician should focus on finding and reading Patient-Oriented Evidence That Matters (*POEM*) studies, especially POEMs that are highly relevant to his or her clinical practice. The clinician should read POEMs that are not as relevant to his or her clinical practice only if time permits. DOE studies should receive a lower priority when allocating time to read the medical literature. DOE studies that do not pertain to commonly encountered medical problems should be read only if the clinician is extremely interested in the study and has extra reading time. (Adapted with permission from Slawson DC, Shaughnessy AF, Bennett JH. Becoming a medical information master: Feeling good about not knowing everything. J Fam Pract 1994;38:505–513.)

Now supposed a study measures the effect of a new antibiotic compared to a standard antibiotic for reducing hospitalizations secondary to CAP in a large patient sample. The study clearly shows that the novel antibiotic is statistically and clinically better than the standard antibiotic for reducing hospitalizations. This study would be considered a POEM because it meets the three criteria; it focuses on POE, CAP is a common health issue, and the study provides valid findings that require the clinician to change his or her clinical practice to recommend the novel antibiotic instead of the standard antibiotic.

Unfortunately, in the vast jungle of medical literature, POEMs are rarer than DOEs and POEs. A search of 85 journals containing > 8000 original research articles over a 6-month period found that only 211 (2.6%) of those articles were POEMs. Of the POEMs, 50% were contained in 10 of the 85 journals searched, which included the *Journal of the American Medical Association, New England Journal of Medicine, Archives of Internal Medicine, Lancet,* and *British Medical Journal.*[17]

Although rare, POEM studies provide information of greater relevance to the pharmacist's practice than do DOE studies and should be high-priority reading material. The journals just listed are good places to start a search. Figure 12-1 provides a scheme for using a patient-centered approach for choosing studies to read. The clinician should focus on finding and reading POEMs, especially those that are highly relevant to his or her clinical practice. The clinician should read POEMs that are less relevant to his or her clinical practice only if time permits. DOE studies should receive a lower priority when allocating time to reading the medical literature. DOE studies that do not pertain to commonly encountered medical problems should be read only if the clinician is extremely interested in the study and has spare time.

In summary, the pharmacist should make time to read studies that are highly relevant to his or her practice and that measure Patient-Oriented Evidence That Matters.

VALIDITY AND WORK

In addition to relevance, two other components of the usefulness equation are validity and work (Table 12-1). Previous chapters outlined how studies should be assessed for validity, or the truthfulness of the findings. RCTs that employ rigorous scientific methods and are well designed to minimize bias and the potential for chance findings are more likely to provide valid evidence than are observational studies, for example.

The final component of the usefulness equation involves the concept of work. Work refers to the amount of time, money, or effort required for obtaining, evaluating, and integrating a study into clinical practice. The more work involved, the less useful the evidence.

However, it is important to remember that pharmacists need to find a balance among relevance, validity, and work when searching for articles to read. Using a patient-centered information-management system is one effective way of keeping up with the medical literature.

Foraging Through the Medical Literature

Now that a strategy for selecting articles is in place—a patient-centered approach is needed to effectively and efficiently find information—how does the pharmacist actually go about obtaining the new information? Every clinician needs a system for keeping current with the medical literature. And such a system can generally includes a foraging tool and a hunting tool. A **foraging tool** is a means of being alerted to new information as it becomes available. A **hunting tool** is a method for finding the information again if and when needed. An information master must have and use both foraging and hunting tools.[18] Without foraging and hunting systems, the pharmacist will not be aware of new information and may not be able to find older information when it's needed to answer a clinical question.

FORAGING TOOLS

A wide variety of foraging tools exists to help clinicians become aware of new evidence as it becomes available. InfoPOEMs (www.infopoems.com), developed by Slawson and Shaughnessy (two widely recognized authorities on **information mastery** whose work provided a basis for this chapter), is available on the World Wide Web by subscription only. The service offers a free month-long trial so a clinician can try the tool before buying a subscription.

The DailyInfoPOEMs service lists valid, relevant research via an e-mail summary sent to subscribers every weekday. Using a systematic approach and explicit selection criteria, the service probes > 100 biomedical journals each month. Although POEMs are of highest priority, POE and DOE studies are often listed as well. For each article found, the service provides a summary of key findings along with recommendations on how the study results can be applied to clinical practice. At present, this foraging tool is broadly applicable to clinicians who practice in primary care, although the service is expanding into other clinical specialties, such as pediatrics.

Journal Watch (www.jwatch.org) is another popular and well-respected foraging tool available online or in print. Journal Watch is published twice a month in print and is updated twice a week on the Web site. To take advantage of the full service, the clinician must subscribe. However, the Web site offers a free registration, which allows the user to view the current issue's table of contents and all content older than 6 months. Journal Watch covers both general medicine and various specialty areas, such as cardiology, dermatology, emergency medicine, women's health, psychiatry, and infectious disease.

The American College of Physicians (ACP) Journal Club (www.acpjc.org/index.html) offers a foraging tool that is available in print and online by subscription only. The general purpose of ACP Journal Club is to select original studies and systematic reviews that warrant attention by clinicians who want to keep pace with important advances in internal medicine. These articles are summarized in "value-added abstracts" and commented on by clinical experts. Information is gleaned from > 100 journals.

InfoPOEMs, Journal Watch, and the ACP Journal Club are invaluable tools for keeping current with the medical literature. They are useful not only because they alert the clinician to newly available evidence but also because they provide some critique of the literature. However, to have full access to these foraging tools, the pharmacist must pay a subscription fee.

Other foraging tools are available without a subscription. The Turning Research into Practice (TRIP) Database (www.tripdatabase.com/index.html) reviews these five leading general medicine journals: *Journal of the American Medical Association*, *New England Journal of Medicine*, *Archives of Internal Medicine*, *Lancet*, and *British Medical Journal*. The service provides updates on new important research and issues alerts to new practice guidelines (from the United States and elsewhere) and systematic reviews. The system also contains an archive of frequently asked questions (FAQs) concerning clinical issues and offers evidence-based answers.

PubMed's National Center for Biotechnology Information (NCBI; www.ncbi.nlm.nih.gov/entrez/query.fcgi?DB = pubmed) is a free service that can be used for foraging. After completing the registration form, the pharmacist can perform a search in MEDLINE (see Chapter 2). The search results can be saved and can be amended by e-mail updates as new evidence appears in the MEDLINE database. For example, suppose a pharmacist wants to be alerted when new evidence pertaining to rosiglitazone for the treatment of diabetes becomes available from an RCT. The pharmacist first executes a MEDLINE search, then saves the search, and finally chooses to receive updates on any new related evidence that gets indexed in MEDLINE. Figure 12-2 presents a screen shot of this foraging tool.

Medscape (www.medscape.com/home) is freely available via the World Wide Web. It provides in-depth coverage of recent medical association conferences, continuing-education opportunities, and access to selected journal content from prominent medical publishers. The Medscape Web site can be customized to provide medical news and updates tailored to the clinician's specialty.

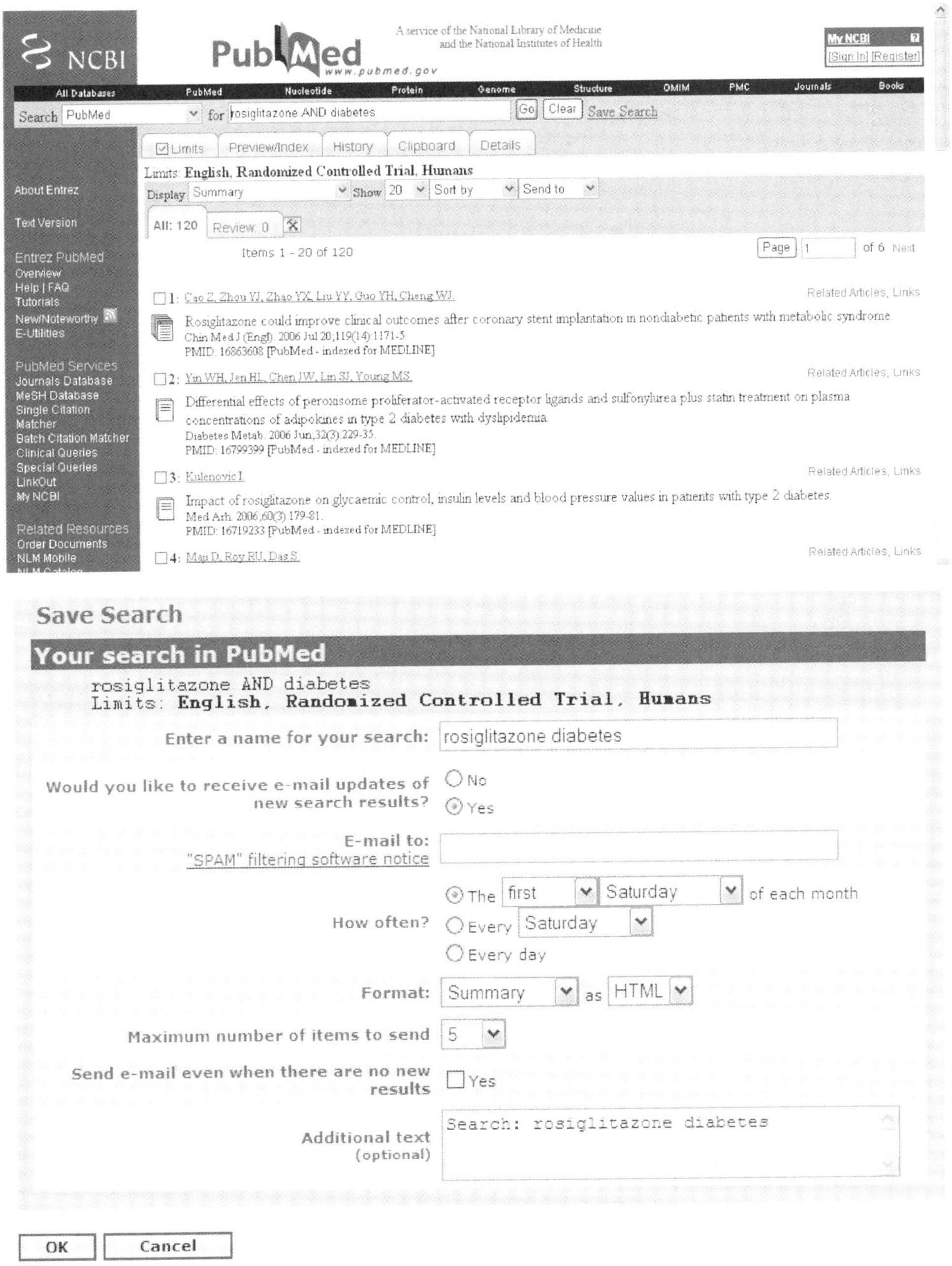

FIGURE 12-2 PubMed NCBI Foraging Tool. **A.** Screen shot of a PubMed search for "rosiglitazone AND diabetes" with the following limits: English language, randomized controlled trials, and humans. **B.** If the pharmacist clicks "Save Search" (seen in part **A**), this PubMed NCBI form is seen. By completing the form, the pharmacist can receive updates whenever newly indexed literature that meets the search specifications is added to the MEDLINE database.

News wires and the tables of contents of journals provide additional foraging tools. Clinicians can access health news feeds from Reuters or HealthDay news services on various Web sites. For example, the popular Internet search engine Yahoo! (www.yahoo.com) provides access to both these news feeds. The Yahoo! Web site home page can be customized to display news updates related to recently published studies. The pharmacist can also register

TABLE 12-3	Foraging Tools	
TOOL	**ACCESS**	**SUBSCRIPTION**
InfoPOEMs—The Clinical Awareness System	www.infopoems.com/	Yes
Journal Watch Online	www.jwatch.org/	Yes
American College of Physicians (ACP) Journal Club	www.acpjc.org/index.html	Yes
Turning Research into Practice (TRIP) Database	www.tripdatabase.com/index.html	No
PubMed NCBI	www.ncbi.nlm.nih.gov/entrez/query.fcgi?DB = pubmed	No
Medscape	www.medscape.com/home	No

for tables of contents to various medical journals. For example, *New England Journal of Medicine* offers a cost-free service consisting of a weekly e-mail that contains the current issue's table of contents. Often, links to free, full-text landmark clinical trials contained in the journal are provided in the e-mail.

These no-cost foraging tools are important for alerting the clinician to just-this-minute information. However, their value is limited because the focus is not as narrowly aimed at identifying POEMs as are some of the subscription services, such as Journal Watch, InfoPOEMs, and ACP Journal Club. In addition, some freely available tools provide only alerts and do not provide critical evaluation of the literature. Common foraging tools are summarized in Table 12-3.

When evaluating a foraging system, remember that the best systems provide evidence updates that have been critically evaluated for validity and that are highly relevant to clinical practice. The evidence should be presented in a clear and easily understandable manner to reduce the reader's workload. Thus a good foraging tool for the busy practicing clinician fits nicely with the usefulness equation given in Table 12-1. The downside to good foraging systems is that they can be costly and provide only summaries of the clinical evidence. For a complete evaluation of the study, an in-depth analysis of the original article is still necessary.

Pharmacists should critically appraise any foraging system before paying for a subscription or using the service. Some points to consider are the following:[18]

- The information filtering process employed
- Validity determinations for the summarized information
- The writing quality of the information summary
- Breadth of biomedical journals covered and their application to clinical practice
- The specific recommendations made

Information Filtering

As discussed earlier in this chapter, clinicians need to keep up with studies that are highly relevant to their own clinical practice. Thus the pharmacist should select a foraging service that focuses on identifying and summarizing articles that pertain to his or her interest area. The pharmacist must also evaluate the foraging system to determine whether it provides patient-oriented evidence. The service should weed out less useful studies and focus mainly on POEMs.

Determining Validity

To be useful, the information provided has to be valid. Thus a foraging system needs to share explicitly and transparently the manner by which the article was selected and reviewed. The clinician should seek labels that indicate the level of evidence for the summarized study (see Chapter 11). For example, InfoPOEMs uses the levels of evidence developed by the Oxford Centre for Evidence-Based Medicine.[19] In this scheme, for example, level 1a designates the highest level of evidence, indicating that the evidence was obtained from a homogeneous systematic review of RCTs. In contrast, the lowest level, level 5, means that the summary was based on expert opinion without explicit critical appraisal.

Writing Quality

Editors at any foraging service are distilling studies that can be 10 pages or more in length into 200- to 300-word summaries. Thus the quality of writing and communication skills of the writing staff are of paramount importance. Editors need to capture the most important points from the study and communicate them to reader in a clear, concise, accurate, and understandable manner. When evaluating a foraging service, the pharmacist should view examples of study summaries to make sure they are well written.

Comprehensiveness of Literature Search

Another aspect of a foraging service is the breadth of biomedical journals reviewed. Are the journals reviewed comprehensive enough to meet the clinician's needs? To be useful, the foraging service should include biomedical journals pertinent to the clinician's specific discipline, specialty, or practice area. This should be evident from the listing of biomedical journals routinely reviewed by the foraging service. It is important to remember that the foraging tool is only as good as the literature search executed by the service.

Recommendations Made

To be truly useful to the clinician, the foraging service should not only summarize the evidence from a relevant study but also help the clinician place the information into the general POEM context. This is accomplished by relating specific study results to current treatment strategies and by providing specific recommendations for clinical practice.

HUNTING TOOLS

In addition to a high-quality foraging tool, an information master must also have a high-quality hunting tool to help him or her find the information again when it is needed. Often, a foraging tool is integrated or coordinated with a hunting tool. For example, InfoPOEMs Clinical Awareness System has both a foraging tool (DailyInfoPOEMs) and a hunting tool (InfoRetriever). The hunting tool allows the clinician to search the InfoPOEMs database online or via a handheld personal data device. Journal Watch also offers an online search function for finding evidence summaries.

Retrieving articles with an abstracting database is also an option. Secondary databases, such as MEDLINE, EMBASE, and International Pharmaceutical Abstracts (IPA), were discussed in detail in Chapter 2. In addition, some Internet search engines offer effective ways to find information. Google Scholar (scholar.google.com) is one such search engine, and it provides a simple way to look for esearch literature. The clinician can search across many disciplines and sources, including peer-reviewed papers, abstracts, and research articles. Google Scholar can help the clinician quickly find the most relevant research. Finally, personal electronic folders or hard copy files of frequently used studies and medical information that pertain to the clinician's practice can be refreshed periodically.

As with a foraging tool, a hunting tool needs to be assessed for quality. The hunting tool should be easily accessible and efficient to use. The hunting tool should quickly and efficiently lead the pharmacist to valid, relevant, key evidence and recommendations that can be applied at the point of patient care.

Maintaining Literature Evaluation Skills

Although foraging and hunting tools provide an efficient and effective way to keep up with the medical literature, pharmacists should also take time to hone and maintain literature evaluation skills. Some foraging tools provide critical evaluation of the medical literature, but others serve only to alert the clinician to the newly available evidence. In addition, as stated before, pharmacists must not rely solely on the foraging service's evaluation of the study but must critically evaluate the study for themselves

Literature evaluation is a key to keeping current with the literature. It has been suggested that a clinician should devote at least 1 to 2 hr each week to finding and reviewing primary literature highly relevant to his or her scope of practice.[20] Because this may be a difficult habit to acquire and maintain individually, many clinicians form journal club groups in which participants take turns critically evaluating a study for the other members. Both the study and the critical evaluation are discussed at group meetings.

It is particularly advantageous to include healthcare practitioners other than pharmacists in such journal clubs. This practice not only enhances the pharmacist's perspective on the needs and expertise of the other members of the healthcare team but also provides teaching moments from the pharmacist's perspective.

Not keeping current with the medical literature will reflect poorly on the competency of the practitioner. For example, how will the pharmacist recommend new drug therapies if he or she is unaware of them or hasn't evaluated the drugs' safety and effectiveness? Evidence on drug safety and efficacy comes directly from the primary literature.

Furthermore how will a community pharmacist handle situations in which patients bring in news stories relating to a recently published study? For example, the September 13, 2006, issue of *Journal of the American Medical Association* contained a study conducted in Japan showing that green tea prolongs life.[21] The study hit the news wires, patients learn of it, and someone is bound to ask the pharmacist if it is a good idea to take green tea extract supplements. How will the pharmacist help the patient make a decision about using the extract if he or she hasn't read and evaluated the study?

Literature appraisal skills are a key step to engaging in self-directed learning. Being a life-long self-learner is necessary if the pharmacist wants to maintain professional competency. If literature evaluation skills are not practiced regularly, they can be quickly lost. Setting aside time each week to focus on honing these skills while keeping up with the medical literature is a good approach and is needed when providing pharmaceutical care in the evidence-based model of medicine.

Summary

Developing and maintaining skills to keep current with the medical literature is an essential component for an information master. This chapter outlines a patient-centered approach for keeping current with the medical literature, including the use of various foraging and hunting tools.

Recall from Chapter 1 that information mastery is the ability to efficiently and effectively forage through vast amounts of available information, find and critically assess the best and most pertinent pieces of information, and apply information to the clinical situation. To be an integral member of the healthcare team working under the evidence-based medicine paradigm, pharmacists must become information masters. Pharmacists need to know what information to look for, how to efficiently and effectively search for and find information, and how to critically appraise that information to answer clinical questions and to practice in the evidence-based model of medicine. The information contained in this book provides a solid foundation for that effort. Good luck!

STUDY PROBLEMS

1. Label the following study outcomes as DOE or POE:
   Hemoglobin A_{1c}
   Systolic blood pressure
   Risk of myocardial infarction
   Total cholesterol
   Survival rates
   Pain improvement

2. List the three criteria that define a POEM. Find a POEM in the medical literature.

3. Compare and contrast InfoPOEMs and Journal Watch. Search for other information-management tools. Register for any free online services.

4. Interview a pharmacist to learn how he or she keeps current with the medical literature.

5. Develop an argument to refute the following statement: "Pharmacists do not need to become information masters."

6. Develop a plan for how you will keep current with the medical literature. Contrast your ideas with those of the pharmacist you interviewed for question 4.

7. Examine several foraging and hunting tools described in this chapter. Find out which seem to best suited to your intended area of practice. Select a topic that is being discussed currently in one of your other classes and compare several tools to find out which provides the best current information.

REFERENCES

1. Slawson DC, Shaughnessy AF, Bennett JH. Becoming a medical information master: Feeling good about not knowing everything. J Fam Pract 1994;38:505–513.
2. Davis DA, Thomson MA, Oxman AD, et al. Evidence for the effectiveness of CME: A review of 50 randomized controlled trials. JAMA 1992;268:1111–1117.
3. Evidence-Based Medicine Working Group. Evidence-based medicine: A new approach to teaching the practice of medicine. JAMA 1992;268.2420–2425.
4. Arndt KA. Information excess in medicine. Overview, relevance to dermatology, and strategies for coping. Arch Dermatol 1992;128:1249–1256.
5. Curley SP, Connelly DP, Rich EC. Physician's use of medical knowledge resources: Preliminary theoretical framework and findings. Med Decis Making 1990;10:231–241.
6. Temple RJ. A regulatory authority's opinion about surrogate endpoints. In: Nimmo WS, Tucker GT, eds., Clinical Measurement in Drug Evaluation. New York: Wiley, 1995.

7. The Long-Term Intervention with Pravastatin in Ischaemic Disease (LIPID) Study Group. Prevention of cardiovascular events and death with pravastatin in patients with coronary heart disease and a broad range of initial cholesterol levels. N Engl J Med 1998;339:1349–1357.

8. Downs JR, Clearfield M, Weis S, et al. Primary prevention of acute coronary events with lovastatin in men and women with average cholesterol levels. Results of AFCAPS/TexCAPS. JAMA. 1998;279:1615–1622.

9. Heart Protection Study Collaborative Group. MRC/BHF Heart Protection Study of cholesterol lowering with simvastatin in 20,536 high-risk individuals: A randomised placebo controlled trial. Lancet 2002;360:7–22.

10. Davidson M, Ma P, Stein EA, et al. Comparison of effects on low-density lipoprotein cholesterol and high-density lipoprotein cholesterol with rosuvastatin versus atorvastatin in patients with type IIa or IIb hypercholesterolemia. Am J Cardiol 2002;89:268–275.

11. Paoletti R, Fahmy M, Mahla G, et al. Rosuvastatin demonstrates greater reduction of low-density lipoprotein cholesterol compared with pravastatin and simvastatin in hypercholesterolaemic patients: A randomized, double-blind study. J Cardiovasc Risk 2001;8:383–390.

12. McFarlane SI, Muniyappa R, Francisco R, et al. Pleiotropic effects of statins: lipid reduction and beyond. J Clin Endrocrinol Metab 2002;87:1451–1458.

13. Gotzsche PC, Liberati A, Torri V, et al. Beware of surrogate outcome measures. Int J Technol Assess Health Care 1996;12:238–246.

14. Hulley S, Grady D, Bush T, et al. Randomized trial of estrogen plus progestin for secondary prevention of coronary heart disease in postmenopausal women. JAMA 1998;280:605–613.

15. Bucher HC, Guyatt GH, Cookl DJ, et al. Users' guides to the medical literature: Applying clinical trial results—How to use an article measuring the effect of an intervention on surrogate endpoints. JAMA 1999;282:771–778.

16. Slawson DC, Shaughnessy AF. Obtaining useful information from expert based sources. Br Med J 1997;314:947–949.

17. Ebell MH, Barry HC, Slawson DC, et al. Finding POEMs in the medical literature. J Fam Pract 1999;48:350–355.

18. Slawson DC, Shaughnessy AF. Teaching evidence-based medicine: Should we be teaching information management instead? Acad Med 2005;80:685–689.

19. Phillips B, Ball C, Sackett D et al. Levels of Evidence and Grades of Recommendation. Centre for Evidence-Based Medicine, Oxford, UK. Available at www.cebm.net/levels_of_evidence.asp#levels. Accessed Feb 2007.

20. Oxman AD, Sackett DL, Guyatt GH. Users' guides to the medical literature. I. How to get started. JAMA 1993;270:2093–2095.

21. Kuriyama S, Shimazu T, Ohmori K, et al. Green tea consumption and mortality due to cardiovascular disease, cancer, and all causes in Japan. JAMA 2006;296:1255–1265.

Appendix

A

Drug Information Tables

TABLE A.1	Example Drug Information Question Classifications Based on Type of Information Requested[a]

- ☐ Adult drug dosing/administration
- ☐ Adverse drug reactions
- ☐ Approved drug indications/uses
- ☐ Bioequivalence
- ☐ Chemical data
- ☐ Compounding/formulation
- ☐ Drug—Drug interactions
- ☐ Drug—Food interactions
- ☐ Drug—Natural product interactions
- ☐ Drug compatibility and stability
- ☐ Drug cost/pricing
- ☐ Drug identification
- ☐ Drug use in pregnancy and lactation
- ☐ Foreign drug products
- ☐ Geriatric drug dosing/administration
- ☐ Hepatic drug dosing
- ☐ Manufacturer information
- ☐ Natural products/complementary or alternative medicine
- ☐ Nutrition
- ☐ Patient counseling
- ☐ Pediatric drug dosing/administration
- ☐ Pharmacokinetics
- ☐ Renal drug dosing
- ☐ Therapeutics
- ☐ Toxicology/poisoning
- ☐ Unapproved/investigational uses of drugs

[a]This classification scheme is only an example. Other schemes are available. Some drug information centers or pharmacies have classification schemes tailored specifically for their institution.

TABLE A.2	Commonly Used Secondary Resources
DATABASE	**DESCRIPTION**
Cochrane Library	By subscription only
	Three components:
	a) Cochrane Database of Systematic Reviews (CDSR)
	• Provides access to high-quality systematic reviews of specific clinical questions
	b) Database of Abstracts of Reviews of Effectiveness (DARE)
	• Abstracts of published systematic reviews on the effects of healthcare from around the world that have been critically analyzed according to a high standard of criteria; provides access to quality reviews in subjects for which a full Cochrane review may not yet exist
	c) Controlled Clinical Trials Registry
	• A bibliography of controlled trials identified by contributors to the Cochrane Collaboration and others as part of an international effort to hand search the world's journals and create an unbiased source of data for systematic reviews; includes reports published in conference proceedings and in many other sources not currently listed in MEDLINE or other bibliographic databases
Current Contents	By subscription only
	• From Thomas Scientific
	• Offers subgroups, such as life science and clinical medicine
	• The Clinical Medicine database provides access to complete bibliographic information from articles, editorials, meeting abstracts, commentaries, and all other significant items in recently published editions of > 1120 of the world's leading clinical medicine journals and books in a broad range of categories
EMBASE	By subscription only
	• Similar to MEDLINE except it covers a wider array of international journals and meeting abstracts
	• Contains > 11 million records from 1974 to present plus > 7 million unique MEDLINE records from 1966 to present; records are from > 5000 journals; ~ 600,000 records added annually; $> 80\%$ of recent records contain full abstracts
	• Includes drug research; pharmacology; pharmaceutics; pharmacy; side effects and interactions; toxicology; pharmacoeconomics; human medicine (clinical and experimental); basic biomedical sciences; biotechnology; biomedical engineering and instrumentation; health policy and management; public, occupational and environmental health; pollution; substance dependence and abuse; psychiatry; and forensic medicine
	• Updated daily; records processed in 10 working days (on average)
	• Tutorials and instructions available at www.info.embase.com/embase_com/user/learning_tools/index.shtml or via a free interactive training CD

TABLE A.2	**Commonly Used Secondary Resources, cont.**

International Pharmaceutical Abstracts (IPA) — By subscription only

- Developed by the American Society of Health-System Pharmacists (ASHP)
- The most comprehensive abstracting service for domestic and international information relevant to pharmacy and pharmaceutical sciences
- Covers 850 pharmaceutical, medical, and health-related journals published worldwide from 1970 to present
- Includes state pharmacy journals that deal with state regulations, salaries, guidelines, manpower studies, laws and more
- Scope of the database ranges from the clinical, practical, and theoretical to the economic and scientific aspects of the literature
- Updated monthly

Iowa Drug Information Service (IDIS) — By subscription only

- From the College of Pharmacy at the University of Iowa
- Indexing service that allows for access to complete, full-text journal articles from ~ 200 biomedical journals

MEDLINE

- Multiple publishers, including OVID (by subscription) and PubMed (free: www.pubmed.gov)
- Developed by the National Center for Biotechnology Information (NCBI) at the National Library of Medicine (NLM), which is located at the National Institutes of Health (NIH)
- One of the most expansive and accessible databases of biomedical information
- Covers ~ 4300 biomedical journals published in the United States and 70 other countries
- Scope includes biomedicine and health—covering medicine, dentistry, nursing, veterinary medicine, healthcare systems, and preclinical sciences
- Database file contains > 11 million citations dating back to the mid-1960s; coverage is worldwide, but most records are from English-language sources or have English abstracts
- Bibliographies, abstracts, and (in some cases) links to full-text articles
- Medical subject headings (MeSH) database—the controlled vocabulary for searching
- Updated daily

TABLE A.3	**Commonly Used Tertiary References for Answering Drug Information Questions**[a]

ADULT DRUG DOSING/ADMINISTRATION
- DRUGDEX System (Thomson Micromedex)
- American Society of Health-System Pharmacists (ASHP) AHFS Drug Information
- Facts & Comparisons (Wolters Kluwer)
- Product package insert and prescribing information
- *Drug Information Handbook* (Lexi-Comp)
- *Clinical Pharmacology* (Gold Standard)

ADVERSE DRUG REACTIONS
- DRUGDEX System (Thomson Micromedex)
- American Society of Health-System Pharmacists (ASHP) AHFS Drug Information
- *Davies's Textbook of Adverse Drug Reactions* (Oxford University Press)
- Product package insert and prescribing information
- *Meyler's Side Effects of Drugs* (Elsevier)
- *Clinical Pharmacology* (Gold Standard)

APPROVED DRUG INDICATIONS/USES
- Facts & Comparisons (Wolters Kluwer)
- American Society of Health-System Pharmacists (ASHP) AHFS Drug Information
- *Drug Information Handbook* (Lexi-Comp)
- *Physician's Desk Reference* (*PDR;* Thomson Healthcare)
- *USP DI. Volume I: Drug Information for the Health Care Professional* (Thomson Healthcare)

BIOEQUIVALENCE
- Approved Drug Products with Therapeutic Equivalence Evaluations. Orange Book (www.fda.gov/cder/orange/default.htm)
- *USP DI. Volume III: Approved Drug Products and Legal Requirements* (Thomson Healthcare)
- *Physician's Desk Reference* (*PDR;* Thomson Healthcare)

CHEMICAL DATA
- *Remington: The Science and Practice of Pharmacy* (Lippincott Williams & Wilkins)
- *Merck Index* (Merck Publishing)
- *Martindale's: The Complete Drug Reference* (Pharmaceutical Press; Thomson Micromedex)

COMPOUNDING AND FORMULATION
- *Children's Hospital of Philadelphia Extemporaneous Formulations* (American Society of Health-System Pharmacists)
- *Trissel's Stability of Compounded Formulations* (American Pharmacist Association)
- *Remington: The Science and Practice of Pharmacy* (Lippincott Williams & Wilkins)
- *A Practical Guide to Contemporary Pharmacy Practice* (Lippincott Williams & Wilkins)

DRUG COMPATIBILITY AND STABILITY
- *Trissel's Stability of Compounded Formulations* (American Pharmacist Association)
- *King Guide to Parenteral Admixtures* (King Guide Publications)
- American Society of Health-System Pharmacists (ASHP) AHFS Drug Information
- *Clinical Pharmacology* (Gold Standard)

DRUG COST AND PRICING
- *Red Book* (Thomson Healthcare)
- *Price-Chek PC* (Medi-Span; Wolters Kluwer)

| **TABLE A.3** | **Commonly Used Tertiary References for Answering Drug Information Questions**[a], cont. |

DRUG IDENTIFICATION
- IDENTIDEX System (Thomson Micromedex)
- *Ident-A-Drug* (Therapeutic Research Center)
- Facts & Comparisons (Wolters Kluwer)
- *Physician's Desk Reference* (*PDR;* Thomson Healthcare)
- *American Drug Index* (Facts & Comparisons)
- *USP Dictionary of USAN and International Drug Names* (U.S. Pharmacopeia)
- *Clinical Pharmacology* (Gold Standard)

DRUG INTERACTIONS
- *Drug Interaction Facts* (Facts and Comparisons)
- *Hansten and Horn's Drug Interactions Analysis and Management* (Facts & Comparisons)
- *Evaluations of Drug Interactions* (First DataBank)
- DRUG-REAX System; AltMed-REAX System (Thomson Micromedex)
- *Stockley's Drug Interactions* (Pharmaceutical Press)

DRUG USE IN PREGNANCY AND LACTATION
- *Drugs in Pregnancy and Lactation* (Lippincott Williams & Wilkins)
- REPRORISK System (Thomson Micromedex)
- *Medications and Mother's Milk: A Manual of Lactational Pharmacology* (Pharmasoft Medical)
- Product package insert and prescribing information

FOREIGN DRUG PRODUCTS
- *Index Nominum: The International Drug Directory* (Medpharm Scientific)
- *European Drug Index* (Elsevier)
- *Martindale: The Complete Drug Reference* (Pharmaceutical Press; Thomson Micromedex)
- *Drug Information Handbook International* (Lexi-Comp)

GERIATRIC DRUG DOSING AND ADMINISTRATION
- *Geriatric Dosage Handbook* (Lexi-Comp)
- American Society of Health-System Pharmacists (ASHP) AHFS Drug Information
- DRUGDEX System (Thomson Micromedex)
- Facts & Comparisons (Wolters Kluwer)

HEPATIC DRUG DOSING
- DRUGDEX System (Thomson Micromedex)
- Facts & Comparisons (Wolters Kluwer)
- *Geriatric Dosage Handbook* (Lexi-Comp)
- American Society of Health-System Pharmacists (ASHP) AHFS Drug Information
- *Clinical Pharmacology* (Gold Standard)

MANUFACTURER INFORMATION
- *American Drug Index* (Facts and Comparisons)
- *Red Book* (Thomson Healthcare)
- Facts & Comparisons (Wolters Kluwer)
- *Physician's Desk Reference* (PDR; Thomson Healthcare)

NATURAL PRODUCTS AND COMPLEMENTARY OR ALTERNATIVE MEDICINE
- Natural Medicines Comprehensive Database (Therapeutic Research Center)
- *The Review of Natural Products* (Facts & Comparisons)
- The Complete German Commission E Monographs (American Botanical Counsel)
- AltMedDex System and AltMed-REAX System (Thomson Micromedex)
- *Physician's Desk Reference for Herbal Medicines* (Medical Economics)

| **TABLE A.3** | **Commonly Used Tertiary References for Answering Drug Information Questions**[a]**, cont.** |

PATIENT COUNSELING
- *USP DI, Volume II: Advice for the Patient* (Thomson Healthcare)
- AltCareDex System and CareNotes System (Thomson Micromedex)
- *Medication Teaching Manual* (American Society of Hospital Pharmacists)
- *Patient Counseling Handbook* (American Pharmaceutical Association)
- *Professional's Guide to Patient Drug Facts* (Facts & Comparisons)

PEDIATRIC DRUG DOSING AND ADMINISTRATION
- *Harriet Lane Handbook* (Mosby)
- *Pediatric Dosage Handbook* (Lexi-Comp)
- *Drug Information Handbook* (Lexi-Comp)
- American Society of Health-System Pharmacists (ASHP) AHFS Drug Information
- DRUGDEX System (Thomson Micromedex)
- Facts & Comparisons (Wolters Kluwer)

PHARMACOKINETICS
- KINETIDEX System (Thomson Micromedex)
- *Applied Pharmacokinetics: Principles of Therapeutic Drug Monitoring* (Lippincott Williams & Wilkins)
- *Basic Clinical Pharmacokinetics* (Lippincott Williams & Wilkins)
- American Society of Health-System Pharmacists (ASHP) AHFS Drug Information
- *Clinical Pharmacokinetics: Concepts and Applications* (Lippincott Williams & Wilkins)
- Product package insert and prescribing information

RENAL DRUG DOSING
- Bennett's tables
- *Drug Prescribing in Renal Failure* (American College of Physicians)
- DRUGDEX System (Thomson Micromedex)
- *Geriatric Dosage Handbook* (Lexi-Comp)
- American Society of Health-System Pharmacists (ASHP) AHFS Drug Information
- Product package insert and prescribing information
- *Clinical Pharmacology* (Gold Standard)

THERAPEUTICS
- *Pharmacology: A Pathophysiologic Approach* (McGraw-Hill)
- *Applied Therapeutics: The Clinical Use of Drugs* (Lippincott Williams & Wilkins)
- *Harrison's Principles of Internal Medicine* (McGraw-Hill)
- *Cecil's Textbook of Medicine* (Saunders)

TOXICOLOGY AND POISONING
- POISONDEX System (Thomson Micromedex)
- *Goldfrank's Toxicologic Emergencies* (McGraw-Hill)
- *Ellenhorn's Medical Toxicology: Diagnosis and Treatment of Human Poisoning* (Lippincott Williams & Wilkins)
- *Casarett & Doull's Toxicology: The Basic Science of Poisons* (McGraw-Hill)
- *Poisoning and Toxicology Handbook* (Lexi-Comp)

UNAPPROVED AND INVESTIGATIONAL USES OF DRUGS
- DRUGDEX System (Thomson Micromedex)
- American Society of Health-System Pharmacists (ASHP) AHFS Drug Information
- Facts & Comparisons (Wolters Kluwer)
- *USP DI. Volume I: Drug Information for the Health Care Professional* (Thomson Healthcare)
- U.S. Food and Drug Administration (www.fda.gov)
- Clinical Pharmacology (Gold Standard)

[a]Always use the latest edition or version of the reference.

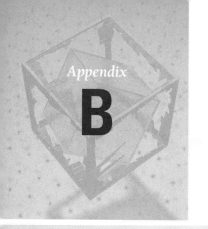

Appendix

B

Statistical Tables

Table B.1. Combinations of Binomial Events: The Number of Ways in Which *j* Outcomes Can Be Obtained with *n* Total Events.

n	0	1	2	3	4	5	6	7	8	9	10	11	12	13	14	15
1																
2	1	2	1													
3	1	3	3	1												
4	1	4	6	4	1											
5	1	5	10	10	5	1										
6	1	6	15	20	15	6	1									
7	1	7	21	35	35	21	7	1								
8	1	8	28	56	70	56	28	8	1							
9	1	9	36	84	126	126	84	36	9	1						
10	1	10	45	120	210	252	210	120	45	10	1					
11	1	11	55	165	330	462	462	330	165	55	11	1				
12	1	12	66	220	495	792	924	792	495	220	66	12	1			
13	1	13	78	286	715	1287	1716	1716	1287	715	286	78	13	1		
14	1	14	91	364	1001	2002	3003	3432	3003	2002	1001	364	91	14	1	
15	1	15	105	455	1365	3003	5005	6435	6435	5005	3003	1365	455	105	15	1

Table B.2. Areas associated with different values of the standard normal distribution. The value in the body of the table is the area under the curve between - infinity and the indicated value of z. To find the area of the normal curve between - ∞ and z = 0.63, for example, find the row identified as "0.6" in the z column identifies as "0.03." The area under the curve is the value at the intersection of the row and column numbers: 0.7357. Thus, 73.57% of the area under the curve is located between - ∞ and z = 0.63

z	0.00	0.01	0.02	0.03	0.04	0.05	0.06	0.07	0.08	0.09
−3.0	0.0130	0.0013	0.0013	0.0012	0.0012	0.0011	0.0011	0.0011	0.0010	0.0010
−2.9	0.0019	0.0018	0.0018	0.0017	0.0016	0.0016	0.0015	0.0015	0.0014	0.0014
−2.8	0.0026	0.0025	0.0024	0.0023	0.0023	0.0022	0.0021	0.0021	0.0020	0.0019
−2.7	0.0035	0.0034	0.0033	0.0032	0.0031	0.0030	0.0029	0.0028	0.0027	0.0026
−2.6	0.0047	0.0045	0.0044	0.0043	0.0041	0.0040	0.0039	0.0038	0.0037	0.0036
−2.5	0.0062	0.0060	0.0059	0.0057	0.0055	0.0054	0.0052	0.0051	0.0049	0.0048
−2.4	0.0082	0.0080	0.0078	0.0075	0.0073	0.0071	0.0069	0.0068	0.0066	0.0064
−2.3	0.0107	0.0104	0.0102	0.0099	0.0096	0.0094	0.0091	0.0089	0.0087	0.0084
−2.2	0.0139	0.0136	0.0132	0.0129	0.0125	0.0122	0.0119	0.0116	0.0113	0.0110
−2.1	0.0179	0.0174	0.0170	0.0166	0.0162	0.0158	0.0154	0.0150	0.0146	0.0143
−2.0	0.0228	0.0222	0.0217	0.0212	0.0207	0.0202	0.0197	0.0192	0.0188	0.0183
−1.9	0.0287	0.0281	0.0274	0.0268	0.0262	0.0256	0.0250	0.0244	0.0239	0.0233
−1.8	0.0359	0.0351	0.0344	0.0336	0.0329	0.0322	0.0314	0.0307	0.0301	0.0294
−1.7	0.0446	0.0436	0.0427	0.0418	0.0409	0.0401	0.0392	0.0384	0.0375	0.0367
−1.6	0.0548	0.0537	0.0526	0.0516	0.0505	0.0495	0.0485	0.0475	0.0465	0.0455
−1.5	0.0668	0.0655	0.0643	0.0630	0.0618	0.0606	0.0594	0.0582	0.0571	0.0559
−1.4	0.0808	0.0793	0.0778	0.0764	0.0749	0.0735	0.0721	0.0708	0.0694	0.0681
−1.3	0.0968	0.0951	0.0934	0.0918	0.0901	0.0885	0.0869	0.0853	0.0838	0.0823
−1.2	0.1151	0.1131	0.1112	0.1093	0.1075	0.1056	0.1038	0.1020	0.1003	0.0985
−1.1	0.1357	0.1335	0.1314	0.1292	0.1271	0.1251	0.1230	0.1210	0.1190	0.1170
−1.0	0.1587	0.1562	0.1539	0.1515	0.1492	0.1469	0.1446	0.1423	0.1401	0.1379
−0.9	0.1841	0.1814	0.1788	0.1762	0.1736	0.1711	0.1685	0.1660	0.1635	0.1611
−0.8	0.2119	0.2090	0.2061	0.2033	0.2005	0.1977	0.1949	0.1922	0.1894	0.1867
−0.7	0.2420	0.2389	0.2358	0.2327	0.2296	0.2266	0.2236	0.2206	0.2177	0.2148
−0.6	0.2743	0.2709	0.2676	0.2643	0.2611	0.2578	0.2546	0.2514	0.2483	0.2451
−0.5	0.3085	0.3050	0.3015	0.2981	0.2946	0.2912	0.2877	0.2843	0.2810	0.2776
−0.4	0.3446	0.3409	0.3372	0.3336	0.3300	0.3264	0.3228	0.3192	0.3156	0.3121
−0.3	0.3821	0.3783	0.3745	0.3707	0.3669	0.3632	0.3594	0.3557	0.3520	0.3483
−0.2	0.4207	0.4168	0.4129	0.4090	0.4052	0.4013	0.3974	0.3936	0.3897	0.3859
−0.1	0.4602	0.4562	0.4522	0.4483	0.4443	0.4404	0.4364	0.4325	0.4286	0.4247
0.0	0.500	0.4960	0.4920	0.4880	0.4840	0.4801	0.4761	0.4721	0.4681	0.4641

Table B.2. Areas associated with different values of the standard normal distribution, cont.

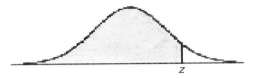

	0.00	0.01	0.02	0.03	0.04	0.05	0.06	0.07	0.08	0.09
0.0	0.5000	0.5040	0.5080	0.5120	0.5160	0.5199	0.5239	0.5279	0.5319	0.5359
0.1	0.5398	0.5438	0.5478	0.5517	0.5557	0.5596	0.5636	0.5675	0.5714	0.5753
0.2	0.5793	0.5832	0.5871	0.5910	0.5948	0.5987	0.6026	0.6064	0.6103	0.6141
0.3	0.6179	0.6217	0.6255	0.6293	0.6331	0.6368	0.6406	0.6443	0.6480	0.6517
0.4	0.6554	0.6591	0.6628	0.6664	0.6700	0.6736	0.6772	0.6808	0.6844	0.6879
0.5	0.6915	0.6950	0.6985	0.7019	0.7054	0.7088	0.7123	0.7157	0.7190	0.7224
0.6	0.7257	0.7291	0.7324	0.7357	0.7389	0.7422	0.7454	0.7486	0.7517	0.7549
0.7	0.7580	0.7611	0.7642	0.7673	0.7704	0.7734	0.7764	0.7794	0.7823	0.7852
0.8	0.7881	0.7910	0.7939	0.7967	0.7995	0.8023	0.8051	0.8078	0.8106	0.8133
0.9	0.8159	0.8186	0.8212	0.8238	0.8264	0.8289	0.8315	0.8340	0.8365	0.8389
1.0	0.8413	0.8438	0.8461	0.8485	0.8508	0.8531	0.8554	0.8577	0.8599	0.8621
1.1	0.8643	0.8665	0.8686	0.8708	0.8729	0.8749	0.8770	0.8790	0.8810	0.8830
1.2	0.8849	0.8869	0.8888	0.8907	0.8925	0.8944	0.8962	0.8980	0.8997	0.9015
1.3	0.9032	0.9049	0.9066	0.9082	0.9099	0.9115	0.9131	0.9147	0.9162	0.9177
1.4	0.9192	0.9207	0.9222	0.9236	0.9251	0.9265	0.9279	0.9292	0.9306	0.9319
1.5	0.9332	0.9345	0.9357	0.9370	0.9382	0.9394	0.9406	0.9418	0.9429	0.9441
1.6	0.9452	0.9463	0.9474	0.9484	0.9495	0.9505	0.9515	0.9525	0.9535	0.9545
1.7	0.9554	0.9564	0.9573	0.9582	0.9591	0.9599	0.9608	0.9616	0.9625	0.9633
1.8	0.9641	0.9649	0.9656	0.9664	0.9671	0.9678	0.9686	0.9693	0.9699	0.9706
1.9	0.9713	0.9719	0.9726	0.9732	0.9738	0.9744	0.9750	0.9756	0.9761	0.9767
2.0	0.9772	0.9778	0.9783	0.9788	0.9793	0.9798	0.9803	0.9808	0.9812	0.9817
2.1	0.9821	0.9826	0.9830	0.9834	0.9838	0.9842	0.9846	0.9850	0.9854	0.9857
2.2	0.9861	0.9864	0.9868	0.9871	0.9875	0.9878	0.9881	0.9884	0.9887	0.9890
2.3	0.9893	0.9896	0.9898	0.9901	0.9904	0.9906	0.9909	0.9911	0.9913	0.9916
2.4	0.9918	0.9920	0.9922	0.9925	0.9927	0.9929	0.9931	0.9932	0.9934	0.9936
2.5	0.9938	0.9940	0.9941	0.9943	0.9945	0.9946	0.9948	0.9949	0.9951	0.9952
2.6	0.9953	0.9955	0.9956	0.9957	0.9959	0.9960	0.9961	0.9962	0.9963	0.9964
2.7	0.9965	0.9966	0.9967	0.9968	0.9969	0.9970	0.9971	0.9972	0.9973	0.9974
2.8	0.9974	0.9975	0.9976	0.9977	0.9977	0.9978	0.9979	0.9979	0.9980	0.9981
2.9	0.9981	0.9982	0.9982	0.9983	0.9984	0.9984	0.9985	0.9985	0.9986	0.9986
3.0	0.9987	0.9987	0.9987	0.9988	0.9988	0.9989	0.9989	0.9989	0.9990	0.9990

Table B.3. Probability distributions of the statistic _t_. Values in the left-most column are degrees of freedom (df), other column headings indicate the proportion of the distribution with more extreme values than the value of _t_ located in the body of the table. Values shown are for a one-tailed (directional) and a two-tailed (nondirectional) hypothesis. For example, with $\alpha=0.05$, df = 10 and a nondirectional hypothesis, values of _t_ greater than +2.228 delineate the upper and lower 2.5% extremes of the _t_ distribution for a total a area of 5%. For a directional test with $\alpha = 0.05$ and df = 10., and assuming the mean difference is hypothesized to be positive, the critical value of t is 1.812. The entire α area is located in the uppper extreme of the distribution.

DEGREES OF FREEDOM (df)	PROBABILITIES						WAY
	0.1	0.05	0.025	0.0125	0.01	0.0005	ONE
	0.2	0.1	0.05	0.025	0.02	0.001	TWO
1	3.078	6.314	12.706	25.452	31.821	636.619	
2	1.886	2.920	4.303	6.205	6.965	31.599	
3	1.638	2.353	3.182	4.177	4.541	12.924	
4	1.533	2.132	2.776	3.495	3.747	8.610	
5	1.476	2.015	2.571	3.163	3.365	6.869	
6	1.440	1.943	2.447	2.969	3.143	5.959	
7	1.415	1.895	2.365	2.841	2.998	5.408	
8	1.397	1.860	2.306	2.752	2.896	5.041	
9	1.383	1.833	2.262	2.685	2.821	4.781	
10	1.372	1.812	2.228	2.634	2.764	4.587	
11	1.363	1.796	2.201	2.593	2.718	4.437	
12	1.356	1.782	2.179	2.560	2.681	4.318	
13	1.350	1.771	2.160	2.533	2.650	4.221	
14	1.345	1.761	2.145	2.510	2.624	4.140	
15	1.341	1.753	2.131	2.490	2.602	4.073	
16	1.337	1.746	2.120	2.473	2.583	4.015	
17	1.333	1.740	2.110	2.458	2.567	3.965	
18	1.330	1.734	2.101	2.445	2.552	3.922	
19	1.328	1.729	2.093	2.433	2.539	3.883	
20	1.325	1.725	2.086	2.423	2.528	3.850	
21	1.323	1.721	2.080	2.414	2.518	3.819	
22	1.321	1.717	2.074	2.405	2.508	3.792	
23	1.319	1.714	2.069	2.398	2.500	3.768	
24	1.318	1.711	2.064	2.391	2.492	3.745	
25	1.316	1.708	2.060	2.385	2.485	3.725	
26	1.315	1.706	2.056	2.379	2.479	3.707	
27	1.314	1.703	2.052	2.373	2.473	3.690	
28	1.313	1.701	2.048	2.368	2.467	3.674	
29	1.311	1.699	2.045	2.364	2.462	3.659	
30	1.310	1.697	2.042	2.360	2.457	3.646	
40	1.303	1.684	2.021	2.329	2.423	3.551	
50	1.299	1.676	2.009	2.311	2.403	3.496	
100	1.290	1.660	1.984	2.276	2.364	3.390	
150	1.287	1.655	1.976	2.264	2.351	3.357	
200	1.286	1.653	1.972	2.258	2.345	3.340	
10000	1.282	1.645	1.960	2.242	2.327	3.291	

Table B.4. Critical values of *F* distributions for alpha = 0.05. The critical value is determined by the degrees of freedom (df) for the numerator (column header) and the df for the denominator (row header). For example, the critical value of *F* for df numerator = 5 and df denominator = 10 is 3.326. This is a one-tailed test.

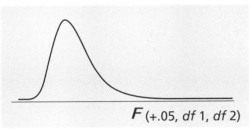

F (+.05, df 1, df 2)

DENOMINATOR df	NUMERATOR df					
	1	2	5	10	15	20
1	161.448	199.500	230.162	241.882	245.950	248.013
2	18.513	19.000	19.296	19.396	19.429	19.446
5	6.608	5.786	5.050	4.735	4.619	4.558
10	4.965	4.103	3.326	2.978	2.845	2.774
15	4.543	3.682	2.901	2.544	2.403	2.328
20	4.351	3.493	2.711	2.348	2.203	2.124
25	4.242	3.385	2.603	2.236	2.089	2.007
30	4.171	3.316	2.534	2.165	2.015	1.932
40	4.085	3.232	2.449	2.077	1.924	1.839
60	4.001	3.150	2.368	1.993	1.836	1.748
120	3.920	3.072	2.290	1.910	1.750	1.659
1000	3.851	3.005	2.223	1.840	1.676	1.581

DENOMINATOR df	NUMERATOR df					
	25	30	40	60	120	1000
1	249.260	250.095	251.143	252.196	253.253	254.187
2	19.456	19.462	19.471	19.479	19.487	19.495
5	4.521	4.496	4.464	4.431	4.398	4.369
10	2.730	2.700	2.661	2.621	2.580	2.543
15	2.280	2.247	2.204	2.160	2.114	2.072
20	2.074	2.039	1.994	1.946	1.896	1.850
25	1.955	1.919	1.872	1.822	1.768	1.718
30	1.878	1.841	1.792	1.740	1.683	1.630
40	1.783	1.744	1.693	1.637	1.577	1.517
60	1.690	1.649	1.594	1.534	1.467	1.399
120	1.598	1.554	1.495	1.429	1.352	1.267
1000	1.517	1.471	1.406	1.332	1.239	1.110

Table B.5. Critical values of chi-square distributions. Degrees of freedom (df) are indicated in the left-most column. For example, the critical value of chi-square with 5 df and an α level of 0.05 is 11.070. This test is one-tailed.

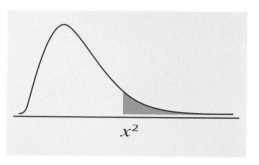

DEGREES of FREEDOM (df)	PROBABILITIES ASSOCIATED WITH VALUES OF χ^2					
	0.2	0.1	0.05	0.025	0.01	0.001
1	1.642	2.706	3.841	5.024	6.635	10.828
2	3.219	4.605	5.991	7.378	9.210	13.816
3	4.642	6.251	7.815	9.348	11.345	16.266
4	5.989	7.779	9.488	11.143	13.277	18.467
5	7.289	9.236	11.070	12.833	15.086	20.515
6	8.558	10.645	12.592	14.449	16.812	22.458
7	9.803	12.017	14.067	16.013	18.475	24.322
8	11.030	13.362	15.507	17.535	20.090	26.124
9	12.242	14.684	16.919	19.023	21.666	27.877
10	13.442	15.987	18.307	20.483	23.209	29.588
11	14.631	17.275	19.675	21.920	24.725	31.264
12	15.812	18.549	21.026	23.337	26.217	32.909
13	16.985	19.812	22.362	24.736	27.688	34.528
14	18.151	21.064	23.685	26.119	29.141	36.123
15	19.311	22.307	24.996	27.488	30.578	37.697
16	20.465	23.542	26.296	28.845	32.000	39.252
17	21.615	24.769	27.587	30.191	33.409	40.790
18	22.760	25.989	28.869	31.526	34.805	42.312
19	23.900	27.204	30.144	32.852	36.191	43.820
20	25.038	28.412	31.410	34.170	37.566	45.315
21	26.171	29.615	32.671	35.479	38.932	46.797
22	27.301	30.813	33.924	36.781	40.289	48.268
23	28.429	32.007	35.172	38.076	41.638	49.728
24	29.553	33.196	36.415	39.364	42.980	51.179
25	30.675	34.382	37.652	40.646	44.314	52.620
26	31.795	35.563	38.885	41.923	45.642	54.052
27	32.912	36.741	40.113	43.195	46.963	55.476
28	34.027	37.916	41.337	44.461	48.278	56.892
29	35.139	39.087	42.557	45.722	49.588	58.301
30	36.250	40.256	43.773	46.979	50.892	59.703
40	47.269	51.805	55.758	59.342	63.691	73.402
50	58.164	63.167	67.505	71.420	76.154	86.661
60	68.972	74.397	79.082	83.298	88.379	99.607
70	79.715	85.527	90.531	95.023	100.425	112.317
80	90.405	96.578	101.879	106.629	112.329	124.839
90	101.054	107.565	113.145	118.136	124.116	137.208
100	111.667	118.498	124.342	129.561	135.807	149.449

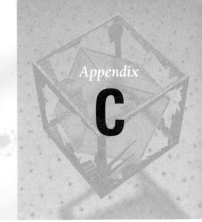

Reprints of Critiqued Articles

This appendix consists of reprints of many of the articles reviewed in detail in this text (in alphabetical order by first author's last name). Unfortunately, the policies of several journals precluded the inclusion of their articles, so those papers must be obtained from the journals themselves.

Bent S, Kane D, Shinohara K, et al. Saw palmetto for benign prostatic hyperplasia. N Engl J Med 2006;354:557–566. Copyright © 2006 Massachusetts Medical Society. All rights reserved. *Reprinted with permission. Chapter 8.*

Boer R, de Koning HJ, van der Maas PJ. A longer breast carcinoma screening interval for women age older than 65 years? Cancer 1999;86:1506–1510. Copyright © 1999 American Cancer Society. *Reprinted with permission of Wiley-Liss, Inc., a subsidiary of John Wiley & Sons, Inc. Chapter 9.*

Simpson SH, Eurich DT, Majumdar SR, et al. A meta-analysis of the association between adherence to drug therapy and mortality. Br Med J 2006;333:15. Copyright © 2006 BMJ Publishing Group Ltd. *Reprinted with permission. Chapter 10.*

Sud A. et al., Adherence to medications by patients after acute coronary syndrome. Ann Pharmacother 2005;39:1792–1797. *Reprinted with permission. Chapter 7.*

The NEW ENGLAND
JOURNAL *of* MEDICINE

ESTABLISHED IN 1812   FEBRUARY 9, 2006   VOL. 354   NO. 6

Saw Palmetto for Benign Prostatic Hyperplasia

Stephen Bent, M.D., Christopher Kane, M.D., Katsuto Shinohara, M.D., John Neuhaus, Ph.D.,
Esther S. Hudes, Ph.D., M.P.H., Harley Goldberg, D.O., and Andrew L. Avins, M.D., M.P.H.

ABSTRACT

BACKGROUND

Saw palmetto is used by over 2 million men in the United States for the treatment of benign prostatic hyperplasia and is commonly recommended as an alternative to drugs approved by the Food and Drug Administration.

METHODS

In this double-blind trial, we randomly assigned 225 men over the age of 49 years who had moderate-to-severe symptoms of benign prostatic hyperplasia to one year of treatment with saw palmetto extract (160 mg twice a day) or placebo. The primary outcome measures were changes in the scores on the American Urological Association Symptom Index (AUASI) and the maximal urinary flow rate. Secondary outcome measures included changes in prostate size, residual urinary volume after voiding, quality of life, laboratory values, and the rate of reported adverse effects.

RESULTS

There was no significant difference between the saw palmetto and placebo groups in the change in AUASI scores (mean difference, 0.04 point; 95 percent confidence interval, −0.93 to 1.01), maximal urinary flow rate (mean difference, 0.43 ml per minute; 95 percent confidence interval, −0.52 to 1.38), prostate size, residual volume after voiding, quality of life, or serum prostate-specific antigen levels during the one-year study. The incidence of side effects was similar in the two groups.

CONCLUSIONS

In this study, saw palmetto did not improve symptoms or objective measures of benign prostatic hyperplasia. (ClinicalTrials.gov number, NCT00037154.)

From the Osher Center for Integrative Medicine, Department of Medicine (S.B., A.L.A.), the Division of General Internal Medicine, Department of Medicine (S.B., A.L.A.), and the Departments of Epidemiology and Biostatistics (J.N., E.S.H., A.L.A.) and Family Practice (H.G.), University of California, San Francisco, San Francisco; the General Internal Medicine Section, Department of Medicine (S.B., A.L.A.), and the Urology Section (C.K., K.S.), San Francisco Veterans Affairs Medical Center, San Francisco; and the Division of Research, Kaiser Permanente Northern California, Oakland (H.G., A.L.A.). Address reprint requests to Dr. Bent at San Francisco VAMC, 111-A1, 4150 Clement St., San Francisco, CA 94121 or at bent@itsa.ucsf.edu.

N Engl J Med 2006;354:557-66.
Copyright © 2006 Massachusetts Medical Society.

The NEW ENGLAND JOURNAL *of* MEDICINE

EXTRACTS OF THE SAW PALMETTO BERRY are widely used for the treatment of benign prostatic hyperplasia, often as an alternative to pharmaceutical agents. In a national survey conducted in 2002, 1.1 percent of the adult population in the United States, or approximately 2.5 million adults, reported using saw palmetto.[1] The herb is widely used in Europe, where half of German urologists prefer prescribing plant-based extracts to synthetic drugs.[2] Although most prior randomized trials of saw palmetto have reported small improvements in the symptoms of benign prostatic hyperplasia or in urinary flow rates, these studies are limited by the small numbers of subjects enrolled, their short duration, their failure to use standard outcome measures, and the lack of information from participants concerning how effectively the placebo was blinded.[3-20] Using widely accepted outcome measures and a matched placebo capsule, we conducted a randomized, double-blind trial to determine the efficacy of saw palmetto for the treatment of benign prostatic hyperplasia.

METHODS

PARTICIPANTS

The study protocol and all procedures were approved by the committee on human research at the University of California, San Francisco, and the Kaiser Foundation Research Institute, Oakland, California. The study took place between July 2001 and May 2004. All participants provided written informed consent. Men over the age of 49 years who had moderate-to-severe symptoms of benign prostatic hyperplasia, as defined by a score on the American Urological Association Symptom Index (AUASI) of at least 8 and a peak urinary flow rate of less than 15 ml per second, were recruited from the San Francisco Veterans Affairs Medical Center, Kaiser Permanente Northern California, and the surrounding community by direct mailings to patients, letters to primary care providers, posters, and newspaper and local radio advertisements. All potential participants were screened by means of a telephone interview to identify exclusion criteria. Men who passed the screening interview were asked to come for a clinic visit; those who declined or did not appear at the clinic were classified as having declined to participate. Men were ineligible if they were at high risk for urinary retention (defined by a peak urinary flow rate of less than 4 ml per second or a residual volume of more than 250 ml after voiding); had a history of prostate cancer, surgery for benign prostatic hyperplasia, urethral stricture, or neurogenic bladder; had a creatinine level of more than 2.0 mg per deciliter (177 μmol per liter); had a prostate-specific antigen (PSA) level of more than 4.0 ng per deciliter; were using medications known to affect urination; or had a severe concomitant disease. Patients were eligible to participate if they had stopped taking an alpha-blocker at least one month before randomization or discontinued taking saw palmetto or a 5α-reductase inhibitor six months before randomization. All potentially eligible participants were assigned to a one-month, single-blind, placebo run-in period and were excluded if their rate of adherence was less than 75 percent, as measured by a capsule count.

INTERVENTION

Eligible patients were randomly assigned to receive a saw palmetto extract, 160 mg twice daily, or a similar-appearing placebo in soft brown gelatin capsules. This regimen was selected because it had been used in the vast majority of prior clinical trials.[21] An advisory committee chartered by the National Center for Complementary and Alternative Medicine (NCCAM) conducted a competitive process to select the saw palmetto product to be used in this trial, a proprietary carbon dioxide extract from Indena USA in a soft gelatin capsule furnished by Rexall-Sundown. The extract was manufactured in one batch to optimize product consistency. High-performance gas chromatography of samples of the extract revealed that it contained 92.1 percent total fatty acids just before the initiation of the study; a subsequent analysis at the midpoint of the study revealed that the extract contained 90.7 percent total fatty acids and 0.33 percent total sterols. Placebo capsules contained polyethylene glycol-400, a bitter-tasting liquid with an oily appearance and no free fatty acids, and a brown coloring agent to produce a placebo with the appearance of saw palmetto. Patients were advised to take the study medication twice a day with meals and to bring all unused capsules to each study visit. Patients made eight visits to the study clinic over a period of 14 months, including 12 months of post-randomization follow-up.

OBJECTIVES AND OUTCOMES

The primary objectives of the study were to determine whether the daily use of saw palmetto extract reduces the symptoms of benign prostatic hyperplasia, as measured by the AUASI or objective measures of urinary obstruction (urinary flow rates), as compared with placebo. The AUASI is a validated seven-item, self-administered questionnaire that measures symptoms referable to urinary obstruction, with scores ranging from 0 to 35 according to symptom severity: scores of 0 to 7 indicate mild symptoms; scores of 8 to 19, moderate symptoms; and scores of 20 to 35, severe symptoms.[22] Secondary objectives included an examination of changes in the quality of life specific to benign prostatic hyperplasia and overall quality of life (assessed by two self-administered questionnaires, the Benign Prostatic Hyperplasia [BPH] Impact Index[23] and the Medical Outcomes Study 36-Item Short-Form General Health Survey [SF-36[24]]); prostate size, measured by transrectal ultrasonography; residual volume after voiding, measured by BladderScan (Diagnostic Ultrasound); self-reported side effects; and changes in levels of PSA, creatinine, testosterone, and other laboratory values. The SF-36 consists of 36 items, 35 of which are aggregated to evaluate eight dimensions of health: physical function, pain, general and mental health, vitality, social function, and physical and emotional health.

RANDOMIZATION

Participants who satisfied all eligibility criteria, including completion of the run-in period, underwent randomization in equal proportions to the saw palmetto and placebo groups. Randomization was stratified according to the category of AUASI score (moderate [8 to 19] vs. severe [20 to 35])[22] and blocked with the use of randomly chosen even-numbered block sizes of less than 10 according to the ralloc.ado procedure in Stata, a software module used to design randomized, controlled trials.[25] The randomization list was created by personnel who were not associated with the study. The study medication was dispensed in numbered bottles (provided by the manufacturer), according to the randomization sequence. All study participants and all study personnel who administered interventions, assessed outcomes, or performed data analysis were unaware of the treatment assignment and the randomized sequence list.

STATISTICAL ANALYSIS

The study was designed to have a statistical power of 90 percent to detect a difference between groups of 3.0 in the AUASI score,[26] on the basis of a published standard deviation of 6.0 in the AUASI[27,28] and a two-sided alpha value of 0.04 (set below 0.05 to allow for possible interim analyses). These calculations and values required the enrollment of 178 men, and the number was increased to a target enrollment of 224 to account for a potential dropout rate of up to 20 percent.

The primary efficacy analyses were the comparisons of the change over time in the AUASI scores and the peak urinary flow rate between the saw palmetto and placebo groups. We assessed the significance of these differences in changes in outcomes over time using linear mixed-effects models.[29] These models included random intercepts to accommodate the repeated measures gathered from each study participant as well as terms for the fixed effects of time, study group, and the interaction between time and study group, the effects of interest in our analyses. We assessed the functional form of the effect of time within each study group using likelihood-ratio tests and found that for most outcomes, linear time effects fit the data well. However, for the AUASI scores and testosterone levels, a model with quadratic time effects fit the data significantly better, and our models for these outcomes included these nonlinear effects of time. We specified the linear mixed-effects model analytic strategy, including the assessment of the functional form of the effect of time, before analyzing the study data. For each outcome, we present estimated treatment effects, which we calculated as the difference in the predicted change in the response over a period of 12 months between the two study groups. The linear mixed-effects model analyses provide these estimates along with associated standard errors, which were used to construct 95 percent confidence intervals for treatment effects. We fit the linear mixed-effects model using the XTREG procedure in Stata software (version 8.0).[30] The overall differences in the total response curves between the two groups were tested with likelihood-ratio tests. The data and safety monitoring board (composed of experts selected by the National Institutes of Health who were not affiliated with the study) elected not to perform interim analyses of efficacy.

Baseline variables were compared between

The NEW ENGLAND JOURNAL *of* MEDICINE

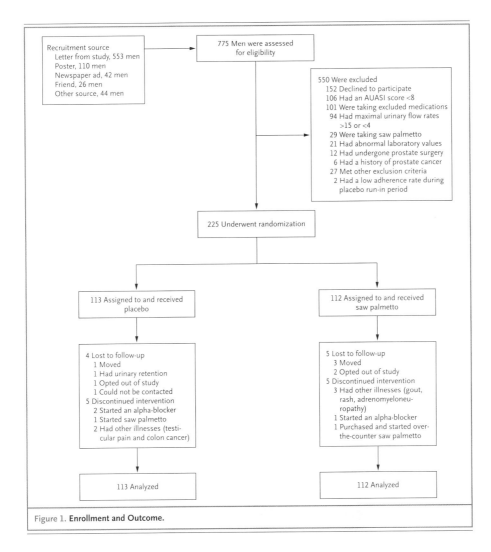

Figure 1. **Enrollment and Outcome.**

groups with the use of Student's t-test for continuous variables and chi-square tests for categorical variables. All analyses were conducted according to the intention-to-treat principle, so that all data obtained from men who did not complete the study were included in the final analyses. All reported P values are two-sided and have not been adjusted for multiple testing.[31]

Three subgroup analyses were planned a priori on the basis of baseline data: an examination of changes in the primary outcome measures among men with moderate symptoms as compared with men with severe symptoms, men with a high prostate volume as compared with those with a low prostate volume (dichotomized at 40 ml),[32] and men with high PSA levels as compared with men with low levels (dichotomized at 1.4 ng per deciliter).[32]

The funding organizations (the National Institute of Diabetes and Digestive and Kidney Diseases and the National Center for Complementary and Alternative Medicine) and the supplier of saw palmetto had no role in the design or conduct of the study, the collection, management, analysis, and interpretation of the data, or the preparation, review, and approval of the manuscript.

Table 1. Baseline Characteristics of 225 Men with Benign Prostatic Hyperplasia.*

Characteristic	All Men (N=225)	Saw Palmetto (N=112)	Placebo (N=113)
Age — yr	63.0±7.7	62.9±8.0	63.0±7.4
Race or ethnic group — no. (%)			
White	183 (82)	94 (84)	89 (79)
Black	12 (5)	4 (4)	8 (7)
Asian or Pacific Islander	15 (7)	7 (6)	8 (7)
Hispanic	11 (5)	6 (5)	5 (4)
Other	3 (1)	1 (1)	2 (2)
Education — yr	16.5±3.5	16.5±3.3	16.6±3.6
AUASI score†	15.4±5.5	15.7±5.7	15.0±5.3
BPH Impact Index score‡	3.1±2.1	3.4±2.2	2.8±2.1
SF-36 score§			
Physical subscale	49.5±8.5	49.0±8.2	50.0±8.9
Mental subscale	52.9±7.9	52.5±7.8	53.3±8.0
Sexual function (O'Leary scale)¶	2.1±1.0	2.2±1.1	2.0±1.0
Prostate volume — ml‖	34.2±14.5	34.7±13.9	33.9±15.2
Prostate transitional-zone volume — ml‖	12.9±10.7	13.2±10.4	12.5±11.0
Maximal urinary flow rate — ml/sec	11.5±3.9	11.4±3.5	11.6±4.3
Residual volume after voiding — ml	82.3±58.2	80.0±51.9	84.5±63.8
PSA — ng/dl	1.7±1.4	1.8±1.4	1.6±1.4
Creatinine — mg/dl	1.0±0.17	1.0±0.16	1.0±0.18
Testosterone — ng/dl	374±135	375±128	373±142

* Plus–minus values are means ±SD. There were no significant differences in baseline characteristics between the groups except in the BPH Impact Index (P=0.02 by Wilcoxon's test). To convert creatinine values to micromoles per liter, multiply by 88.4. PSA denotes prostate-specific antigen. Race and ethnic group were self-reported.
† Scores on the AUASI can range from 0 (no symptoms) to 35 (severe symptoms).
‡ Scores on the BPH Impact Index can range from 0 (no symptoms) to 13 (severe symptoms).
§ Scores on the SF-36 can range from 0 to 100; higher scores indicate a better quality of life.
¶ Overall scores on the O'Leary Scale of Sexual Function can range from 0 to 4, with higher scores indicating better function.
‖ Prostate volume was measured by transrectal ultrasonography.

RESULTS

Of 775 men who were screened for eligibility, 225 satisfied all eligibility criteria and underwent randomization, 112 to saw palmetto and 113 to placebo, between July 2001 and May 2003. Figure 1 shows the source of recruitment for potential participants and reasons for exclusion. Five men in the saw palmetto group and four men in the placebo group were lost to follow-up, for a completion rate of 96 percent. An additional five men in each group discontinued the study medication but completed all outcome assessments. The adherence rate was high, with 92 percent of all study medicine consumed and no significant difference in adherence between groups. The baseline characteristics of the treatment groups were similar, with the exception of the scores on the BPH Impact Index (P=0.02) (Table 1).

There was a small but significant decrease (improvement) in the AUASI score during the single-blind, placebo run-in period in both groups (mean change among all participants, –1.49; 95 percent confidence interval, –0.96 to –2.02) (Fig. 2). Both groups also had a small decrease in the AUASI score during the one-year study: the score decreased by 0.68 in the saw palmetto group (95 percent confidence interval, –1.37 to 0.01) and by

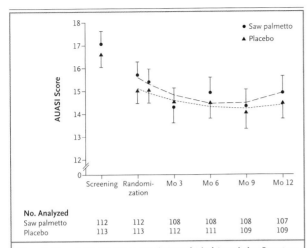

No. Analyzed

	Screening	Randomization	Mo 3	Mo 6	Mo 9	Mo 12
Saw palmetto	112	112	108	108	108	107
Placebo	113	113	112	111	109	109

Figure 2. Mean (±SE) Change in American Urological Association Symptom Index (AUASI) Scores in the Saw Palmetto and Placebo Groups.

Values at screening represent prerandomization screening values. The full range of the scale is from 0 to 35, with higher numbers indicating more severe symptoms.

0.72 in the placebo group (95 percent confidence interval, −1.40 to −0.04) (Table 2). There was, however, no significant difference between groups in the mean change in AUASI scores over time (difference in mean change, 0.04 point; 95 percent confidence interval, −0.93 to 1.01). Figure 2 shows that the fitted curves for the saw palmetto and placebo groups nearly coincide, indicating similar changes in AUASI scores over time in the two groups (likelihood-ratio chi-square test, 0.62 with 2 degrees of freedom; P=0.73).

Similarly, there was no significant difference between groups in the change in the peak urinary flow rate during the one-year study period. The peak urinary flow rate changed by 0.42 ml per minute (95 percent confidence interval, −0.25 to 1.10) in the saw palmetto group and by −0.01 ml per minute (95 percent confidence interval, −0.68 to 0.66) in the placebo group (mean difference, 0.43 ml per minute; 95 percent confidence interval, −0.52 to 1.38). Figure 3 shows that the fitted curves for the saw palmetto and placebo groups nearly coincide, indicating similar changes in the

Table 2. Changes in Primary and Secondary Outcome Measures.*

Measure	Saw Palmetto (N=112)	Placebo (N=113)	Difference between Groups (95% CI)
	mean (±SE) change		
Primary outcomes			
AUASI score†	−0.68±0.35	−0.72±0.35	0.04 (−0.93 to 1.01)
Peak urinary flow rate (ml/sec)	0.42±0.34	−0.01±0.34	0.43 (−0.52 to 1.38)
Secondary outcomes			
Prostate volume (ml)	3.76±0.98	4.98±0.96	−1.22 (−3.90 to 1.47)
Prostate transitional-zone volume (ml)	3.26±1.03	2.01±1.01	1.25 (−1.57 to 4.07)
Residual volume after voiding (ml)	14.10±7.24	18.62±7.14	−4.51 (−24.44 to 15.42)
BPH Impact Index score‡	−0.33±0.13	−0.09±0.13	−0.24 (−0.60 to 0.13)
SF-36 score§			
Mental subscale	−0.72±0.72	0.47±0.71	−1.18 (−3.16 to 0.79)
Physical subscale	0.10±0.67	−0.51±0.66	0.61 (−1.24 to 2.45)
Sexual function (O'Leary scale)¶	−0.06±0.10	0.07±0.10	−0.13 (−0.40 to 0.14)
Laboratory values			
Creatinine (mg/dl)	0.002±0.01	−0.004±0.01	0.006 (−0.02 to 0.03)
Testosterone (ng/dl)	−16.82±8.74	−1.42±8.64	−15.40 (−39.49 to 8.69)
PSA (ng/dl)	−0.005±0.07	0.15±0.07	−0.16 (−0.36 to 0.04)

* Plus–minus values are means ±SE. To convert creatinine values to micromoles per liter, multiply by 88.4. CI denotes confidence interval, and PSA prostate-specific antigen.
† Scores on the AUASI can range from 0 (no symptoms) to 35 (severe symptoms).
‡ Scores on the BPH Impact Index can range from 0 (no symptoms) to 13 (severe symptoms).
§ Scores on the SF-36 can range from 0 to 100; higher scores indicate a better quality of life.
¶ Overall scores on the O'Leary Scale of Sexual Function can range from 0 to 4, with higher scores indicating better function.

peak urinary flow rate over time in the two groups (likelihood-ratio chi-square test, 0.87 with 2 degrees of freedom; P=0.65).

Examination of the secondary outcome measures also revealed no significant difference between treatment groups (Table 2). Changes in prostate size, residual volume after voiding, the BPH Impact Index, the overall quality of life as measured by the SF-36, and serum PSA, creatinine, and testosterone levels did not differ significantly between the two groups. The preplanned subgroup analyses also showed no benefit for any of the subgroups: for the AUASI outcome, there were no significant differences in response between the groups when stratified according to the baseline AUASI score (P=0.32), prostate size (P=0.23), or PSA level (P=0.86). Similarly, for the peak urinary flow rate, there were no interactions with the baseline AUASI score (P=0.13), prostate size (P=0.63), or PSA level (P=0.87).

A total of 26 serious adverse events occurred in 17 participants during the study: 8 in men assigned to saw palmetto and 18 in men assigned to placebo (Table 3). The risk of at least one serious adverse event did not differ significantly between the two groups (P=0.31 by Fisher's exact test). There were also no significant differences in the mean number of nonserious adverse events per participant in the saw palmetto and placebo groups (0.51 vs. 0.47, P=0.72 by Student's t-test) (Table 4) or in the change in laboratory values, including testosterone, PSA, and creatinine levels (Table 2).

The adequacy of blinding was assessed by asking participants whether they believed they were taking saw palmetto or placebo capsules. At 12 months, 40 percent of men in the saw palmetto group believed they were taking the herbal extract, as compared with 46 percent of men in the placebo group (P=0.38).

DISCUSSION

In this year-long randomized trial, we found that saw palmetto was not superior to placebo for improving urinary symptoms and objective measures of benign prostatic hyperplasia. The confidence intervals around the finding of no effect were narrow, excluding clinically important effects. For example, the 95 percent confidence interval for the difference in the change in the AUASI score between groups (–0.93 to 1.01) is

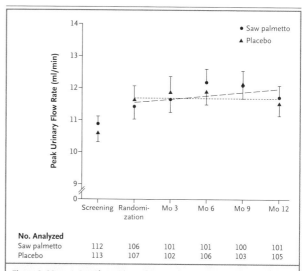

No. Analyzed

	Screening	Randomization	Mo 3	Mo 6	Mo 9	Mo 12
Saw palmetto	112	106	101	101	100	101
Placebo	113	107	102	106	103	105

Figure 3. Mean (±SE) Change in Peak Urinary Flow Rates in the Saw Palmetto and Placebo Groups.

Values at screening represent prerandomization screening values.

Table 3. Serious Adverse Events.

Variable	Saw Palmetto (N=112)	Placebo (N=113)
	number	
Events		
Cardiovascular event	2	7
Elective orthopedic surgery	3	3
Gastrointestinal bleeding	2	1
Bladder cancer	0	1
Colon cancer	0	1
Elective hernia repair	0	1
Hematoma	0	1
Melanoma	1	0
Prostate cancer	0	1
Shortness of breath	0	1
Rhabdomyolysis	0	1
Total	8	18
Patients with ≥1 event	6	11

consistent with only a 1-point improvement in the AUASI score. Previous research has suggested that a clinically meaningful change in symptoms of benign prostatic hyperplasia requires a change in the AUASI score of at least 3 points.[26] Also, all symptomatic measures (including the AUASI and

Table 4. **The 10 Most Commonly Reported Nonserious Adverse Events.**

Variable	Saw Palmetto (N = 112)	Placebo (N = 113)
	number	
10 Most common events		
Upper respiratory tract infection	12	10
Back pain	4	4
Rash	1	3
Diarrhea	2	2
Gout	2	2
Gastroesophageal reflux disease	0	3
Abdominal pain	2	1
Joint pain or swelling	2	1
Trauma	2	1
Cough	1	2
Patients with any adverse event	39	34

the BPH Impact Index) and all objective measures (including urinary flow rates, residual volume after voiding, and prostate size) were consistent in showing no evidence of an effect. The subgroup analyses indicated that there was no benefit among patients with either more or less severe symptoms or among patients with either small or large prostate glands.

In 2001, a systematic review identified 21 randomized, placebo-controlled trials of saw palmetto, of which 18 were double-blind and 13 compared saw palmetto alone with placebo. Only one of the studies of saw palmetto alone used a symptom scale equivalent to the AUASI (the International Prostate Symptom Scale); it found that saw palmetto improved symptom scores by 2.2 points, as compared with placebo (95 percent confidence interval, 0.3 to 4.4).[13] In nine of the studies that compared saw palmetto with placebo, the summary estimate showed that saw palmetto increased the peak urinary flow rate by 1.86 ml per second more than placebo (95 percent confidence interval, 0.60 to 3.12).[21] The studies included in this review had a number of methodologic limitations, including a mean duration of 13 weeks, a failure to use validated symptom scores, and inadequate concealment of treatment assignment in 10 of the 21 studies.[21] Nonetheless, the weight of the prior evidence suggested that saw palmetto may induce mild-to-moderate improvements in urinary symptoms and flow measures.

Several factors can explain the discrepancy between our negative study and the summary of prior evidence. We measured the adequacy of blinding, and we found that blinding was effective, with a similar percentage of men in the saw palmetto and placebo groups reporting that they believed they were taking the active extract. Since other studies did not assess the adequacy of blinding, and since saw palmetto has such a strong, pungent odor, many prior studies may not have achieved adequate blinding. Inadequate blinding has the potential to reduce the response in men who are given placebo (who may be aware they are taking placebo), artificially increasing the comparative efficacy of saw palmetto.

It is also possible that the participants in this study had attributes that made them less likely to have a response to saw palmetto. However, the baseline characteristics of participants in our trial with regard to age, symptom scores, prostate volume, and peak urinary flow rate were similar to those of men in previous trials of herbs or pharmaceutical agents for benign prostatic hyperplasia.[21,28,32-34]

The level of active ingredient in the extract may not have been sufficient to produce a measurable effect. We cannot completely address this possibility, because the active ingredient in saw palmetto, if one exists, is not known. However, prior in vitro studies suggest that the active ingredient is contained within the fatty-acid fraction.[35] Although there are no widely accepted guidelines on the contents of saw palmetto extract, authorities have recommended that the extract contain either 80 to 95 percent combined fatty acids and sterols[36-38] or 85 to 95 percent fatty acids and greater than 0.2 percent sterols.[39] The U.S. Pharmacopeia states that the product should contain 70 to 95 percent fatty acids and 0.2 to 0.5 percent sterols.[40] The extract we used (which, on separate measurements, had 90.7 to 92.1 percent fatty acids and 0.33 percent sterols) meets all the criteria proposed by the various authorities and was selected by an expert advisory committee chartered by the NCCAM.

The saw palmetto extract we used also had characteristics similar to those of other commonly used products in the United States. A reference laboratory that provides Web-based information tested the majority of saw palmetto products available in the United States and found that 17 of 22 tested products had fatty acid levels of 85 to 95 percent and sterol levels of more than 0.2 percent.[39] The saw palmetto extract in our study had the same range of values for these ingredients and is therefore similar to the majority of currently available products. In summary, we found that 160 mg of saw palmetto given twice daily for one year does not improve lower urinary tract symptoms caused by benign prostatic hyperplasia.

Supported by a grant (1 RO1 DK56199-01, to Dr. Avins) from the National Institute of Diabetes and Digestive and Kidney Diseases and by a grant (1 K08 ATO1338-01, to Dr. Bent) from the National Center for Complementary and Alternative Medicine.

Dr. Kane reports having received consulting fees from both American Medical Systems and Intuitive Surgical, and having received lecture fees from Merck and TAP. Dr. Shinohara reports having received lecture fees from GlaxoSmithKline and Pfizer. Dr. Avins reports receiving grant support from Merck. No other potential conflict of interest relevant to this article was reported.

We are indebted to the study team — Drs. Suzanne Staccone and Evelyn Badua, Amy Padula, Bertina Lee, and Arleen Sakamoto — as well as to Drs. Henry Leung (research pharmacy) and Howard Leong (laboratory sciences) for providing outstanding clinical care; and to Dr. Joseph Presti for his help in the initial planning of the study.

REFERENCES

1. Barnes PM, Powell-Griner E, McFann K, Nahin RL. Complementary and alternative medicine use among adults: United States, 2002. Adv Data 2004;343:1-19.
2. Lowe FC, Ku JC. Phytotherapy in treatment of benign prostatic hyperplasia: a critical review. Urology 1996;48:12-20.
3. Champault G, Patel JC, Bonnard AM. A double-blind trial of an extract of the plant Serenoa repens in benign prostatic hyperplasia. Br J Clin Pharmacol 1984;18:461-2.
4. Tasca A, Barulli M, Cavazzana A, Zattoni F, Artibani W, Pagano F. Treatment of obstructive symptomatology caused by prostatic adenoma with an extract of Serenoa repens: double-blind study vs. placebo. Minerva Urol Nefrol 1985;37:87-91. (In Italian.)
5. Reece Smith H, Memon A, Smart CJ, Dewbury K. The value of permixon in benign prostatic hypertrophy. Br J Urol 1986;58:36-40.
6. Carbin BE, Larsson B, Lindahl O. Treatment of benign prostatic hyperplasia with phytosterols. Br J Urol 1990;66:639-41.
7. Bauer HW, Casarosa C, Cosci M, Fratta M, Blessmann G. Saw palmetto fruit extract for treatment of benign prostatic hyperplasia: results of a placebo-controlled double-blind study. MMW Fortschr Med 1999;141:62. (In German.)
8. Metzker H, Kieser M, Holscher U. Wirksamkeit eines Sabal-Urtica-kombinationspraparates bei der behandlung der benignen prostatahyperplasie (BPH). Urologe [B] 1996;36:292-300.
9. Descotes JL, Rambeaud JJ, Deschaseaux P, Faure G. Placebo-controlled evaluation of the efficacy and tolerability of Permixon in benign prostatic hyperplasia after the exclusion of placebo responders. Clin Drug Invest 1995;9:291-7.
10. Mandressi A, Tarallo U, Maggioni A, Tombolini P, Rocco F, Quadraccia S. Medical treatment of benign prostatic hyperplasia: efficacy of the extract of Serenoa repens (Permixon) compared to that of the extract of Pygeum africanum and a placebo. Urologia 1983;50:752-8.
11. Emili E, Lo Cigno M, Petrone U. Risultati clinici su un nuovo farmaco nella terapia dell'ipertofia della prostata (Permixon). Urologia 1983;50:1042-8.
12. Boccafoschi C, Annoscia S. Confronto fra estratto di serenoa repens e placebo mediante prova clinica controllata in pazienti con adenomatosi prostatica. Urologia 1983;50:1257-68.
13. Gerber GS, Kuznetsov D, Johnson BC, Burstein JD. Randomized, double-blind, placebo-controlled trial of saw palmetto in men with lower urinary tract symptoms. Urology 2001;58:960-4.
14. Willetts KE, Clements MS, Champion S, Ehsman S, Eden JA. Serenoa repens extract for benign prostate hyperplasia: a randomized controlled trial. BJU Int 2003;92:267-70.
15. Marks LS, Partin AW, Epstein JI, et al. Effects of a saw palmetto herbal blend in men with symptomatic benign prostatic hyperplasia. J Urol 2000;163:1451-6.
16. Cukier J, Ducassou J, Le Guillou M, et al. Permixon versus placebo: results of a multicenter study. C R Ther Pharmacol Clin 1985;4:15-21.
17. Gabric V, Miskic H. Behandlung des benignen Prostata-adenoms und der chronischen prostatitis. Therapiewoche 1987;37:1775-88.
18. Mattei FM, Capone M, Acconcia A. Medikamentose therapie der benignen prostatahyperplasie mit einem extrakt der sagepalme. T W Urologie Nephrologie 1990;2:346-50.
19. Braeckman J, Denis L, De Leval J, et al. A double-blind placebo-controlled study of the plant extract Serenoa repens in the treatment of benign hyperplasia of the prostate. Eur J Clin Res 1997;9:247-59.
20. Lobelenz J. Extractum Sabal fructus bei benigner prostatahyperplasie (BPH). Klinische prufung im stadium I und II. Therapeutikon 1992;6:34-7.
21. Wilt T, Ishani A, Mac Donald R. Serenoa repens for benign prostatic hyperplasia. Cochrane Database Syst Rev 2002;3:CD001423.
22. American Urological Association guideline on the management of benign prostatic hyperplasia. Linthicum, Md.: American Urological Association Education and Research, 2003.
23. Fowler FJ Jr, Barry MJ. Quality of life assessment for evaluating benign prostatic hyperplasia treatments: an example of using a condition-specific index. Eur Urol 1993;24:Suppl 1:24-7.
24. Ware JE, Snow KK, Kosinski M, Gandek B. SF-36 health survey manual and interpretation guide. Boston: New England Medical Center Health Institute, 1993.
25. Barry MJ, Williford WO, Chang Y, et al. Benign prostatic hyperplasia specific health status measures in clinical research: how much change in the American Urological Association symptom index and the benign prostatic hyperplasia impact index is perceptible to patients? J Urol 1995;154:1770-4.
26. Lepor H, Williford WO, Barry MJ, et al. The efficacy of terazosin, finasteride, or both in benign prostatic hyperplasia. N Engl J Med 1996;335:533-9.
27. McConnell JD, Bruskewitz R, Walsh P, et al. The effect of finasteride on the risk of acute urinary retention and the need for surgical treatment among men with benign prostatic hyperplasia. N Engl J Med 1998;338:557-63.
28. Ryan P. RALLOC: Stata module to design randomized controlled trials: Statistical Software Components s319901. Boston: Boston College Department of Economics, 2000.
29. McCulloch CE, Searle SR. Generalized, linear, and mixed models. New York: John Wiley, 2001.
30. Stata statistical software. College Station, Tex.: Stata Corporation, 2003.
31. Rothman KJ. No adjustments are needed for multiple comparisons. Epidemiology 1990;1:43-6.
32. Boyle P, Gould AL, Roehrborn CG. Prostate volume predicts outcome of treatment of benign prostatic hyperplasia with finasteride: meta-analysis of randomized clinical trials. Urology 1996;48:398-405.
33. Roehrborn CG, Siegel RL. Safety and efficacy of doxazosin in benign prostatic hyperplasia: a pooled analysis of three double-blind, placebo-controlled studies. Urology 1996;48:406-15.
34. McConnell JD, Roehrborn CG, Bautista OM, et al. The long-term effect of doxazosin, finasteride, and combination therapy on the clinical progression of be-

nign prostatic hyperplasia. N Engl J Med 2003;349:2387-98.

35. Niederprum HJ, Schweikert HU, Zanker KS. Testosterone 5 alpha-reductase inhibition by free fatty acids from Sabal serrulata fruits. Phytomedicine 1994;1: 127-33.

36. Saw palmetto. In: Ulbricht CE, Basch EM. Natural standard herb and supplement reference: evidence-based clinical reviews. St. Louis: Elsevier/Mosby, 2005: 651-66.

37. Rotblatt M, Irvin Z. Evidence-based herbal medicine. Philadelphia: Hanley & Belfus, 2002.

38. Fugh-Berman A. The 5-minute herb and dietary supplement consult. Philadelphia: Lippincott Williams & Wilkins, 2003.

39. Product review: saw palmetto. (Accessed January 13, 2006, at http://www.consumerlab.com/results/sawpalmetto.asp.)

40. Saw palmetto extract. In: Expert Committee. United States pharmacopeial forum: (DSB) dietary supplement: botanicals. Vol. 28. No. 2. Rockville, Md.: Pharmacopeial Convention, 2005:425. (USP28-NF23.)

A Longer Breast Carcinoma Screening Interval for Women Age Older than 65 Years?

Rob Boer, M.Sc.
Harry J. de Koning, M.D., Ph.D.
Paul J. van der Maas, M.D., Ph.D.

Department of Public Health, Erasmus University Rotterdam, Rotterdam, the Netherlands.

BACKGROUND. The observed increase in sojourn time for preclinical breast carcinoma raises the question of whether women age $\geq$ 65 years can be screened less frequently than younger women.

METHODS. A cost-utility analysis using a computer model that simulates the demography, epidemiology, and natural history of breast carcinoma to estimate expected life-years gained, extra incidence, extra life-years with disease, and costs incurred by different breast carcinoma screening programs in the general population was conducted.

RESULTS. The estimated ratio of favorable/unfavorable effects was lower for longer screening intervals compared with shorter screening intervals. The cost-effectiveness ratio was much less favorable in shorter screening intervals.

CONCLUSIONS. The results of the current analysis showed that although a longer sojourn time for preclinical breast carcinoma should not necessarily be accompanied by a longer screening interval, a shorter screening interval was not very efficient. *Cancer* **1999;86:1506–10.** © *1999 American Cancer Society.*

KEYWORDS: breast neoplasms, cost-benefit analysis, mammography, mass screening, quality-adjusted life-years.

N ow that the U.S. government has decided to encourage breast carcinoma screening among women age $\geq$ 65 years by providing Medicare coverage for yearly mammography screening,[1,2] the next step is to determine what is the best screening interval for this group of women.

The screen-detectable preclinical period of breast carcinoma increases with age, as shown in an earlier model-based study on the HIP trial.[3] This is at least due in part to the growth rate of preclinical tumors decreasing with women's age.[4] The question therefore is whether it would be appropriate to apply a longer screening interval to women age > 65 years compared with those ages 50–64 years. In the past, we noted that the balance between the favorable and unfavorable effects of breast carcinoma screening in women age > 70 years is very complex.[5] We believe a longer screening interval does not necessarily affect this balance favorably, as will be shown in this article.

Unfavorable Effects

The two main unfavorable effects on the quality of life of screened women are extra incidence (defined as a detection of cases of breast carcinoma that would not have been diagnosed without screening because the woman would have died of other causes before a clinical diagnosis was made) and a longer period of knowledge of and follow-up for breast carcinoma because of lead time. A slow-growing

Address for reprints: Rob Boer, M.Sc., Department of Public Health, Erasmus University Rotterdam, P. O. Box 1738, 3000 DR Rotterdam, the Netherlands.

Received August 10, 1998; revisions received November 20, 1998, March 8, 1999, and May 10, 1999; accepted May 10, 1999.

tumor is more likely to cause both types of unfavorable effects than a fast-growing tumor. With an increasing growth rate, the probability of screen detection of a tumor that would not be diagnosed without screening approaches zero. Women with a fast-growing, screen-detected tumor have a greater chance that clinical diagnosis (due to symptoms if there was no screening) would occur before death of other causes, and the lead time for the tumor can only be short. A long screening interval will cause the majority of slowly growing tumors to be detected, thereby generating the majority of the potentially unfavorable effects of screening. The additional screen detected tumors yielded by reducing the screening interval from, for example, 3 to 2 years will be relatively fast-growing tumors that otherwise would have become manifest as interval tumors in the third year after screening. These cases hardly contribute to an extra incidence and have a lead time of < 3 years because very few women die in the period between 2 and 3 years after the previous screening, whereas their early detection may well lead to the prevention of breast carcinoma deaths.

Model Assumptions

We used the MISCAN program[6] to analyze the consequences of several screening policies.

The most relevant assumptions for this research are as follows. The model assumes an exponential distribution of preclinical disease states and an average duration of the screen-detectable period that shows in detection rates at first screenings divided by the incidence in a situation in which no screening is performed, increasing from 2.0 years in the 50–54 years age group to 3.7 years in the 65–69 years age group and 8.7 years in the 80–84 years age group.[2,7] The screening policies analyzed comprise a basic program of screening at intervals of 2 years in the group ages 50–64 years, possibly extended to include the 65–94 years age group with screening intervals of 1, 2, or 3 years.

Other assumptions in the model include the following. The natural history of breast carcinoma is modeled as a progression through a number of states. The first state is "no breast carcinoma,," in which women remain until a transition occurs to one of the preclinical states when the tumor becomes detectable by screening. In the model there is one ductal carcinoma in situ (DCIS) state and four invasive carcinoma states according to T classification (T1a, T1b, T1c, and T2+). The duration of each of the different states follows an exponential distribution. The transition to the clinically diagnosed states (with the same subdivision) is governed by the rate of incidence and clinical stage distribution data. In the case of early detec-

tion women will enter the screen-detected states (again with the same subdivision). The two end-states of the model are death from breast carcinoma and death from other causes, as based on mortality data.

Age specific assumptions on the mean duration of the (five preceding) screen-detectable preclinical states of breast carcinoma and the sensitivity of screening had been validated using all data from the Dutch screening projects (age ≥ 35 years in Nijmegen and age ≥ 40 years in Utrecht) covering different periods and screening intervals.[2,8] Sensitivity is state-dependent: 0.4, 0.65, 0.8, 0.9, and 0.95 (age 50+ years) for DCIS, T1a, T1b, T1c, and T2+ disease, respectively. The mean duration of the preclinical screen-detectable period was approximately 1.8 years at age 35 years to 6.2 years at age 70 years. These assumptions resulted in a good fit between model predictions and observed detection rates and interval tumors (both by age, stage, screening round, and interval) in the Dutch screening projects.[2] The estimated mean dwelling times from the validation procedure later were adjusted slightly based on the more recent experience concerning detection rates at first screenings from the Dutch national screening program. Other epidemiologic parameters such as rate of incidence, stage distribution, and mortality in the situation without screening were based on Dutch data.

Applying screening to a population causes a shift from diagnosing relatively large clinical tumors toward earlier (screen-detected) disease stages resulting in a decrease in breast carcinoma mortality rates, as shown in the randomized screening trials. Women with screen-detected tumors can have a reduced risk of dying from breast carcinoma in the model depending on the tumor size at the time of detection. The probability of this improvement in prognosis after early detection has been estimated from the Swedish randomized trials.[7]

Balance of Favorable and Unfavorable Effects

Tables 1 and 2 show the expected effects of a screening program with 100% attendance, comparing the basic scenario of 2-year screening intervals only in the 50–64 years age group with scenarios including the additional effects of also screening in the 65–82 years age group at intervals of 1, 2, and 3 years.

Table 1 shows the most significant effects due to the entire screening program expressed per 1000 members of the total female population alive at the start of the program. Each addition to the program increased both favorable and unfavorable effects. The expected number of deaths prevented per 1000 women increased from 2.9 to 6.2 when adding yearly screening of women age > 65 years to the basic sce-

TABLE 1

Expected Favorable and Unfavorable Effects from a Total Screening Starting at Age 50 Years and with a Screening Interval of 1, 2, and 3 Years in the Age Group 65–82 Years Compared with the Basic Screening Program in the Age Group 50–64 Years with an Interval of 2 Years

	Screening interval > age 65 yrs			Basic program
	1 yr	2 yrs	3 yrs	
Per 1000 women at start of program				
Screens	6200	4400	3800	2600
Breast carcinoma	6.2	5.5	5.0	2.9
Deaths prevented				
Life-years gained	83	76	71	54
Extra incidence	6.5	5.8	5.4	0.6
Extra life-years with disease	140	125	114	41

TABLE 2

Expected Favorable and Unfavorable Effects of Extending a Screening Program to Ages 65–82 Years with an Interval of 1, 2, and 3 Years, Relative to the Basic Program

	Screening interval over age 65 yrs			Basic program
	1 yr	2 yrs	3 yrs	
Per 1000 screens				
Breast carcinoma	0.9	1.5	1.8	1.1
Deaths prevented				
Life-years gained	8	12	15	21
Extra incidence	1.7	3.0	4.2	0.2
Extra life-years with disease	28	48	64	15
Per life-year gained				
Extra incidence	0.21	0.24	0.27	0.01
Extra life-years with disease	3.5	3.8	4.2	0.7

TABLE 3

Roughly Estimated Marginal Cost-Effectiveness Ratios with 3% Yearly Discount Rate

Screening interval > age 65 yrs	Extra cost per extra life-year gained in U.S. $
3 yrs	9600
2 yrs	19,700
1 yr	38,600
Basic program (average cost per life-year gained)	8300

nario. Similarly, the extra incidence increased from 0.6 to 6.5 per 1000 women.

The first section of Table 2 describes the expected effects expressed per 1000 screens in the basic scenario and expected extra effects per 1000 extra screens relative to the basic scenario in the scenarios with screening in women age > 65 years. "Extra" in this case means that Table 2 presents the differences in effects and in the number of screenings between a scenario with screening in women age > 65 years and the basic scenario.

The last section of Table 2 presents the balance of favorable and unfavorable effects by dividing the expected unfavorable effects by the life-years gained from the basic scenario and the extra effects from the other scenarios relative to the basic scenario.

A screening interval of 3 years in women age > 65 years already yields a large proportion of the maxi-

mum possible reduction in the breast carcinoma mortality rate. Increasing the screening frequency therefore will yield no substantial increase in the number of breast carcinoma deaths prevented. The expected number of life-years gained per 1000 women using the every-3- years scenario was 71 and increased to only 83 for the yearly screening scenario (Table 1). This means that shortening the screening interval resulted in a lower number of life-years gained per 1000 screenings, a decrease from 15 to 8 life-years gained per 1000 screenings when the interval was changed from 3 years to 1 year.

Screening women ages ≥ 65 years is expected to result in more unfavorable effects due to early detection (extra incidence and extra life-years with disease) than screening in women age < 65 years. However, increasing the screening frequency leads to a less than proportional increase in negative effects (a decrease from 4.2 to 1.7 of extra incidence per 1000 screenings). Because these negative effects increase even less than the positive effects, a higher screening frequency yields a more favorable ratio between the two. Hence, weighing the favorable health effects against the unfavorable health effects provides ratios for the extra incidence and extra life-years with disease per life-year gained of 0.27 respectively 4.2 for a 3-year screening interval decreasing to 0.21 respectively 3.5 for yearly screening. Thus, analyzing the balance between favorable and unfavorable effects, there would appear to be no reason for a longer screening interval in women of older ages.

Balance of Cost and Life-Years Gained

From the perspective of efficiency the question of whether a screening interval of 1 year is worthwhile certainly is a legitimate one. Table 3 presents a cost-effectiveness estimate. Highly simplified cost assumptions were used because further precision has no relevance for this particular discussion. The cost per screening was set at U.S. $100 with a net zero balance of other costs induced and saved by screening such as diagnostics, primary therapy, and (prevented) palliative care. The expected cost of reducing the screening interval from 2 years to 1 year was estimated as $38,000 per extra life-year gained, or 4.6 times the cost incurred in the case of a screening interval of 2 years in the 50–64 years age group.

DISCUSSION

This article presents two findings: 1) the balance of favorable and unfavorable effects of breast carcinoma screening improves with increasing screening frequency, and 2) the cost per life-year gained increases rapidly with increasing screening frequency. The second finding is not surprising because similar results have been presented for other age ranges in breast carcinoma screening[8] as well as for cervical carcinoma screening.[9,10] We present that finding primarily to moderate what possibly may be too much enthusiasm for a very short screening interval. Our examination of the strength of our outcomes therefore concentrates on the first finding.

First we limited the influence of extending the age range from an upper age of 82 years to practically all women in the Medicare system by choosing age 94 years as the upper limit. As could be expected, this led to a greater increase of unfavorable effects than of life-years gained.[5] For screening intervals of 2 years the extra rate of incidence per life-year gained increased from 0.24 to 0.52 and the number of extra life-years with diagnosed breast carcinoma per life-years gained increased from 3.8 to 5.1. However, improvement in the balance of favorable and unfavorable effects remains the extra incidence and number of extra life-years with disease per life-year gained decreased from 0.59 resp. 5.5 for screening intervals of 3 years to 0.45 resp. 4.5 for a 1-year screening interval.

Another strong influence on the balance of favorable and unfavorable effects is the duration of the screen-detectable preclinical period. For the approximately 50–69 years age range, this duration has been well established due to the many screening studies that have taken place in this age group. It can be argued that the apparent increase in the mean duration does not extend to women of older ages.[5] A model in which the mean duration of the screen-detectable preclinical period does not increase further after age 65 years expects much lower rates of unfavorable effects because stable rather than increasing lead times after age 65 years result in a lower probability of dying from causes other than breast carcinoma during the period of lead time after screen detection. This effect appears most clearly when considering an upper age limit of 94 years. For screening intervals of 2 years the extra incidence per life-year gained decreases from 0.52 to 0.12 and the number of

extra life-years with disease per life-years gained increases from 5.1 to 2.0. However, also in this scenario, the improvement in the balance between favorable and unfavorable effects remains; the extra incidence and number of extra life-years with disease per life-year gained decreases from 0.14 respectively 2.2 for the 3-year screening interval to 0.11 respectively 1.9 for the 1-year screening interval.

The different alternative scenarios concerning the upper age limit and the duration of the screen-detectable preclinical period appear to have little influence on the cost-effectiveness ratios. The expected cost per life-year gained is slightly higher for the alternative scenarios than for the basic scenario, but the cost of the 3-year screening interval does not exceed U.S. $10,800 per life-year gained and the cost of a 1-year screening interval does not exceed U.S. $40,700 per life-year gained. This is not intended to show that the cost-effectiveness ratios presented in the current study are highly accurate, but rather to show the robustness of the finding that an increasing screening frequency entails a strong increase in cost per life-year gained.

We expect that our finding of an improved balance between favorable and unfavorable effects with an increased screening frequency, combined with an increasing cost per life-year gained, extrapolates to all cancer screening with the goal of detection of invasive disease. One example might be prostate carcinoma screening. The principal finding possibly does not apply to cervical carcinoma screening or to endoscopic colorectal carcinoma screening. In these malignancies very frequent screening perhaps ultimately only leads to more early detection of the precursors of invasive disease, which would not lead to further improvements in prognosis, whereas the probability of finding regressive lesions (an unfavorable effect) still may increase.

CONCLUSIONS

In striving to optimize health effects, a longer sojourn time of preclinical breast carcinoma should not necessarily be accompanied by a longer screening interval. However, frequent screening is not likely to be an attractive option from the point of view of efficiency. Breast carcinoma screening in women age $\geq$ 65 years thus involves making a particularly difficult trade-off between effectiveness and efficiency.

REFERENCES

1. Eastman P. NCI adopts new mammography screening guidelines for women. *J Natl Cancer Inst* 1997;89(8):538–9.
2. van Oortmarssen GJ, Habbema JD, van der Maas PJ, de Koning HJ, Collette HJ, Verbeek AL, et al. A model for breast cancer screening. *Cancer* 1990;66(7):1601–12.

3. van Oortmarssen GJ, Habbema JD, Lubbe JT, van der Maas PJ. A model-based analysis of the HIP project for breast cancer screening. *Int J Cancer* 1990;46(2):207–13.

4. Peer PG, van Dijck JA, Hendriks JH, Holland R, Verbeek AL. Age-dependent growth rate of primary breast cancer. *Cancer* 1993;71(11):3547–51.

5. Boer R, de Koning HJ, van Oortmarssen GJ, van der Maas PJ. In search of the best upper age limit for breast cancer screening. *Eur J Cancer* 1995;31A(12):2040–3.

6. Habbema JD, van Oortmarssen GJ, Lubbe JT, van der Maas PJ. The MISCAN simulation program for the evaluation of screening for disease. *Comput Methods Programs Biomed* 1985;20(1):79–93.

7. de Koning HJ, Boer R, Warmerdam PG, Beemsterboer PM, van der Maas PJ. Quantitative interpretation of age-specific mortality reductions from the Swedish breast cancer-screening trials. *J Natl Cancer Inst* 1995;87(16):1217–23.

8. de Koning HJ, van Ineveld BM, van Oortmarssen GJ, de Haes JC, Collette HJ, Hendriks JH, et al. Breast cancer screening and cost-effectiveness; policy alternatives, quality of life considerations and the possible impact of uncertain factors. *Int J Cancer* 1991;49(4):531–7.

9. Eddy DM. Screening for cervical cancer. *Ann Intern Med* 1990;113(3):214–26.

10. van Ballegooijen M, Habbema JD, van Oortmarssen GJ, Koopmanschap MA, Lubbe JT, van Agt HM. Preventive Pap smears: balancing costs, risks and benefits. *Br J Cancer* 1992;65(6):930–3.

Research

BMJ

A meta-analysis of the association between adherence to drug therapy and mortality

Scot H Simpson, Dean T Eurich, Sumit R Majumdar, Rajdeep S Padwal, Ross T Tsuyuki, Janice Varney, Jeffrey A Johnson

Abstract

Objective To evaluate the relation between adherence to drug therapy, including placebo, and mortality.
Design Meta-analysis of observational studies.
Data sources Electronic databases, contact with investigators, and textbooks and reviews on adherence.
Review methods Predefined criteria were used to select studies reporting mortality among participants with good and poor adherence to drug therapy. Data were extracted for disease, drug therapy groups, methods for measurement of adherence rate, definition for good adherence, and mortality.
Results Data were available from 21 studies (46 847 participants), including eight studies with placebo arms (19 633 participants). Compared with poor adherence, good adherence was associated with lower mortality (odds ratio 0.56, 95% confidence interval 0.50 to 0.63). Good adherence to placebo was associated with lower mortality (0.56, 0.43 to 0.74), as was good adherence to beneficial drug therapy (0.55, 0.49 to 0.62). Good adherence to harmful drug therapy was associated with increased mortality (2.90, 1.04 to 8.11).
Conclusion Good adherence to drug therapy is associated with positive health outcomes. Moreover, the observed association between good adherence to placebo and mortality supports the existence of the "healthy adherer" effect, whereby adherence to drug therapy may be a surrogate marker for overall healthy behaviour.

Introduction

About one in four people do not adhere well to prescribed drug therapy.[1] Following principles of evidence based medicine, clinicians use the most relevant and available evidence to guide decisions on drug therapy. Once the prescription is written, however, the fate of drug therapy is with the patient. Poor adherence is considered a critical barrier to treatment success and remains one of the leading challenges to healthcare professionals.[2]

Much of the literature on adherence focuses on methods for measuring adherence and identification of risk factors for poor adherence,[3-6] with the premise that good adherence must be associated with good health outcomes.[7] Although the most detailed systematic review on adherence in the literature included a wide array of disease states, drug therapy was only one element within a range of therapeutic interventions.[7] Combining adherence to drug therapy with adherence to other behavioural and therapeutic interventions limits the ability to examine specifically the relation between adherence to drug therapy and health outcomes.

Ideally the effect of adherence should be measured on an objective health outcome, such as mortality. Individual studies have reported that good adherence to prescribed drug therapy—even to placebo—was associated with a lower risk of mortality.[w1-w3] This is contrary to the proposition that a placebo has little effect on health outcomes[8] and has led to speculation that adherence to drug therapy may act as an identifiable marker for overall healthy behaviour, the so called healthy adherer effect.[w1-w4 8-10] We tested this hypothesis by summarising published observations of the relation between adherence to drug therapy and mortality, with a particular interest in placebo arms of controlled studies.

Methods

We used standard systematic review methods.[11] Eligible for inclusion in our study were randomised controlled trials, retrospective analyses of data from randomised controlled trials, and observational studies evaluating the association between adherence to drug therapy and mortality. We applied no language restrictions.

A professional librarian (JV) carried out the literature search. She searched several electronic databases from inception date to 20 June 2005: Allied and Complementary Medicine (AMED), Cumulative Index to Nursing and Allied Health Literature (CINAHL), Embase, Educational Research Information Center (ERIC), HealthSTAR, Medline, PsycINFO, and the Web of Science. Articles were identified using synonyms for adherence and mortality as database specific subject headings and keywords. We also checked references from textbooks[12-14] and review articles[1 7 9 10 15-17] on adherence for additional articles.

After excluding editorials, conference proceedings, letters, news articles, government reports, and practice guidelines, two investigators (SHS, DTE) independently screened titles and abstracts to identify potentially relevant citations. A citation was retained for further evaluation if either investigator selected it. Citations were excluded that did not report original data, have human participants, evaluate drug adherence, or report patient adherence.

Each potentially relevant article was reviewed to determine if it met the following inclusion criteria: described original research, explained the method used to measure adherence (for example, self report, electronic drug event monitoring system, pharmacy refill data, clinician estimation, tablet count), provided a clear definition for good adherence, stratified patients into good and poor adherence groups, and reported mortality

Web references w1-w22 and author details are on bmj.com

according to adherence groups. Discrepancies were resolved by majority vote after review by a third investigator (JAJ).

Inter-reviewer agreement was measured during the initial screen to identify potentially relevant citations and on review of the full articles for study inclusion.[18] We characterised level of agreement using a qualitative scale developed by Landis and Koch.[19]

Data collection and outcome measures

Two investigators (DTE, RSP) used standardised forms to extract data from the included articles for disease state, drug therapy groups, methods used to measure adherence, definition for good adherence, and mortality. Accuracy of data collection was verified by comparing forms. We used the study authors' definition to stratify participants into good and poor adherence groups. When the number of deaths according to adherence group was not specifically stated in the article, we calculated this value from available information. If there was insufficient information in the article to calculate mortality according to adherence group, we contacted the corresponding author. The study was excluded if we were unable to obtain from the authors the number of deaths in each adherence group.

Statistical analysis

We analysed data using Rev Man 4.2.7. Each treatment arm in a randomised controlled trial was considered a discrete analysis of the relation between adherence and mortality. We used a random effects model to calculate pooled odds ratios and 95% confidence intervals.[20] Given the inclusion criteria, we anticipated including studies of a variety of diseases; therefore we examined heterogeneity using the Q and I^2 statistics.[20 21] We used a variation of Tobias' method to evaluate changes to the pooled odds ratio and tests for heterogeneity.[22] Rather than removing one study at a time, we used predetermined subgroups to identify potential sources of heterogeneity. For example, to test the theory of a healthy adherer effect,[w1-w4 8-10] we constructed a separate model to summarise the association between adherence to placebo and mortality. A priori subgroups included the effect of active treatment compared with placebo, study design, disease state,

method used to measure adherence, and definition for good adherence.

Results

Overall, 6231 unique citations were identified and 1140 ones related to non-studies were removed. In total, 5012 citations were excluded after review of the title and abstract (fig 1). Agreement to identify potentially relevant articles was 0.68, which is considered "substantial."[19] From the 79 potentially relevant articles, 21 studies with 46 847 participants met the inclusion criteria.[w1-w21] Agreement at this stage was 0.97, considered "almost perfect."[19]

Supplemental information on mortality was obtained from multiple sources for some studies. In the University Group Diabetes Program, mortality for participants with good adherence was available in a paper on statistical methods.[w18 w22] Supplemental mortality data according to adherence group were obtained from five corresponding authors.[w5 w7 w9 w10 w15]

Eight studies were randomised, placebo controlled trials (37 701 participants) reporting mortality according to adherence group for each treatment arm in a retrospective analysis.[w1-w4 w8 w16-w18 w22] Thirteen cohort studies (9146 participants) reported mortality according to adherence groups.[w5-w7 w9-w15 w19-w21] Table 1 lists the characteristics of the included studies. Eight studies evaluated drug therapy in participants with a recent myocardial infarction,[w1-w8] seven studies were in patients infected with HIV,[w9-w15] and two studies were in primary prevention of heart disease.[w16 w17] The remaining studies evaluated adherence to drug therapy for patients with type 2 diabetes,[w18 w22] hyperlipidaemia,[w19] heart failure,[w20] and immune suppression after heart transplant.[w21] Fifteen studies reported an adherence rate threshold to define good adherence.[w1-w5 w7 w8 w11 w13-w19 w22] All cause mortality was the primary outcome in nine studies[w2 w3 w9-w13 w15 w19] and a secondary outcome in 12.[w1 w4 w5-w8 w14 w16-w18 w20-w22] The adherence substudy for the cardiac arrhythmia suppression trial reported arrhythmic mortality according to adherence group.[w4] Although 67% of the deaths in this trial were attributable to an arrhythmia, data for all cause mortality were not available.[w4 23]

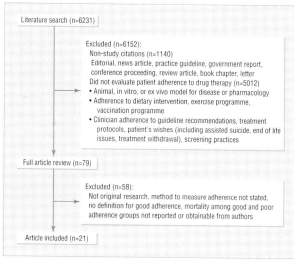

Fig 1 Flow of articles identified and studies included in review

Table 1 Characteristics of included studies in meta-analysis of adherence to drug therapy and mortality

Study	Study type	Treatment groups (No of participants)	Adherence measures	Threshold for good adherence	Observation period
Post-myocardial infarction management:					
Coronary Drug Project Research Group 1980[w1]	Randomised controlled trial	Placebo (2695), clofibrate (1065)	Pill count, clinician's impression	≥80%	≥5 years
Wei et al 2002[w5]	Cohort	Statins (427)	Pharmacy refill	≥80%	Average 2.4 years
Cotter et al 2004[w6]	Cohort	Acetylsalicylic acid (64)	Thromboxane blood level	Less than healthy volunteer	1 year
β blocker heart attack trial (men) 1990[w2]	Randomised controlled trial	Placebo (1094), propranolol (1081)	Pill count	>75%	1 year
β blocker heart attack trial (women) 1993[w3]	Randomised controlled trial	Placebo (240), propranolol (265)	Pill count	≥75%	Median 26 months
Wei et al 2004[w7]	Cohort	β blockers (386)	Pharmacy refill	≥80%	Median 3.7 years
Canadian amiodarone myocardial infarction arrhythmia trial 1999[w8]	Randomised controlled trial	Placebo (538), amiodarone (573)	Pill count	≥66%	2 years
Cardiac arrhythmia suppression trial 1996[w4]	Randomised controlled trial	Placebo (579), encainide or flecainide (574)	Pill count	>80%	Average 10 months
HIV infection:					
San Andres Rebollo et al 2004[w9]	Cohort	Antiretroviral therapy (950)	Self report	Continued use	8 years
Cohn et al 2002[w10]	Cohort	Antiretroviral therapy (626)	Self report	No missed doses in previous 48 hours	56 weeks
Garcia de Olalla et al 2002[w11]	Cohort	Antiretroviral therapy (1219)	Self report and pharmacy refill	≥90%	3 years
Grimwade et al 2005[w12]	Cohort	Cotrimoxazole prophylaxis (1288)	Self report and frequency of clinic visits	Continued use, collection of new tablet supply, and ongoing attendance at clinic	6 months
Hogg et al 2002[w13]	Cohort	Antiretroviral therapy (1282)	Pharmacy refill	≥75%	1 year
Paterson et al 2000[w14]	Cohort	Protease inhibitors (81)	Medication event monitoring system	≥95%	Median 6 months
Wood et al 2003[w15]	Cohort	Antiretroviral therapy (1422)	Pharmacy refill	≥75%	4 years
Primary prevention of cardiovascular disease:					
Physicians' health study 1994[w16]	Randomised controlled trial	Placebo (10 989), acetylsalicylic acid (11 004)	Self report	≥95%	Average 60.2 months
West of Scotland prevention study 1997[w17]	Randomised controlled trial	Placebo (3293), pravastatin (3302)	Pill count	≥75%	Mean 4.9 years
Other disease states:					
University Group Diabetes Project 1970[w22] 1971[w18] (type 2 diabetes)	Randomised controlled trial	Placebo (205), tolbutamide (204)	Clinician's impression	≥75%	≥75% followed for ≥5 years
Howell et al 2004[w19] (hypercholesterolaemia)	Cohort	Statins (869)	Pharmacy refill	≥80%	11 years
Miura et al 2001[w20] (heart failure)	Cohort	Digoxin (431)	Blood levels of drug	Therapeutic range	72 months
Dobbels et al 2004[w21] (heart transplant)	Cohort	Immunosuppressive regimen(101)	Medication event monitoring system (for cyclosporin use)	No variation in dose compliance and no drug holidays	5 years

The primary analysis of mortality risk according to adherence group was based on 2779 (5.9%) deaths in 46 847 participants. Overall, 1462 (4.7%) deaths occurred in 31 439 participants with good adherence to drug therapy and 1317 (8.5%) deaths in 15 408 participants considered to have poor adherence. The pooled odds ratio for mortality for good adherence compared with poor adherence was 0.56 (95% confidence interval 0.50 to 0.63). Some degree of heterogeneity was found: Q statistic P = 0.08 and I^2 = 28.6%.

The placebo arms from eight studies contained 19 633 participants and reported 996 (5.1%) deaths.[w1-w4 w8 w16-w18 w22] Overall, good adherence to placebo was associated with a lower risk of mortality: pooled odds ratio 0.56, 0.43 to 0.74 (fig 2). Some heterogeneity of effect was found in this analysis: Q statistic P = 0.05 and I^2 = 51.2%. A subgroup analysis restricted to studies of drug therapy after myocardial infarction reduced variance substantially: Q statistic P = 0.79 and I^2 = 0%.[w1-w4 w8] The pooled odds ratio of these five studies was 0.45 (0.38 to 0.54).

Two studies were identified in which active drug therapy increased the risk of mortality compared with placebo.[w22 w23] Therefore separate models were constructed to summarise the effect of adherence to active drug therapy found to be harmful compared with beneficial (fig 3). The two studies evaluating adherence to harmful drug therapy reported 53 (6.8%) deaths in 778 participants.[w4 w18 w22] The pooled odds ratio for mortality was 2.90 (1.04 to 8.11) for participants with good compared with poor adherence to the active treatment (fig 3).

The association between adherence to proved beneficial drug therapy and mortality was reported in 19 studies involving 26 436 participants and 1730 (6.5%) deaths.[w1-w3 w5-w17 w19-w21] The pooled odds ratio from these studies was 0.55 (0.49 to 0.62) for mortality in participants with good adherence compared with poor adherence (fig 3). These observations were homogeneous (Q statistic P = 0.71 and I^2 = 0%) and further stratification by study characteristics did not result in substantive changes to these relations (table 2). However, moderate variance of the observed effects was found among the seven HIV studies (I^2 = 50.2%) and among the four studies that used subjective methods to measure adherence (I^2 = 61.0%).[21] Minor variance (I^2 = 8.6%) was found among the 13 cohort studies (table 2).[21]

Discussion

This meta-analysis of 21 studies, involving 46 847 participants, showed a consistent association between adherence to drug therapy and mortality. For participants with good adherence to placebo or beneficial drug therapy, the risk of mortality was about half that of participants with poor adherence. Conversely, the risk of mortality was more than doubled for participants with good adherence to proved harmful drug therapy compared with participants with poor adherence.

Study	Good adherence to drug therapy	Poor adherence to drug therapy	Odds ratio (random) (95% CI)	Weight (%)	Odds ratio (random) (95% CI)
Coronary Drug Project Research Group 1980[w1]	274/1813	249/882		27.53	0.45 (0.37 to 0.55)
β blocker heart attack trial (men) 1990[w2]	31/1037	4/57		5.11	0.41 (0.14 to 1.20)
β blocker heart attack trial (women) 1993[w3]	15/219	4/21		4.20	0.31 (0.09 to 1.05)
Canadian amiodarone myocardial infarction arrhythmia trial 1999[w8]	42/447	17/91		11.81	0.45 (0.24 to 0.84)
Cardiac arrhythmia suppression trial 1996[w4]	8/486	1/93		1.54	1.54 (0.19 to 12.46)
Physicians health study 1994[w16]	105/6864	90/4125		23.59	0.70 (0.52 to 0.93)
West of Scotland prevention study 1997[w17]	95/2420	40/873		19.54	0.85 (0.58 to 1.24)
University Group Diabetes Project 1970[w22] 1971[w18]	11/143	10/62		6.69	0.43 (0.17 to 1.08)
Total (95% CI)	**13 429**	**6204**		**100.00**	**0.56 (0.43 to 0.74)**

Total events: 581 (good adherence), 415 (poor adherence)
Test for heterogeneity: $\chi^2 = 14.34$, df = 7 (P = 0.05), $I^2 = 51.2\%$
Test for overall effect: Z = 4.23, P <0.0001

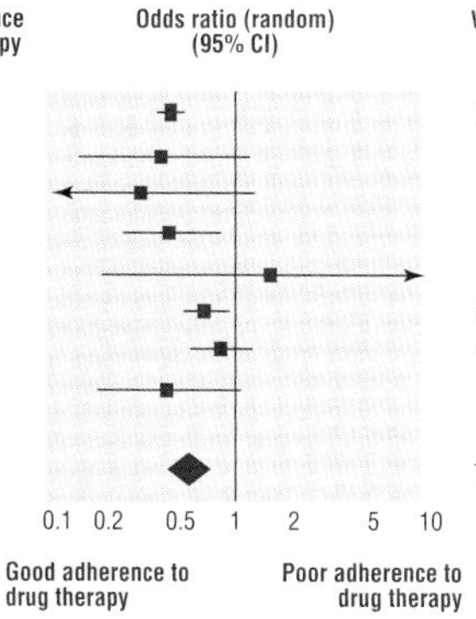

0.1 0.2   0.5   1   2   5   10
Good adherence to drug therapy — Poor adherence to drug therapy

Fig 2   Association between adherence to placebo and mortality

Study	Good adherence to drug therapy	Poor adherence to drug therapy	Odds ratio (random) (95% CI)	Weight (%)	Odds ratio (random) (95% CI)
Harmful drug therapy					
Cardiac arrhythmia suppression trial 1996[w4]	23/505	0/69		13.34	6.77 (0.41 to 112.72)
University Group Diabetes Project 1970[w22] 1971[w18]	26/151	4/53		86.66	2.55 (0.85 to 7.68)
Total (95% CI)	**656**	**122**		**100.00**	**2.90 (1.04 to 8.11)**

Total events: 49 (good adherence), 4 (poor adherence)
Test for heterogeneity: $\chi^2 = 0.43$, df=1, P=0.51, $I^2 = 0\%$
Test for overall effect: z=2.03, P=0.04

Beneficial drug therapy					
Coronary Drug Project Research Group 1980[w1]	106/708	88/357		12.11	0.54 (0.39 to 0.74)
Wei et al 2002[w5]	14/272	14/155		2.06	0.55 (0.25 to 1.18)
Cotter et al 2004[w6]	1/52	1/12		0.15	0.22 (0.01 to 3.72)
β blocker heart attack trial (men) 1990[w2]	14/1009	3/72		0.75	0.32 (0.09 to 1.15)
β blocker heart attack trial (women) 1993[w3]	11/242	2/23		0.49	0.50 (0.10 to 2.41)
Wei et al 2004[w7]	24/226	26/160		3.43	0.61 (0.34 to 1.11)
Canadian amiodarone myocardial infarction arrhythmia trial 1999[w8]	33/445	19/128		3.35	0.46 (0.25 to 0.84)
San Andres Rebollo et al 2004[w9]	69/197	300/753		11.39	0.81 (0.59 to 1.13)
Cohn et al 2002[w10]	8/585	2/41		0.49	0.27 (0.06 to 1.32)
Garcia de Olalla et al 2002[w11]	156/831	105/388		15.13	0.62 (0.47 to 0.83)
Grimwade et al 2005[w12]	12/743	27/545		2.56	0.31 (0.16 to 0.63)
Hogg et al 2002[w13]	62/955	44/327		7.29	0.45 (0.30 to 0.67)
Paterson et al 2000[w14]	0/23	1/58		0.12	0.82 (0.03 to 20.75)
Wood et al 2003[w15]	117/1067	76/355		12.04	0.45 (0.33 to 0.62)
Physicians health study 1994[w16]	89/6608	102/4396		14.80	0.57 (0.43 to 0.77)
West of Scotland prevention study 1997[w17]	66/2435	40/867		7.59	0.58 (0.39 to 0.86)
Howell et al 2004[w19]	24/654	14/215		2.65	0.55 (0.28 to 1.08)
Miura et al 2001[w20]	17/218	32/213		3.15	0.48 (0.26 to 0.89)
Dobbels et al 2004[w21]	9/84	2/17		0.46	0.90 (0.18 to 4.59)
Total (95% CI)	**17 354**	**9082**		**100.00**	**0.55 (0.49 to 0.62)**

Total events: 832 (good adherence), 898 (poor adherence)
Test for heterogeneity: $\chi^2 = 14.34$, df=18, P=0.71, $I^2 = 0\%$
Test for overall effect: z=10.54, P<0.0001

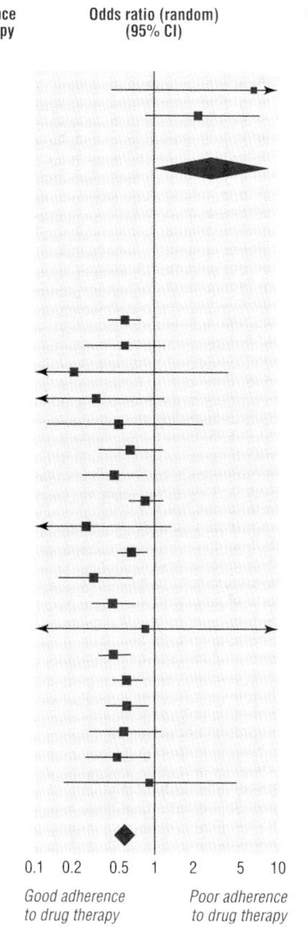

0.1 0.2   0.5   1   2   5   10
Good adherence to drug therapy — *Poor adherence to drug therapy*

Fig 3   Association between adherence to harmful or beneficial drug therapy and mortality

Table 2 Subgroup analysis of active treatment arms considered beneficial

Analysis group	No of studies	Pooled odds ratio (95% CI)	Tests for heterogeneity	
			P value (Q statistic)	I² (%)
Active treatment arm considered beneficial	19	0.55 (0.49 to 0.62)	0.71	0
Post-myocardial infarction studies only[w1-w3 w5-w8]	7	0.52 (0.41 to 0.66)	0.96	0
HIV studies only[w9-w15]	7	0.53 (0.41 to 0.69)	0.06	50.2
Primary prevention studies only[w16 w17]	2	0.58 (0.46 to 0.73)	0.99	0
Method used to measure adherence:				
Objective method (pill count, pharmacy refill, blood level, medication event monitor system)[w1-w3 w5-w8 w11 w13-w15 w17 w19-w21]	15	0.53 (0.46 to 0.60)	0.99	0
Subjective method (patient self report, clinician impression)[w9 w10 w12 w16]	4	0.55 (0.37 to 0.83)	0.05	61.0
Threshold used to define good adherence group:				
≥75%[w1-w3 w5 w7 w11 w13-w17 w19]	12	0.54 (0.48 to 0.61)	0.97	0
≥80%[w1 w5 w7 w11 w14 w16 w19]	7	0.58 (0.50 to 0.68)	1.00	0
≥90%[w11 w14 w16]	3	0.60 (0.49 to 0.73)	0.91	0
Study design:				
Randomised controlled studies only[w1-w3 w8 w16 w17]	6	0.55 (0.46 to 0.65)	0.95	0
Cohort studies only[w5-w7 w9-w15 w19-w21]	13	0.55 (0.47 to 0.64)	0.36	8.6

The association between adherence to harmful therapy and mortality is important in the light of recent issues of patient safety and post-marketing drug surveillance. Our observation suggests that stratification by adherence group may facilitate earlier identification of harmful therapies if the rate of adverse events is higher in participants with good adherence. According to the consolidated standards of reporting trials statement, investigators should, at a minimum, report the number of participants receiving the intended treatment.[24] Although randomised clinical trials will often measure adherence—either through pill count from returned vials or information on frequency of refills—this information is usually reported only as an overall adherence rate.[25] Many authors have identified that an array of adherence rates can confound the association between treatment and response and substantially affect generalisability.[25-27] Therefore we would encourage clinical trialists to consider reporting treatment effects stratified by adherence group.

In 1997 McDermott and colleagues reviewed the literature on cardiovascular disease that reported admission to hospital and mortality according to adherence groups.[9] They found that seven of 12 studies had a significant association between adherence and outcomes and noted that adherence to placebo was associated with improved outcomes in three studies. More recently DiMatteo and colleagues determined that the risk of a poor health outcome was 26% lower in participants with good adherence.[7] Although that meta-analysis included studies from a wide range of medical conditions, drug therapy was included with a variety of other healthcare interventions. In addition, the placebo arms from controlled trials were excluded from their analysis. Our study confirms, updates, and extends these observations by including studies from across several disease states and summarises the observations between adherence to drug therapy (both active drug and placebo) and mortality.

Our study shares limitations inherent with meta-analyses in general and with studies of adherence specifically. Firstly, important studies relevant to the research question may have been missed during the literature search, although this was unlikely. Secondly, as with previous reviews,[7 9] our data sources were observational studies, thus restricting our ability to explore fully the influence of unmeasured confounding variables. For example, participants with good adherence to study drugs (even placebo) may also have good adherence to other healthy behaviours such as diet, exercise, regular follow-up with healthcare professionals, immunisations, screening, and use of other drugs.[w1-w4 8-10] All of these could independently affect the risk of mortality. Conversely, participants with poor adherence may have consciously chosen to use a lower dosage[28 29] or have other conditions, such as depression, that affect adherence.[10 30] In the absence of individual patient data to control for these factors, we tested the healthy adherer effect hypothesis and assumed that the presence of good adherence is a marker for overall healthy behaviour.[w1-w4 8-10] Thirdly, in the absence of an ideal method to measure adherence,[31] we observed a wide variety of measurement methods and definitions for good adherence. Grouping studies according to measurement method and definition for good adherence did not, however, result in substantive changes to our overall observation. Finally, with the exception of two studies,[w6 w20] all studies used indirect methods to measure adherence. These methods are limited by the assumption that drug acquisition is a reasonable surrogate for consumption. This assumption would, however, overestimate exposure and bias our observation towards the null.

With these limitations in mind, our findings support the tenet that good adherence to drug therapy is associated with positive health outcomes. Moreover, the observed association between good adherence to placebo and lower mortality also supports the existence of the healthy adherer effect, whereby adherence to drug therapy may be a surrogate marker for overall healthy behaviour. Our findings set the stage for future studies to address the causal relation between adherence and health outcomes but, more importantly, quantify for patients and providers how important it is to take drugs of proved efficacy as prescribed.

We thank the individual trialists for providing information from their study databases and Maria Santana, who translated three Spanish papers.

Contributors: SHS had the idea for the article. All authors took part in the planning and design of the study. SHS, DTE, RSP, and JV did the data collection. MS (listed in the acknowledgements) assisted in data collection from articles printed in Spanish. SHS carried out the statistical analyses. SHS,

What is already known on this topic

About one in four people do not adhere well to prescribed drug therapy

Poor adherence is considered a critical barrier to treatment success and remains an important challenge to healthcare professionals

What this study adds

Good adherence to drug therapy is associated with positive health outcomes

The observed association between adherence to placebo and mortality supports the premise of a healthy adherer effect, where adherence to drug therapy may be a surrogate marker for overall healthy behaviour

DTE, SRM, RSP, RTT, and JAJ had access to the data and participated in the interpretation of the data. SHS wrote the first draft of the paper. SHS provided leadership for the study and is guarantor.

Funding: None.

Competing interests: None declared.

1 DiMatteo MR. Variations in patients' adherence to medical recommendations: a quantitative review of 50 years of research. *Med Care* 2004;42:200-9.
2 Miller NH, Hill M, Kottke T, Ockene IS. The multilevel compliance challenge: recommendations for a call to action. A statement for healthcare professionals. *Circulation* 1997;95:1085-90.
3 Morris LS, Schulz RM. Patient compliance—an overview. *J Clin Pharm Ther* 1992;17:283-95.
4 Donovan JL. Patient decision making. The missing ingredient in compliance research. *Int J Technol Assess Health Care* 1995;11:443-55.
5 Ellis S, Shumaker S, Sieber W, Rand C. Adherence to pharmacological interventions. Current trends and future directions. The Pharmacological Intervention Working Group. *Control Clin Trials* 2000;21:S218-25.
6 Osterberg L, Blaschke T. Adherence to medication. *N Engl J Med* 2005;353:487-97.
7 DiMatteo MR, Giordani PJ, Lepper HS, Croghan TW. Patient adherence and medical treatment outcomes: a meta-analysis. *Med Care* 2002;40:794-811.
8 Czajkowski SM, Chesney MA, Smith AW. Adherence and the placebo effect. In: Shumaker SA, Schron EB, Ockene JK, eds. *The handbook of health behavior change.* New York: Springer, 1990:515-34.
9 McDermott MM, Schmitt B, Wallner E. Impact of medication nonadherence on coronary heart disease outcomes. A critical review. *Arch Intern Med* 1997;157:1921-9.
10 Hays RD, Kravitz RL, Mazel RM, Sherbourne CD, DiMatteo MR, Rogers WH, et al. The impact of patient adherence on health outcomes for patients with chronic disease in the medical outcomes study. *J Behav Med* 1994;17:347-60.
11 In: Higgins JPT, Green S, eds. *Cochrane handbook for systematic reviews of interventions 4.2.5* [updated May 2005]. www.cochrane.dk/cochrane/handbook/hbook.htm (accessed 3 Apr 2006).
12 Shumaker SA, Schron EB, Ockene JK. *The handbook of health behavior change.* New York: Springer, 1990.
13 Cramer JA, Spilker B. *Patient compliance in medical practice and clinical trials.* New York: Raven, 1991.
14 Myers LB, Midence K. *Adherence to treatment in medical conditions.* Australia: Harwood Academic, 1998.
15 Cramer JA. A systematic review of adherence with medications for diabetes. *Diabetes Care* 2004;27:1218-24.
16 Fogarty L, Roter D, Larson S, Burke J, Gillespie J, Levy R. Patient adherence to HIV medication regimens: a review of published and abstract reports. *Patient Educ Couns* 2002;46:93-108.
17 Simoni JM, Frick PA, Pantalone DW, Turner BJ. Antiretroviral adherence interventions: a review of current literature and ongoing studies. *Top HIV Med* 2003;11:185-98.
18 Cohen JA. A coefficient of agreement for nominal scales. *Educ Psychol Meas* 1960;20:37-46.
19 Landis JR, Koch GG. The measurement of observer agreement for categorical data. *Biometrics* 1977;33:159-74.
20 DerSimonian R, Laird N. Meta-analysis in clinical trials. *Control Clin Trials* 1986;7:177-88.
21 Higgins JP, Thompson SG, Deeks JJ, Altman DG. Measuring inconsistency in meta-analyses. *BMJ* 2003;327:557-60.
22 Tobias A. Assessing the influences of a single study in meta-analysis. *Stata Tech Bull* 1999;47:15-7.
23 Echt DS, Liebson PR, Mitchell LB, Peters RW, Obias-Manno D, Barker AH, et al. Mortality and morbidity in patients receiving encainide, flecainide, or placebo. The cardiac arrhythmia suppression trial. *N Engl J Med* 1991;324:781-8.
24 Moher D, Schulz KF, Altman D. The CONSORT statement: revised recommendations for improving the quality of reports of parallel-group randomized trials. *JAMA* 2001;285:1987-91.
25 Boudes P. Drug compliance in therapeutic trials: a review. *Control Clin Trials* 1998;19:257-68.
26 Haynes RB, Dantes R. Patient compliance and the conduct and interpretation of therapeutic trials. *Control Clin Trials* 1987;8:12-9.
27 Efron B, Feldman D. Compliance as an explanatory variable in clinical trials. *J Am Stat Assoc* 1991;86:9-26.
28 Weintraub M. Intelligent noncompliance with special emphasis on the elderly. *Contemp Pharm Pract* 1981;4:8-11.
29 Conrad P. The meaning of medications: another look at compliance. *Soc Sci Med* 1985;20:29-37.
30 Ciechanowski PS, Katon WJ, Russo JE. Depression and diabetes: impact of depressive symptoms on adherence, function, and costs. *Arch Intern Med* 2000;160:3278-85.
31 Rudd P. In search of the gold standard for compliance measurement. *Arch Intern Med* 1979;139:627-8.

(Accepted 21 April 2006)

doi 10.1136/bmj.38875.675486.55

Faculty of Pharmacy and Pharmaceutical Sciences, University of Alberta, Edmonton, AB, Canada T6G 2N8
Scot H Simpson *assistant professor*

Institute of Health Economics, Edmonton, AB
Dean T Eurich *research associate*
Janice Varney *librarian*

Division of Internal Medicine, Department of Medicine, Faculty of Medicine and Dentistry, University of Alberta
Sumit R Majumdar *associate professor*
Rajdeep S Padwal *assistant professor*

Division of Cardiology, Department of Medicine, Faculty of Medicine and Dentistry, University of Alberta
Ross T Tsuyuki *professor*

Department of Public Health Sciences, Faculty of Medicine and Dentistry, University of Alberta
Jeffrey A Johnson *professor*

Correspondence to: S H Simpson ssimpson@pharmacy.ualberta.ca

Cardiology

Adherence to Medications by Patients After Acute Coronary Syndromes

Anchal Sud, Eva M Kline-Rogers, Kim A Eagle, Jianming Fang, David F Armstrong, Krishna Rangarajan, Richard F Otten, Dana R Stafkey-Mailey, Stephanie D Taylor, and Steven R Erickson

BACKGROUND: Nonadherence to medication may lead to poor medical outcomes.

OBJECTIVE: To describe medication-taking behavior of patients with a history of acute coronary syndromes (ACS) for 4 classes of drugs and determine the relationship between self-reported adherence and patient characteristics.

METHODS: Consenting patients with the diagnosis of ACS were interviewed by telephone approximately 10 months after discharge. The survey elicited data characterizing the patient, current medication regimens, beliefs about drug therapy, reasons for discontinuing medications, and adherence. The survey included the Beliefs About Medicine Questionnaire providing 4 scales: Specific Necessity, Specific Concerns, General Harm, and General Overuse, and the Medication Adherence Scale (MAS). Multivariate regression was used to determine the independent variables with the strongest association to the MAS. A p value $\leq$ 0.05 was considered significant for all analyses.

RESULTS: Two hundred eight patients were interviewed. Mean $\pm$ SD age was 64.9 $\pm$ 13.0 years, with 60.6% male, 95.7% white, 57.3% with a college education, 87.9% living with $\geq$1 other person, and 42% indicating excellent or very good health. The percentage of patients continuing on medication at the time of the survey category ranged from 87.4% (aspirin) to 66.0% (angiotensin-converting enzyme inhibitors). Reasons for stopping medication included physician discontinuation or adverse effects. Of patients still on drug therapy, the mean MAS was 1.3 $\pm$ 0.4, with 53.8% indicating nonadherence (score >1). The final regression model showed R^2 = 0.132 and included heart-related health status and Specific Necessity as significant predictor variables.

CONCLUSIONS: After ACS, not all patients continue their drugs or take them exactly as prescribed. Determining beliefs about illness and medication may be helpful in developing interventions aimed at improving adherence.

KEY WORDS: acute coronary syndrome, adherence.

Ann Pharmacother 2005;39:1792-7.

Published Online, 4 Oct 2005, *www.theannals.com*, DOI 10.1345/aph.1G249

Cardiovascular disease remains the leading cause of death in the US. In 2001, it was estimated that 22.6% of the population had one or more types of cardiovascular disease, of which >13 million people had coronary heart disease.[1] In spite of the evidence of the value of both primary and secondary intervention, acute coronary syndromes (ACS) continue to be one of the most important causes of morbidity and mortality in the US. The American College of Cardiology and the American Heart Association provide guidelines aimed at improving the use of key therapies in patients with ACS at the time of hospital discharge.[2] The guidelines include the recommendation to utilize 4 classes of evidence-based medications: β-blockers, aspirin and other antiplatelet agents, angiotensin-converting enzyme inhibitors, and lipid-lowering agents.

The ACS guidelines assist the prescriber in identifying appropriate therapies. Once a drug is prescribed, the responsibility to use it then rests on the patient. However, nonadherence to medications is common.[3,4] Medication nonadherence is associated with increased mortality and rehospitalization in patients with heart disease.[5] Studies

Author information provided at the end of the text.

Results of this study were presented by Ms. Kline-Rogers at the American Heart Association 2nd Scientific Conference on Compliance in Healthcare and Research, May 18, 2004, Washington, DC.

have shown that patients who recently experienced a myocardial infarction (MI) and did not adhere closely to their prescribed regimen were 2.6 times more likely to die within a year following the MI compared with those who followed their regimen more closely.[6,7]

Medication adherence has been studied extensively over the past decades. Some of the predictors of nonadherence most often cited include polypharmacy, frequency of medication changes, socioeconomic status, cost, household composition, comorbidity, and accessibility to medical care.[8] Perhaps the most influential variables are the beliefs and attitudes that patients hold about illness and about taking drugs in general as well as those specific to individual agents they are prescribed.[9]

Various social, cognitive, and self-regulatory models have been developed to explain health behaviors, including adherence to treatment recommendations.[10,11] The Self-Regulation model provides a conceptual framework for understanding nonadherence.[9,11] Beliefs about health behaviors play an important role in adherence to prescribed treatment regimens. Using constructs from the Self-Regulation model, Horne et al.[12] developed the Beliefs About Medicine Questionnaire (BMQ). This questionnaire links medication adherence to patients' needs for and concerns about the use of drug therapy.

Healthcare professionals often take for granted that patients understand and believe in the necessity for use of prescribed medicines.[4] They must become more knowledgeable about the nature and causes of patient nonadherence. This study was conducted to systematically assess medication-taking behavior of 4 classes of evidence-based drugs used after ACS. First, continuation rates for the medications were determined and, for patients who appeared to have stopped a drug, reasons for discontinuation were elicited. We further determined adherence to current therapy using a self-reported adherence scale. Lastly, we determined the relationship between patient, disease, and treatment variables with adherence to the 4 classes of medications using multivariate regression modeling.

Methods

SUBJECTS

This study was a cross-sectional survey of patients who had experienced an ACS event surveyed by telephone 6–12 months after discharge. All patients aged ≥18 years discharged from a large Midwestern academic health system from January 2002 to May 2003 with the documented discharge diagnosis of unstable angina or acute MI were potential study subjects. Eligibility criteria included ability to understand English and communicate verbally by telephone. Institutional review board approval was obtained from the university, and each patient consented to participate.

DATA COLLECTION

Data from the hospitalization for the index ACS event were obtained from patients' health system medical records by cardiac fellows using standardized data collection forms. A telephone survey was then administered by trained interviewers between 6 and 12 months after patients' discharge, again using standardized forms and introduction script. At least 3 attempts were made to contact each patient. Initial data collection forms were reviewed by the nurse clinician overseeing the data collection effort for accuracy and completeness.

DATA AND INSTRUMENTS

Patient characteristics were obtained from the medical records or survey and included age, gender, education, household income, and comorbid conditions. A complete list of current medications was obtained from the medical record at the time of discharge and again from patient self-report at the time of the telephone survey. Cardiac-specific medications were categorized as β-blockers, angiotensin-converting enzyme (ACE) inhibitors, lipid-lowering agents, and antiplatelet agents. The antiplatelet category excluded clopidogrel or ticlopidine. At the time of the study, these agents were prescribed most often for a short time and then discontinued.

Overall and cardiac-related health status were determined by asking the patient to rate their status on a 5-point Likert scale (1 = excellent, 2 = very good, 3 = good, 4 = fair, 5 = poor). To determine beliefs toward medication, patients were administered the previously validated BMQ.[12] The BMQ consists of 18 items that generate 4 scale scores: Specific Necessity, Specific Concerns, General Harm, and General Overuse. Each BMQ item uses a 5-point Likert scale (from 1 = strongly agree to 5 = strongly disagree). Each scale score is derived from the mean of the scale items, with a possible score range from 1 to 5. Lower BMQ scale scores indicate stronger agreement with the belief scale. Appendix I presents individual BMQ items (www.hwbooks.com/pdf/appendices/G249.pdf).

The dependent variables included continuation rates for the cardiac-specific medications, reasons for discontinuation, and, for drugs continued at the time of the survey, adherence. Determination of continuation of the cardiac-specific agents was made by comparing the list of drugs obtained at discharge for the index ACS event to the list of drugs reported by the patient at the time of the telephone survey. If a discrepancy existed between the 2 lists, the interviewer prompted the patient during the phone call to provide a reason for discontinuation. Patients were given a set of reasons for discontinuing their medication. They also could provide additional reasons if not included by this list. The list of reasons was derived by the investigators with extensive clinical experience in following ACS patients.

Self-reported adherence was determined using the Medication Adherence Scale (MAS).[13] The 4 items in the scale address reasons for nonadherence such as forgetfulness, carelessness, or stopping medications because they feel better or worse. The items on the MAS use a 5-point Likert scale ranging from 1 = never, 3 = sometimes, and 5 = always. Lower MAS scores indicated better adherence. The MAS was determined for each cardiac-related drug category that the patient indicated they were still taking.

ANALYSIS

Descriptive analyses of patient, disease, treatment, and adherence data are presented as mean ± SD for continuous variables or frequencies and percents for categorical variables. The rate of continuation for each cardiac-related medication category was determined and reported as a frequency and percent. Reasons for discontinuation are also expressed as frequencies and percent.

A mean ± SD MAS score was calculated for each cardiac-related drug class the patient indicated they were still taking. In addition, the frequency and percent of respondents with scores >1 (indicating some level of nonadherence) was reported. An overall MAS score for each patient was derived from the mean of the individual cardiac drug class MAS scores. An overall MAS score >1.0 was considered to indicate nonadherence.

To further examine reasons for less-than-perfect adherence, the mean ± SD responses for each item of the MAS was calculated for each medication category and reported along with the percentage of patients who had scores >1 for the item.

To determine the strength of the relationship between the set of patient, disease, and treatment characteristics and the overall MAS score, multivariate linear regression analysis was conducted. A significance value of $p \leq 0.05$ was used for all analyses. All analyses were performed using SAS version 8.2 (SAS Institute, Cary, NC).

Results

SUBJECTS

A total of 563 potential patients were discharged during the study period. Of these, 208 were contacted and successfully completed the adherence questionnaire. The remaining 355 included 33 patients who died between discharge and the survey and 30 who partially completed the surveys (incomplete medication-taking behavior questionnaire portion of the survey); the remaining patients were either lost to follow-up (n = 72) or were not administered the adherence survey for various reasons (n = 220), of which the primary reason was refusal by the patient to respond to the adherence questions. Nonrespondents did not differ significantly in age, gender, or race from the respondents.

The average follow-up period for this study was 10 months. The study cohort's baseline characteristics are shown in Table 1. Most patients viewed their overall health status and their cardiac-related health status as good to very good. Subjects tended to agree with the statement about the necessity for using drugs (Specific Necessity scale) and disagree with the statement that medications caused harm (General Harm scale). Respondents were, as a group, relatively neutral on their agreement with statements about specific concerns about drugs (Specific Concerns scale) and about overuse of drugs (General Overuse scale).

CONTINUATION

Continuation of the 4 classes of cardiac medications decreased during the time between discharge and the follow-up survey: β-blockers from 90.3% (n = 177) to 80.0% (n = 156), ACE inhibitors from 71.0% (n = 137) to 66.0% (n = 124), lipid-lowering agents from 83.3% (n = 160) to 76.4% (n = 146), and aspirin from 94.7% (n = 184) to 87.3% (n = 172). Table 2 lists the reasons patients gave for not continuing drug therapy. The most common and consistent reason for discontinuation reported by patients was that their physicians did not think the medication was necessary. The next most common and consistent reason was that patients did not tolerate the drugs' adverse effects.

ADHERENCE

The overall mean MAS score was 1.3 ± 0.4 (median 1.1, range 1–3). The MAS score was >1.0 for at least one drug category for 53.8% of patients, indicating some level of nonadherence.

The mean MAS score determined for each drug category is presented in Table 3. For all 4 drug classes, >40% of respondents indicated that they missed taking their cardiac medication to some degree in the previous week. Table 4 presents data from analysis of the scores of each MAS item for each drug category. The MAS item with the highest mean score and most patients choosing a response >1 (indicating poor adherence) was the statement reporting

Table 1. Patient Characteristics[a]	
Variable	**Result**
Age, y, mean (SD)	64.9 (13.0)
Gender, male, n (%)	126 (60.6)
Race, white, n (%)	191 (96.0)
Household size, mean (SD)	1.7 (1.4)
Education, n (%)	
did not finish high school	25 (12.7)
high school graduate/GED	59 (29.9)
some college/technical school	54 (27.4)
college graduate	59 (29.9)
Self-reported health status, mean (SD)	
general health	2.7 (1.1)
cardiac-related health	2.8 (1.1)
excellent	31 (15.4)
very good	52 (25.9)
good	70 (34.8)
fair	32 (15.9)
poor	16 (8.0)
Drugs, mean (SD)	8.1 (3.9)
Comorbid conditions, mean (SD)	3.5 (1.8)
Belief About Medications Scale scores, mean (SD)	
specific necessity	2.2 (0.7)
specific concerns	3.3 (0.8)
general overuse	3.3 (0.7)
general harm	3.8 (0.5)

GED = general equivalency diploma.
[a]N = 208.

Table 2. Reasons for Not Continuing Medication Prescribed at Discharge				
Reason[a]	**β-Blockers (n = 19) n (%)**	**ACE Inhibitors (n = 15) n (%)**	**Lipid-Lowering Agents (n = 18) n (%)**	**Aspirin (n = 16) n (%)**
Physician did not think it was necessary	13 (59.1)	10 (47.6)	9 (50.0)	10 (62.5)
I did not like side effects	4 (18.2)	3 (14.3)	3 (16.7)	
I wanted a different medication	1 (4.5)			
I could not afford it	1 (4.5)	1 (4.8)	1 (5.6)	1 (6.3)
To avoid side effects I heard about		1 (4.8)		
I felt it was unnecessary to continue			1 (5.6)	
My physician switched to a different drug due to the current one not working			1 (5.6)	1 (6.3)
Other			3 (16.7)	4 (25.0)

ACE = angiotensin-converting enzyme.
[a]Subject could provide more than one reason.

being forgetful about taking medicine, followed by being careless when taking medicine.

MULTIVARIATE ANALYSIS OF ADHERENCE

The results of the multivariate regression model are presented in Table 5. The model explained a moderate level of variance in the dependent variable, the MAS score, with an R^2 value for the model of 0.132 (p = 0.01, F = 2.36). The 2 variables with a significant relationship to the MAS score were patient-perceived heart-related health status and the BMQ score Specific Necessity. Patients with better perceived heart-related health status and with the stronger

agreement that medications are a necessity reported better adherence.

Discussion

Four classes of cardiac medicines have been shown to significantly reduce morbidity and mortality in patients diagnosed with ACS. Recent reports have estimated that, collectively, drugs modifying cholesterol, blood pressure, homocysteine, and platelet function may prevent as many as 88% of MIs and 80% of strokes.[14] However, to realize these benefits, patients must adhere to drug therapy to prevent recurrent cardiac events. Our research aimed to determine continuation rates and reasons for discontinuation, along with characterizing adherent medication-taking behavior. We also wanted to understand how behavioral and social factors plus beliefs about medicines influence adherence.

Overall, the continuation rate for cardiac agents in our patients was high. This could be a function of the cohort we studied or a function of the process of care delivered through the use of standardized prescribing protocols for discharge medications in place in our institution. In previous studies, reported continuation rates for cardiac medication have varied. Some have reported continuation rates varying from 65% in patients with heart failure[15] to 40–50% in hypertensive patients.[16] Alternatively, improvements in continuation of medications have been reported in recent years, with rates similar to the ones we have reported, ranging from 70% to 89%.[17-19] These improvements could reflect the widespread acknowledgment of randomized clinical trials, international guidelines on the treatment of heart disease, and quality-improvement initiatives within health systems to improved prescribing of evidence-based therapies.[2]

The main reason given for discontinuation of the drugs at the time of the survey was "my physician did not think it was necessary," indicating patients' perception that, for some reason, physicians were discontinuing drugs prescribed at discharge. Reasons for discontinuation by physicians were not studied due to lack of access to medical

Table 3. Medication Adherence Scale Score for Each Drug Class

Drug Category	Medication Administration Scale Score,[a] mean (SD)	Pts. with Score >1.0,[b] n (%)
β-Blocker (n = 156)	1.27 (0.42)	73 (44.5)
ACE inhibitor (n = 124)	1.26 (0.39)	58 (43.6)
Lipid-lowering agent (n = 146)	1.30 (0.44)	76 (50.3)
Aspirin (n = 172)	1.30 (0.50)	79 (45.9)

ACE = angiotensin-converting enzyme.
[a]Scale: 1 = never occurs, 3 = sometimes occurs, 5 = always occurs.
[b]Indicates some level of nonadherence.

Table 4. Medication Adherence Scale Score for Individual Scale Items

Item	β-Blockers (n = 156)	ACE Inhibitors (n = 124)	Lipid-Lowering Agents (n = 146)	Aspirin (n = 172)
Forget to take medicine, mean (SD), % with score >1 or some degree of nonadherence	1.5 (0.7) 40.7	1.5 (0.7) 37.6	1.6 (0.8) 44.0	1.6 (0.8) 39.2
Careless about taking medicine, mean (SD), % with score >1 or some degree of nonadherence	1.3 (0.7) 19.5	1.3 (0.7) 19.6	1.4 (0.8) 22.5	1.4 (0.8) 21.5
When feel better, stop taking medicine, mean (SD), % with score >1 or some degree of nonadherence	1.1 (0.3) 4.3	1.1 (0.3) 3.1	1.1 (0.3) 4.0	1.1 (0.4) 4.7
If feel worse, stop taking medicine, mean (SD), % with score >1 or some degree of nonadherence	1.2 (0.7) 7.4	1.2 (0.6) 6.1	1.2 (0.7) 8.0	1.2 (0.8) 8.2

ACE = angiotensin-converting enzyme.

Table 5. Multivariate Regression Model Results[a]

Variable	β	p Value
Age	0.022	0.80
Gender	−0.083	0.28
Race	−0.015	0.88
Education	−0.102	0.19
Heart-related health status	0.207	0.009
Number of other people	0.044	0.57
Number of other illnesses	0.128	0.10
Beliefs About Medicine Questionnaire		
Specific Necessity Scale	0.264	0.001
Specific Concerns Scale	−0.033	0.70
General Overuse Scale	0.070	0.45
General Harm Scale	−0.095	0.29

[a]N = 182.

records of other health systems where many of the study patients were followed after discharge. The appropriateness of this reason needs to be further explored in future studies.

Over half of our patients reported some level of nonadherence, mostly due to forgetfulness and carelessness. Forgetfulness has been shown to result in nonadherence rates of 40% in patients taking antihypertensive agents.[20] Practitioners must collaborate with patients to create simple, clearly understood medication schedules that take into account daily activity schedules as well as addressing personal obligations that might lead to forgetfulness.

An association exists between the BMQ Specific Needs scale and adherence. Subjects who agreed with Specific Needs scale statements were more likely to be adherent. Other research has determined that patients' beliefs about drug therapy and about medicine in general have strong influence on adherence.[21] Clinicians may be able to use questions such as these, if not the actual BMQ Specific Needs scale, to screen patients who may be at risk for nonadherent behavior. More research would be required to determine the usefulness of this or similar scales in clinical practice and the type of intervention to use that would be most successful.

Patients reporting good heart-related health status indicated greater self-reported adherence, as patients may feel that medicines are improving their heart condition. Patients' perceptions of the benefit gained by treatment can have a positive influence on medication-taking behavior. Our study confirms previous findings that other variables, such as age, gender, and educational level, are not always associated with self-reported adherence. Effective communication, changing patient beliefs and perceptions of their disorder and medications used, as well as collegial patient–physician interactions, have been shown to improve adherence.[22]

This study, using a sample of patients that was relatively small and who received initial care at only one institution, may not be generalizable to all post-ACS patients. Another potential limitation is that adherence was measured using a self-reported instrument rather than a more objective measure, such as pharmacy claims data or electronic prescription-vial monitoring. The potential to over-report adherent behavior is possible with self-report. However, in this study, the level of nonadherence was >40% for all drug categories, which we interpret as being relatively devoid of response bias. Another potential limitation of using the MAS is that it mentions only 4 types of behaviors, perhaps not capturing other more salient reasons related to medication misadventuring. Further research into the most appropriate set of questions to ask a patient regarding continuation and adherence is important.

Healthcare professionals must understand the many factors affecting medication-taking behavior. It is not enough to simply assume that patients are taking their drugs properly. Physicians, pharmacists, and other health professionals must make a sustained effort to evaluate and educate patients about their medicines. Education and day-to-day support have been shown to reduce poor outcomes by increasing patient participation in the management of chronic illnesses.[23] Unless we identify and alleviate patient concerns or misinformation, adherence and, therefore, patient outcomes will remain less than ideal.

Conclusions

Following an ACS event, not all patients continue their medication or take it exactly as prescribed. Based on the findings of this study, patients' perceptions that their physicians made the decision to discontinue their medication was the most common reason for no longer taking a drug prescribed at discharge. This finding warrants further investigation, perhaps using qualitative survey methods to question patients coupled with review of medical records, to determine the reasons for discontinuation. Patients' beliefs about the necessity for medication and their perception of severity of illness are important variables associated with adherence while actively taking the medication. Further research is necessary to determine how to use this information for screening patients who may be at risk for nonadherence.

Anchal Sud BS, Medical Student, College of Medicine, University of Michigan, Ann Arbor, MI

Eva M Kline-Rogers MS RN, Cardiology Research Nurse, Division of Cardiology, University of Michigan Health System

Kim A Eagle MD, Professor, Division of Cardiology, University of Michigan Health System

Jianming Fang PhD, Statistician, Division of Cardiology, University of Michigan Health System

David F Armstrong MD, General Internal Medicine Resident, Division of Cardiology, University of Michigan Health System

Krishna Rangarajan MD, Undergraduate Research Student, Division of Cardiology, University of Michigan Health System

Richard F Otten MD, General Internal Medicine Resident, Division of Cardiology, University of Michigan Health System

Dana R Stafkey-Mailey PharmD, PhD Candidate, at time of the study, Pharmacoeconomics Fellow, Division of Cardiology, University of Michigan Health System and Pfizer, Inc.; now, Pharmaceutical Economics and Policy, School of Pharmacy, University of Southern California, Los Angeles, CA

Stephanie D Taylor PhD, Assistant Professor, College of Pharmacy, University of Michigan

Steven R Erickson PharmD, Associate Professor, College of Pharmacy, University of Michigan

Reprints: Dr. Erickson, College of Pharmacy, University of Michigan, 428 Church St., Ann Arbor, MI 48109-1065, fax 734/763-2022, serick@umich.edu

References

1. American Heart Association. Heart disease and stroke statistics—2004 update. Dallas, TX: American Heart Association, 2003.
2. Mehta RH, Montoye CK, Gallogy M, Baker P, Blount A, Faul J, et al. GAP Steering Committee of the American College of Cardiology. Improving quality of care for acute myocardial infarction: the Guidelines Applied in Practice (GAP) Initiative. JAMA 2002;287:1269-76.
3. Jackevicius CA, Mamdani M, Tu JV. Adherence with statin therapy in elderly patients with and without acute coronary syndromes. JAMA 2002;288:462-7.
4. Cline CMJ, Björck-Cinné AK, Israelsson BYA, Willenheimer RB, Erhardt LR. Non-compliance and knowledge of prescribed medication in elderly patients with heart failure. Eur J Heart Fail 1999;1:145-9.
5. Dunbar-Jacob J, Bohachick P, Mortimer MK, Sereika SM, Foley SM. Medication adherence in persons with cardiovascular disease. J Cardiovasc Nurs 2003;18:209-18.
6. Gallagher EJ, Viscoli CM, Horwitz RI. The relationship of treatment adherence to the risk of death after myocardial infarction in women. JAMA 1993;270:742-4.

7. Beta-Blocker Heart Attack Trial Research Group. A randomized trial of propranolol in patients with acute myocardial infarction, I: mortality results. JAMA 1982;247:1707-14.

8. Berg JS, Dischler J, Wagner DJ, Raia JJ, Palmer-Shevlin N. Patient compliance: a healthcare problem. Ann Pharmacother 1993;27(9 suppl):S5-19.

9. Horne R. Representations of medication and treatment: advances in theory and measurement. In: Petrie KJ, Weinman J, eds. Perceptions of health and illness: current research and applications. London: Harwood Academic, 1997:155-87.

10. Horne R, Weinman J. Self-regulation and self-management in asthma: exploring the role of illness perceptions and treatment beliefs in explaining nonadherence to preventor medication. Psychol Health 2002;17:17-32.

11. Leventhal H, Cameron L. Behavioural theories and the problem of compliance. Patient Educ Counsel 1987;10:117-38.

12. Horne R, Weinman J, Hankins M. The Beliefs About Medicines Questionnaire: the development and evaluation of a new method for assessing the cognitive representation of medication. Psychol Health 1999;14:1-24.

13. Morisky DE, Green LW, Levine DM. Concurrent predictive validity of a self-reported measure of medication adherence. Med Care 1986;24:67-74.

14. Wald NJ, Law MR. A strategy to reduce cardiovascular disease by more than 80%. BMJ 2003;326:1419-24.

15. Roe CM, Motheral BR, Teitelbaum F, Rich MW. Compliance with and dosing of angiotensin-converting-enzyme inhibitors before and after hospitalization. Am J Health Syst Pharm 2000;57:139-45.

16. Jones JK, Gorkin L, Lian JF, Staffa JA, Fletcher AP. Discontinuation of and changes in treatment after start of new courses of antihypertensive drugs: a study of a United Kingdom population. BMJ 1995;311:293-5.

17. Caro JJ. Stepped care for hypertension: are the assumptions valid? J Hypertens 1997;15(suppl):S35-9.

18. Simpson E, Beck C, Richard H, Eisenberg MJ, Pilote L. Drug prescriptions after acute myocardial infarction: dosage, compliance, and persistence. Am Heart J 2003;145:438-44.

19. Andrade SE, Walker AM, Gottlieb LK, Hollenberg NK, Testa MA, Saperia GM, et al. Discontinuation of antihyperlipidemic drugs—do rates reported in clinical trials reflect rates in primary care settings? N Engl J Med 1995;332:1125-31.

20. Choo PW, Rand CS, Inui TS, Lee ML, Cain E, Cordeiro-Breault M, et al. Validation of patient reports, automated pharmacy records, and pill counts with electronic monitoring of adherence to antihypertensive therapy. Med Care 1999;37:846-57.

21. Vermeire E, Hearnshaw H, VanRoyen P, Denekens J. Patient adherence to treatment: three decades of research. A comprehensive review. J Clin Pharm Ther 2001;26:331-42.

22. Burke LE, Dunbar-Jacob JM, Hill MN. Compliance with cardiovascular disease prevention strategies: a review of the research. Ann Behav Med 1997;19:239-63.

23. Krumholz HM, Amatruda J, Smith GL, Mattera JA, Roumanis SA. Randomized trial of an education and support intervention to prevent readmission of patients with heart failure. J Am Coll Cardiol 2002;39:83-9.

EXTRACTO

ANTECEDENTES: La falta de adherencia al tratamiento puede asociarse a un mal resultado médico.

OBJETIVO: Describir el comportamiento de uso de 4 clases de medicamentos en pacientes con antecedentes de síndrome coronario agudo (SCA) y determinar la relación entre la adherencia al tratamiento notificada por los pacientes y las características de estos.

MÉTODOS: Se entrevistó por teléfono a pacientes con diagnóstico de SCA que aceptaron participar en el estudio, aproximadamente 10 meses después de ser dados de alta del hospital. La encuesta incluía datos sobre características del paciente, regímenes actuales de tratamiento, creencias sobre los medicamentos, razones para abandonarlos, y adherencia a la terapia. La encuesta también incluía el Cuestionario de las Creencias Sobre los Medicamentos, que incluía 4 escalas: Necesidad Específica, Preocupaciones Específicas, Daño General, Sobreutilización General, y Escala de Adherencia a Medicamentos. Se utilizó la regresión multivariada para determinar las variables independientes con la asociación más fuerte con la EAM. Para todos los análisis se consideró significativo un valor de p ≤ 0.05.

RESULTADOS: Se entrevistaron 208 pacientes. La edad promedio fue 64.9 (± 13.0) años, 60.6% eran hombres, 95.7% blanco, 57.3% tenían educación universitaria, 87.9% vivían con más de una persona, y 42% indicaron excelente o muy buena salud. El porcentaje de pacientes que continuaba tomando medicamentos en el momento de la encuesta varió de 87.4% (aspirina) a 66% (inhibidores de ECA). Las razones para abandonar el tratamiento incluían el abandono por el médico o por efectos secundarios. De los pacientes que aún continuaban tomando medicamentos, la EAM promedio fue 1.3 (± 0.4), con 53.8% indicando no adherencia (puntuación >1). El modelo de regresión final tuvo un R^2 = 0.132 e incluyó el estado de salud relacionado con el corazón y NE como variables predictoras significativas.

CONCLUSIONES: Tras el SCA, no todos los pacientes continúan tomando sus medicamentos o los toman exactamente según la prescripción. La determinación de las creencias de los pacientes sobre la enfermedad y medicamentos puede ser útil para desarrollar intervenciones dirigidas a mejorar la adherencia a la terapia.

Juan F Feliú

RÉSUMÉ

OBJECTIF: Décrire les comportements associés à la prise de 4 classes de médicaments chez les patients avec un syndrome coronarien aigu et déterminer s'il existe une relation entre une l'observance déclarée et les caractéristiques des patients.

MÉTHODES: Les patients ayant un diagnostic de syndrome coronarien aigu ont été questionnés par téléphone environ 10 mois après leur congé de l'hôpital. Les données suivantes ont été recueillies soit les médicaments actifs, les raisons pour l'arrêt des médicaments, les croyances concernant les médicaments et l'observance. L'étude incluait un questionnaire des croyances sur les médicaments, qui comprenait 4 échelles: nécessité spécifique, préoccupation spécifique, préjudice général, sur-utilisation générale, et l'échelle d'observance des médicaments. Une régression multi variée a été utilisée pour déterminer les variables indépendantes ayant une association avec l'échelle d'observance médicamenteuse.

RÉSULTATS: Un nombre de 208 patients ont été interrogés. L'âge moyen était de 64.9 ± 13.0 ans avec 60.6% d'hommes, 95.7% de race blanche, 57.3% ayant un niveau d'éducation collégiale, 87.9% demeurant avec ≥1 autre personne, et 42% ayant un niveau de santé excellent ou très bon. Le pourcentage de patients qui ont continué leurs médicaments au moment de l'étude variait entre 87.4% (aspirine) à 66.0% (IECA). Les raisons pour l'arrêt des médicaments étaient les effets indésirables ou un avis du médecin traitant. Chez les patients sous médicaments, la moyenne de l'échelle d'observance des médicaments était de 1.3 ± 0.4, avec 53.8% indiquant la présence de non observance. Le modèle final de régression présentait un R^2 = 0.132 et les variables suivantes soit l'état de santé associé aux problèmes cardiaques et la nécessité spécifique comme étant des éléments pouvant influencer l'observance.

CONCLUSIONS: Suite à un syndrome coronarien aigu, certains patients cessent leurs médicaments ou ne suivent pas les instructions du médecin. Les auteurs mentionnent qu'il s'avère important d'identifier les croyances concernant la maladie et les médicaments afin de développer des interventions pour améliorer l'observance.

Louise Mallet

Glossary of Terms

Absolute risk: see RISK (Chapter 6)

Active controlled trial: an experimental study design used to compare a novel treatment to a standard treatment. (Chapters 3 and 8)

Administrative claims databases: databases that are created when pharmacy and medical insurance claims are processed. The items commonly found on claims in medical claims databases include member identifier, provider identifier, place of service, date of service, procedure code, and financial information. The items commonly found in pharmacy claims databases include member identifier, provider identifier, pharmacy identifier, date of service, prescription number, National Drug Code (NDC) number, quantity dispensed, days supply, and financial information. (Chapter 9)

All-cause mortality: the risk of death for any reason. (Chapter 6)

Allocative efficiency (also known as Pareto efficiency): the distribution of resources that maximizes use or benefit for society. The resources are distributed in such a way that if you changed the distribution, the overall utility or benefit would decrease. (Chapter 9)

α error (type I error): an error in the statistical decision-making process in which a true null hypothesis is rejected. (Chapter 5)

Alternative hypothesis (H_A): the statistical hypothesis that is accepted as being confirmed if the null hypothesis is rejected. (Chapter 5)

Alternatives: the options from which the decision maker must choose. This is the term that describes the options included in an economic analysis. (Chapter 9)

Analysis of variance: a parametric statistical test of differences among two or more group means, carried out in a way that preserves the prespecified α level. (Chapter 7)

Arithmetic mean: an average; the sum of scores in a data set divided by the number of scores. (Chapter 4)

Attack rate: the incidence of mortality or morbidity during an unusually short time interval in a specific group, such as would occur among dormitory residents after the ingestion of tainted food. (Chapter 6)

Attributable risk: see RISK DIFFERENCE. (Chapter 6)

Bayesian analysis: alternative to statistical testing that calculates the chances that previous findings are correct given new data; uses modeling and can be used if some data are missing.

Beneficence: a duty to promote good and act in the best interest of the patient and the health of society. (Chapter 2)

Benefits: positive outcomes produced from an intervention or program. Examples include improved health, cost savings or avoided costs. (Chapter 9)

β error (type II error): an error in the statistical decision-making process in which a false null hypothesis is not rejected. (Chapter 5)

Bias: a systematic error introduced into some aspect of the study by the experimental design or methods. (Chapter 3)

Binomial distribution: a relative frequency distribution characterizing the probability of each possible outcome of a series of binomial events. (Chapter 5)

Binomial event: an event that can have only two outcomes, such as life or death. (Chapter 5)

Biocreep: the tendency of the difference between the treatment effects of a series of noninferiority trials and the original placebo effect to erode to the point at which the treatment effect is no longer different from the original placebo effect. (Chapter 8)

Biostatistics: a set of mathematical tools to classify and analyze health-related data generated through scientific research. (Chapters 1 and 4)

Blinding: a term meaning that the person is unaware of the event, occurrence, treatment, etc. (Chapter 8)

Block randomization: A technique used to control for differences in treatment and other factors at different study sites; it consists of the random assignment of patients to conditions at each individual site to make sure that the proportion of treatment and control patients is similar at each site. (Chapter 8)

Box plot: a graphical display that divides a data set into four parts so that each part contains 25% of the total numbers in the data set. (Chapter 4)

Case-control study: an observational study research paradigm in which the groups are defined in terms of the outcome, and a relationship is sought between the outcome and one or more antecedent exposure variables. (Chapters 3 and 6)

Case-fatality rate: the risk of death from a specific cause. (Chapter 6)

Case series: a summary of the health status of two or more individuals who display a similar or novel condition. (Chapters 3 and 6)

Case study: a brief, informal description of an individual with a novel or unusual condition. (Chapters 3 and 6)

Central limit theorem: Given a population with a mean (μ) and a finite standard deviation (σ), the probability distribution of the means of samples of size n drawn from this population will have a mean of μ, will have a standard deviation of $\sigma/\sqrt{n}$, and will exhibit a normal shape as long as n is large. (Chapter 5)

Chance: the likelihood that an association happened by a random, unpredictable process; also known as luck, providence, destiny, or accident. (Chapter 3)

Clinical practice guidelines: systematically developed statements created to assist practitioner and patient decisions about healthcare for specific circumstances. (Chapter 11)

Coding: a method of cataloging characteristics of research papers according to predefined criteria; also called data extraction. (Chapter 10)

Coefficient of determination: the percent of the total variation in a data set that is attributable to the association between the independent and the dependent variables. (Chapter 7)

Coefficient of variation: measure of relative variability in a data set, expressed as a percent of the mean. (Chapter 4)

Cohort study research design: an observational study research paradigm in which groups are defined with respect to the presence or absence of an exposure, and a relationship is sought between this factor and one or more outcome variables. (Chapters 3 and 7)

Composite outcome: a study outcome consisting of a number of individual outcomes. (Chapter 8)

Concealed allocation: refers to a technique of not revealing the group assignment of a patient to an investigator until the patient is actually assigned to a condition. (Chapter 8)

Confidence interval (CI): a range or interval centered on a measure of central tendency of a sampling distribution that has a given probability of containing the true population parameter. For example, the 95% confidence interval for a sample mean has a 95% chance of containing the value of the population mean. (Chapter 5)

Confounding: contamination of the data by an uncontrolled variable that is correlated with the independent variable and independently associated with the outcome variable. (Chapters 3 and 7)

Consensus development method: a technique to structure the interaction among panel experts who are developing clinical practice guidelines; a selected group (of ~ 10 experts) is brought together to reach consensus about an issue in an open meeting. (Chapter 11)

Continuous scale of measurement: a method of measuring variables quantitatively, in which the interval between adjacent values of the variable depends only on the resolving power of the measuring device. (Chapter 4)

Continuous variables: variables whose values are based on quantitative measurement and may assume any value along the measurement scale, like blood pressure in millimeters of mercury. (Chapter 4)

Control group: subjects in a research study that receive an inactive or standard treatment and whose data provide baseline information from which to compare the effects of an active treatment. (Chapter 3)

Cost: a resource consumed in an attempt to produce a positive outcome. These are usually measured in monetary terms such as dollars. (Chapter 9)

Cost–benefit analysis (CBA): type of economic analysis in which both costs and benefits are in monetary units (dollars). (Chapter 9)

Cost-effectiveness analysis (CEA): an economic analysis comparing the costs and benefits of two or more alternatives; costs are measured in monetary units (dollars) and benefits are measured in natural units (such as hospital days, heart attacks avoided, or number of people with controlled blood pressure). (Chapter 9)

Cost-minimization analysis (CMA): a special form of cost-effectiveness analysis in which the quantity or magnitude of the measured benefits is equal for all alternatives, so the alternative with the lowest cost is the most cost-effective. (Chapter 9)

Cost-of-illness study: a partial economic analysis that measures or estimates the national cost of a disease or condition. The costs included in the analysis may include the cost of diagnosis and treatment as well as lost productivity owing to the disease or condition. (Chapter 9)

Cost–utility analysis (CUA): type of economic analysis by which costs are in monetary units (dollars) and benefits are in utility or value based units (such as QALYs). (Chapter 9)

Cox proportional hazard model: a statistical method used to characterize changes in survival as a function of preexisting conditions. (Chapter 8)

Crossover RCT study design: individuals initially assigned to one condition (or treatment group) are switched to the other condition (or treatment group) at some point in the trial. Cf. PARALLEL-GROUPS RCT STUDY DESIGN. (Chapters 3 and 8)

Cross-sectional study research design: an observational study design used to determine the prevalence of an exposure, an outcome, or an exposure–outcome association at a single point in time or during a brief time interval. (Chapters 3 and 7)

Cumulative frequency distribution: a frequency distribution in which each class interval contains both the present relative frequency and the sum of all previous relative frequencies. (Chapter 4)

Data extraction: see CODING. (Chapter 10)

Decision analysis: a technique to help people make decisions by separating a decision into three components—alternatives, probabilities, and outcomes—and diagramming the decision-making process. (Chapter 9)

Decision tree: a type of decision analysis modeling for linear clinical states or diseases. (Chapter 9)

Degrees of freedom: the number of scores in a sample that may assume more than one value in the calculation of a statistic. (Chapter 4)

Dependent variable: the variable that is measured to assess the effect of the independent variable, often segregated into primary and secondary outcomes. (Chapter 3)

Descriptive research designs: research designs that propose to depict novel or unusual signs, symptoms, or events. (Chapter 3)

Descriptive statistics: the use of statistical tools to summarize or otherwise describe the major characteristics of a data set. (Chapters 4 and 5)

Direct benefits: see DIRECT COSTS

Direct costs: costs (avoided costs = benefits) associated with obtaining medical care (includes medical and nonmedical expenses). (Chapter 9)

Direct medical costs: expenditures for medical products and services. (Chapter 9)

Direct nonmedical costs: expenditures associated with obtaining healthcare but not including the medical products or services (such as travel and childcare). (Chapter 9)

Discounting: adjusting the value, with a specified rate, of a cost or benefit that will occur at some time in the future to its present value. (Chapter 9)

Discrete variables: variables that are expressed in whole numbers, such as counts and ranks. (Chapter 4)

Disease-oriented evidence (DOE): outcomes aimed at increasing understanding of a disease and its incidence and prevalence, diagnosis and treatment, and prognosis. (Chapter 12)

Distributions: a way to organize or arrange data in a manner that makes it easy for an observer to grasp its meaning. (Chapter 4)

Double-blind studies: research protocols in which both the patient and the investigator are unaware of the treatment group assignment. (Chapter 8)

Double-dummy technique: a technique used to maintain blinding under conditions in which treatments differ, such as by route of administration. It consists of preparing both treatment and placebo (or an alternative treatment) in such a manner that such cues do not identify the treatment. (Chapter 8)

Drug information: the provision of information as it relates to any area of pharmacotherapy or pharmacy practice. (Chapter 1)

ECHO model: an integrated model of healthcare interventions, developed by Kozma et al., that divides the outcomes of healthcare into three categories: economic, clinical, and humanistic. (Chapter 9)

Effectiveness: the level of clinical benefit based on real-world use. (Chapter 9)

Effect size: an index used to indicate the magnitude, robustness, or strength of a statistically significant effect. (Chapter 5)

Efficacy: the level of clinical benefit based on controlled trials. (Chapter 9)

Epidemiology: the study of factors that affect health and disease, particularly from a population or public-health perspective. (Chapter 6)

Equivalence trial: a type of active controlled trial designed to indicate whether the effects of two or more active agents are similar in terms of a clinically important outcome. (Chapter 8)

Evidence-based medicine (EBM): the conscientious, explicit, and judicious use of current best evidence along with clinical expertise and patient values in making clinical decisions about the care of individual patients. (Chapters 1 and 3)

Evidence-based method: a procedure for developing clinical practice guidelines that provides more scientific rigor than both informal and formal consensus methods; focus is on using a systematic search of the literature along with transparent methods to appraise the literature and weigh recommendations. (Chapter 11)

Exclusion criteria: attributes of individuals that disqualify them from participation in a study. (Chapter 8)

Exhaustive: a characteristic of a random event in which all potential outcomes are considered. For example, only a head or a tail, but no other outcome, may occur for one any coin flip. (Chapter 5)

Experimental research designs: research designs that involve the active manipulation of one or more independent variables. (Chapter 3)

External validity: the extent to which the evidence provided in a research article is relevant to the patients outside of the study, such as patients in the healthcare provider's clinical practice. This is sometimes referred to as generalizability because the results are applied to the general population. (Chapters 3, 6, and 9)

Extraneous variables: variables that may interfere with the clear observation of the association between the independent and the dependent variable. (Chapter 3)

Face validity: a kind of validity established by consulting likely respondents to ascertain their opinions. (Chapter 7)

File-drawer phenomenon: the tendency of researchers to not publish research efforts that fail to achieve statistical significance. (Chapter 10)

Fixed variable: one whose levels are deliberately selected by the investigator. For example, the different doses of a drug used in a research study. (Chapter 4)

Foraging tool: a method of being alerted to new information as it becomes available. (Chapter 12)

Forest plot: a graphical representation of the point and interval estimates of variables in a research study. (Chapter 10)

Formal consensus method: a procedure for developing clinical practice guidelines that involves a structured 2.5-day conference with recommendations, typically presented to an audience and/or members of the press on the third day; this method provides more structure to the analytic process than the informal consensus method. (Chapter 11)

Frequency charts: used to represent a frequency distribution of values in a data set. (Chapter 4)

Frequency distribution: a way of organizing data by combining adjacent numbers into class intervals and indicating the number of cases included in each interval. (Chapter 4)

Funnel plot: used to examine whether publication bias was a significant factor in the results obtained from a meta-analysis. (Chapter 10)

Gross national product: the value of goods and services produced in a country. (Chapter 9)

Hawthorne effect: a tendency of study subjects to increase performance simply because they have been chosen to participate in a study. (Chapter 8)

Hazard: the risk of an event at a certain instant of time. (Chapters 6 and 8)

Hazard ratio: the ratio of two hazards, interpreted in the same manner as a risk ratio. (Chapter 8)

Health capital: amount of productivity based on full health equaling 100%. (Chapter 9)

Healthy year equivalent (HYE): similar to QALY, but incorporates changes over time and uses values rather than utilities. (Chapter 9)

Heterogeneity: variability, or differences, among treatments, research results, and so on. (Chapter 10)

Hunting tool: a method for refinding published information when needed. (Chapter 12)

Hypothesis testing: a method of using statistical tools to reach a decision about a population based on data from samples drawn from that population. (Chapter 5)

Incidence: in epidemiology, the number of new cases of a disease that occur within a specific time interval. (Chapter 6)

Incidence density: an expression of risk based on person-time. (Chapter 6)

Inclusion criteria: attributes of individuals that qualify them for participation in a research study. (Chapter 8)

Incremental cost-effectiveness analysis: calculating and comparing the incremental cost-effectiveness ratios of two or more alternatives to determine which one is the most cost effective. (Chapter 9)

Incremental cost-effectiveness ratio (ICER): cost of one additional unit of outcome; calculated by dividing the difference in costs by the difference in effects (or benefits) of one alternative compared to the next most effective alternative. (Chapter 9)

Independent variable: exposures, antecedent events, treatments, or interventions that are altered by the investigator to examine their association with the dependent variable. (Chapter 3)

Independent: the outcome of one random event does not affect the outcome of any other random event. (Chapter 5)

Indices of shape: an idea of the shape of the distribution of scores, for example, skewness. (Chapter 4)

Indirect benefits: see INDIRECT COSTS

Indirect costs: costs (avoided costs = benefits) associated with productivity (such as lost workdays and decreased productivity while at work). (Chapter 9)

Inferential statistics: the application of statistical theory and tools to enable generalizing the findings from a smaller subset of patients to all similar patients. (Chapter 4)

Informal consensus method: a procedure for developing clinical practice guidelines in which a group of experts makes recommendations based on a subjective assessment of the evidence, with little description of the specific evidence or process used to derive the recommendations. (Chapter 11)

Information mastery: the ability to forage efficiently through vast amounts of available information, identify and critically assess the best and most pertinent pieces of information, and apply that information to the clinical situation. (Chapters 1 and 12)

Intangible benefits: see INTANGIBLE COSTS

Intangible costs: costs (avoided costs = benefits) that incorporate quality of life. (Chapter 9)

Intention to treat (ITT): a form of data analysis in which the data for each participant who enters the study are included in the final data analysis, even if the person fails to complete the study protocol. This study design provides an estimate of the treatment effect in the treated population. Cf. PER-PROTOCOL ANALYSIS. (Chapter 3)

Interaction: a phenomenon in which two or more treatments produce an effect that is not the simple sum of each individual treatment effect. (Chapter 7)

Internal validity: the veracity of the research, reflecting the general scientific quality of the research study. (Chapters 3 and 6)

Interquartile range (IQR): the central area of a box plot, containing the middle 50% of the scores in a data set. (Chapter 4)

Interval scale of measurement: a quantitative or continuous measurement scale in which the intervals between adjacent levels represent equal quantities across the entire measurement range, but there is no absolute zero. For example, the Celcius temperature scale. (Chapter 4)

Kaplan-Meier survival curve: examines changes in the rate of events over time, either individually or among groups, to associate differences in survival with the presence of independent variables. (Chapter 8)

L'Abbe plot: used to demonstrate the extent of agreement among research papers in estimating the same treatment effect. (Chapter 10)

Last observation carried forward (LOCF): a technique used to fill in missing data for an intention-to-treat analysis that consists of using the last observation from the participant to estimate subsequent missing data points. (Chapter 3)

Life-year: actual amount of life expectancy (quantity) or change in expectancy, in years. (Chapter 9)

Likelihood ratio negative (LR−): an index expressing how much less likely a disease-free person is to test positive on a screening test than is a person with the disease. (Chapter 5)

Likelihood ratio positive (LR+): an index expressing how much more likely a person with the disease is to test positive on a screening test than is a disease-free person. (Chapter 5)

Likert scale: a type of ordinal measurement in which the participant selects the best answer from a list of alternatives. It is frequently used by clinicians to obtain self-reports from patients and to rate signs and symptoms. (Chapters 4 and 7)

Limiters: criteria by which the focus of a literature search can be narrowed. (Chapter 2)

Logistic regression analysis: a form of nonlinear regression analysis in which the goal is to maximize the classification of people into two categories based on the values of one or more independent variables. (Chapter 6)

Marginal cost-effectiveness analysis: calculating and comparing the marginal cost effectiveness ratios of two or more alternatives to determine which one is the most cost effective. For example, the alternatives may relate to conducting the same screening or test a different number of times (alternative 1: five screenings vs. alternative 2: six screenings) for a particular disease or condition. (Chapter 9)

Markov model: type of decision analysis modeling for clinical states or diseases that do not progress linearly; includes time intervals and return to previous states. (Chapter 9)

Matching: a technique for controlling the influence of variables by constructing groups so that each has an equal representation of the variable in question. (Chapter 6)

Mean square regression: an index of the amount of variation in a group of scores that is attributable to the association of the independent and dependent variables. (Chapter 7)

Mean square residual: an index of the average amount of total variation that is attributable to experimental error. (Chapter 7)

Measure of central tendency: an index of the center of the distribution of scores; such as the arithmetic mean, median, and mode. (Chapter 4)

Measure of dispersion: an index of the variability of the scores in the distribution; such as the variance, standard deviation and range. (Chapter 4)

Measurement error: a systematic lack of precision in assessing an outcome variable, such as a body weight scale that reads several kilograms less than the person's true body weight. (Chapter 3)

Median: the middle score of the data set, the 50th percentile. (Chapter 4)

Medical chart review (or chart review): the process of obtaining data from patients' medical chart by reviewing the paper or electronic medical records. (Chapter 9)

Medical subject headings (MeSH): controlled vocabulary for indexing records within the MEDLINE database. (Chapter 2)

Meta-analysis: see QUANTITATIVE SYSTEMATIC REVIEWS. (Chapter 10)

Mode: the most frequent score in a data set. (Chapter 4)

Multivariable linear regression: a method of quantifying of the association between a continuous dependent variable and a set of two or more independent variables. (Chapter 7)

Mutually exclusive: a characteristic of a random event in which the occurrence of one outcome of a random event precludes the simultaneous occurrence of other outcomes. (Chapter 5)

Negative predictive value (NPV): the proportion of subjects who do not have the disease who test negative. (Chapter 5)

Nominal group technique: a technique to structure the interaction among panel experts who are developing clinical practice guidelines; individual panel members privately record his or her judgment and vote for the options; individual judgments are aggregated statistically to derive group judgment. (Chapter 11)

Nominal scale of measurement: the use of numbers as labels, such as designating men as 0 and women as 1. (Chapter 4)

Noninferiority trial: a type of active controlled trial designed to indicate whether the effects of two or more active agents are not worse than each other in terms of a clinically important outcome. (Chapter 8)

Nonmaleficence: a duty to protect and do no harm to patients. (Chapter 2)

Normal distribution: a specialized frequency distribution of continuous variables (technically, therefore, a density function) that can be characterized by its two parameters: the mean and the standard deviation. (Chapter 4)

Nuisance variables: variables that obscure the association between the antecedent and the outcome variables. (Chapter 6)

Null hypothesis (H_0): a statistical hypothesis stating that there is no relationship among independent and dependent variables. (Chapter 5)

Number needed to harm (NNH): the number of people that need to be at risk for a defined period of time for a harm to come to one of them. (Chapter 6)

Number needed to treat (NNT): the number of people that need to be treated for a defined period of time for a benefit to be observed in one person. (Chapter 6)

Observational study research designs: research investigations that examine participants expressly because they exhibit either a specific characteristic or a specific outcome. (Chapters 3 and 6)

Odds: the ratio of the number of ways a desired event can occur divided by the number of ways it cannot occur. (Chapter 6)

Odds ratio: the ratio of two odds. It provides an index of the relative likelihood of one event compared to another. (Chapter 6)

On-treatment analysis: see PER-PROTOCOL ANALYSIS. (Chapter 3)

Open-label studies: research protocols in which there is no attempt to conceal treatment status of the patient. (Chapter 8)

Opportunity costs: costs that could be used for another purpose; usually, the next best purpose. (Chapter 9)

Ordered array: an arrangement of the individual values in a data set in ascending or descending order. (Chapter 4)

Ordinal scale of measurement: a measurement scale used to indicate differences in rank. However, the interval between ranks is not necessarily consistent. (Chapter 4)

Outliers: values in a data set that exceed 1.5 times the IQR. (Chapter 4)

Parallel-groups RCT study design: a randomized controlled trial design in which patients are assigned to one or more treatment and control groups. Patients receive only one treatment during the study. Compare to a crossover RCT study design. (Chapter 3)

Parameters: entities that are used to characterize populations, such as the population mean, μ, and the population standard deviation, σ. They are assumed to be unchanging. (Chapters 4 and 5)

Pareto diagram: combines a relative frequency chart with a cumulative frequency chart. The levels of the independent variable are arranged in descending order on the abscissa. (Chapter 4)

Pareto efficiency: (also known as ALLOCATIVE EFFICIENCY) the distribution of resources that maximizes utility or benefit for society. The resources are distributed in such a way that if you changed the distribution, the overall utility or benefit would decrease. (Chapter 9)

Partial analyses: an economic analysis that examines either the cost of two or more alternatives or interventions or the outcomes of two or more alternatives or interventions. It is a partial analysis because it does not include both the costs and the outcomes of two or more alternatives. (Chapter 9)

Patient-oriented evidence (POE): outcomes that patients care most about—morbidity, mortality, and quality of life. (Chapter 12)

Patient-Oriented Evidence That Matters (POEM): A study that meets the following criteria: (1) it focuses on patient-oriented outcomes; (2) the issue under study is common to clinical practice and the intervention is feasible; and (3) if the information is valid, a change in clinical practice will be required. (Chapter 12)

Pearson product-moment correlation coefficient (r): an index of the linear association between two variables, given that both variables are continuous and normally distributed. (Chapter 7)

Period prevalence: the sum of the number of cases present at the beginning of the measurement interval (i.e., the point prevalence) plus the number of new cases that occur during a specified time period. It is used for diseases (e.g., osteoarthritis) that do not have an abrupt onset. (Chapter 6)

Per-protocol analysis: a form of data analysis that includes data only from participants who completed the entire study protocol. A per-protocol data analysis depicts the efficacy and safety to be expected among patients who comply with the treatment regimen. Compare to an intent-to-treat analysis. (Chapter 3)

Person-time: a measure of a person's participation in units of time, such a person-year. (Chapter 6)

Perspective: the viewpoint of the party interested in the results of the study. (Chapter 9)

Pharmaceutical care: a patient-centered practice in which the practitioner assumes responsibility for a patient's drug-related needs and is held accountable for improvement in patient outcomes. It requires integration of sound therapeutic principles and evidence-based data to render preeminent, patient-centered care. (Chapter 1)

Pharmacoeconomics: the division of health economics or outcomes research dealing with pharmaceuticals and pharmacy services. (Chapter 9)

Pharmacoeconomic studies: research in which the purpose is to provide insight into the costs associated with drug therapy (both benefits and consequences) to individual patients, healthcare systems, and society. (Chapter 3)

Placebo effect: the tendency of those receiving a placebo to demonstrate changes in the dependent variable similar to those in the treatment group. (Chapter 8)

Point prevalence: see PREVALENCE (Chapter 6)

Population: all possible members of a group. (Chapters 4 and 5)

Positive predictive value (PPV): the proportion of subjects who have the disease who test positive on a screening test. (Chapter 5)

Power (1 − β): the probability that a false null hypothesis is rejected. (Chapter 5)

Present value: value of a cost or benefit adjusted with a discount rate to the current year. (Chapter 9)

Prevalence (also called point prevalence): the proportion of the population with the condition at a specific point in time. (Chapter 6)

Primary literature: individual research reports, based on observation or experimentation by the author of the article, that report novel findings or observations. (Chapter 2)

Primary outcomes: the main outcome of a study; the outcome that the study is specifically designed to measure; findings that provide the most direct evidence of an association between an independent and a dependent variable. (Chapters 3 and 8)

Probability: considered as a relative frequency; the ratio of the number of times a specific outcome occurs to the total number of outcomes. (Chapter 5)

Probability distribution: a distribution containing the relative frequency (i.e., the probability) of each possible outcome of a series of events. (Chapter 5)

Prospective cohort study design: an observational study design in which groups are defined in terms of an exposure and are followed to determine differences in an outcome of interest. It is prospective because the follow-up period occurs in the future. (Chapter 7)

Publication bias: the tendency of scientific journals not to publish articles that do not show statistically significant differences. (Chapter 10)

Qualitative systematic reviews: a critical examination of evidence in a specific area of knowledge using rigorous logic and critical thinking methodology to evaluate and synthesize the results of individual investigations to answer a specific question. (Chapters 3 and 10)

Qualitative variables: variables that are used as labels to identify differences in type. (Chapter 4)

Quality-adjusted life-year (QALY): quantity of life in life-years multiplied by the quality of life in utilities. (Chapter 9)

Quality of life (QOL): an individual's perception of the livability of their life; often measured with utility or value instruments (questionnaires). (Chapter 9)

Quantitative systematic reviews: also termed meta-analysis, a critical examination of evidence in a specific area of knowledge using statistical methods to evaluate and synthesize the results of individual investigations to answer a specific question. (Chapters 3 and 10)

Quantitative variables: variables that are used to indicate differences in amount. (Chapter 4)

Quartiles: divisions achieved using the median and two other values that divide the data set into four sections, each containing 25% of the values in the data set. (Chapter 4)

Random event: an outcome whose value cannot be known with certainty until it occurs. (Chapter 5)

Random variable: one whose value cannot be determined with certainty before its actual measurement; for example, the dependent variable. (Chapter 4)

Randomized controlled trial (RCT): a prospective, experimental study design in which the investigator controls the application of the independent variable among two or more groups of individuals to assess its effect on outcome variables. (Chapters 3 and 8)

Range: the difference between the largest and the smallest scores in the data set. (Chapter 4)

Ratio scale of measurement: a quantitative or continuous measurement scale characterized by equal intervals between adjacent levels of the variable. However, its zero is a true null quantity, and the ratio of two values is meaningful. (Chapter 4)

Recall bias: a systematic distortion of the data owing to a difference in the recall abilities of one group compared to the other. (Chapters 3 and 6)

Relative frequency distribution: a frequency distribution in which the proportion (rather than the number) of the total values falling within each class interval is displayed. (Chapter 4)

Relative risk: the ratio of the risk in the treatment group to the risk in the placebo group. (Chapter 6)

Research hypothesis: a conjecture about the way nature works; a proposed relationship between the independent and dependent variables that is tested during the experiment. (Chapters 3 and 5)

Retrospective cohort study design: an observational study design in which groups are defined in terms of an exposure and are followed to determine differences in an outcome of interest. It is retrospective because the follow-up period occurs in the past. (Chapter 7)

Risk: see INCIDENCE. (Chapter 6)

Risk difference (also called attributable risk): the risk in the exposed group minus the risk in the placebo group. The difference is thus the risk attributable to the exposure. (Chapter 6)

Risk ratio: see RELATIVE RISK (Chapter 6)

Robust: no change in the final decision after sensitivity analysis is conducted. (Chapter 9)

Sample: a subset that is obtained from a population. (Chapters 4 and 5)

Sampling distribution of a statistic: The probability distribution of all possible values of a statistic, derived from samples of size n. (Chapter 5)

Sampling error: discrepancy between the value of a sample statistic and that of the population parameter owing to variations in the elements making up the sample. (Chapter 5)

Scatter plot: used to demonstrate the relationship of two variables by plotting their joint occurrences. (Chapter 7)

Search terms: words and phrases used to search secondary databases to identify biomedical literature. (Chapter 2)

Secondary data collection: identifying and obtaining data for a research project that were collected for some other purpose. (Chapter 9)

Secondary Literature: abstracts or summaries of primary literature reports, including bibliographic information of the author, study title, and publication citation (where the study was published). (Chapter 2)

Secondary outcomes: findings that provide supporting evidence of an association between an independent and a dependent variable. (Chapters 3 and 8)

Selection bias: a systematic difference in the way participants are assigned to treatment or control groups. (Chapters 3 and 6)

Sensitivity: a measure of the extent to which the output of a survey instrument changes in response to changes in relevant independent variables. (Chapters 5 and 7)

Sensitivity analysis: the changing of values for estimates (uncertainty) of costs or benefits to test the bounds of the analysis; provides an approach to testing how robust the overall results are relative to key decisions and assumptions that were made in the process of conducting the analysis. (Chapters 9 and 10)

Sensitivity of a screening test: the proportion of subjects with a disease who test positive on the screening test. (Chapter 5)

Simple random assignment: uses the outcome of a random event to determine the allocation of patients to experimental or placebo groups. (Chapter 8)

Simple random sample: a method of obtaining samples from a population in which the selection of each participant is a random event and each participant has a constant probability of being selected from the population. (Chapter 5)

Single-blind studies: research protocols in which the patient is unaware of the treatment group assignment. (Chapter 8)

Spearman rank correlation coefficient: an index of the linear association between two variables, given that both variables are ordinal or that a variable is continuous but not normally distributed. (Chapter 7)

Specificity of a screening test: the proportion of subjects without the disease who test negative on the screening test. (Chapter 5)

Standard deviation: the square root of the variance; a measure of dispersion of the data set. (Chapter 4)

Standard gamble: a method used to obtain utilities based on individual preference for a state of health. (Chapter 9)

Standard normal distribution: a normal distribution of the statistic z, having a mean of 0 and a standard deviation of 1. (Chapter 5)

Statistical estimation: the use of a sample statistic to infer the value of a population parameter. (Chapter 5)

Statistical hypothesis: a formulation of the research hypothesis that can be tested using statistical tools. (Chapter 5)

Statistical modeling: a method that uses mathematical formulas to describe relationships among variables or to control for the effects of potentially confounding variables. (Chapter 5)

Stratification: a method of assigning participants to groups to control for a confounding variable by assigning participants so that a similar proportion of each level of the confounding factor is present in each group. (Chapter 8)

Sum of squares regression: an index of the amount of variation in a group of scores that is attributable to the association of the independent and dependent variables. (Chapter 7)

Sum of squares residual: an index of the amount of total variation in a group of values that is attributable to experimental error. (Chapter 7)

Superiority trial: a type of active controlled trial designed to indicate whether the effects of two or more active agents differ from each other. (Chapter 8)

Surrogate outcome: a laboratory measurement or a physical sign used as a substitute for a clinically meaningful endpoint. (Chapter 12)

Survival analysis: a method of analyzing changes in a variable over time. (Chapter 8)

Systematic review: an objective, rigorous approach to data synthesis that may be either qualitative or quantitative. (Chapters 3 and 10)

Tertiary literature (also called general literature): consists of literature that summarizes, integrates, and evaluates primary research studies—for example, textbooks, compendia, and computer databases. (Chapter 2)

Test–retest reliability: a measure of the extent to which a survey instrument produces the same output with repeated use. (Chapter 7)

Threats to internal validity: potential sources of contamination by factors such as measurement error, bias, confounding, and chance. (Chapter 3)

Time tradeoff: a method used to obtain values based on individual preference for the amount of time in a state of health. (Chapter 9)

Transparency: the completeness of the methods section of a study; provides enough detail to allow the reader to reproduce a study. (Chapter 9)

Treatment group: Subjects in a research study who receive an active therapy. (Chapter 3)

Trial profile: a chart or flow diagram included in the report of an RCT that indicates the fate of each participant who was considered for inclusion in the study; it also presents a concise depiction of the study design. (Chapter 3)

Triple-blind studies: research protocols in which the patient, the investigator, and all other individuals associated with the study are unaware of the study group assignments. (Chapter 8)

2 × 2 contingency table: table consisting of the joint frequency of two variables, each of which has two levels. (Chapter 6)

Type I error: see α error. (Chapter 5)

Type II error: see β error (Chapter 5)

Unbiased estimator: a statistic is an unbiased estimate of the population parameter if the mean of the sampling distribution of that statistic equals the population parameter. (Chapter 5)

Utility: individual preferences related to disease states or treatments under conditions of uncertainty. (Chapter 9)

Validity: a measure of the extent to which a survey instrument measures what it is intended to measure. (Chapter 7)

Value: estimates of individual preferences related to disease states or treatments; controversy exists about whether these are utilities. (Chapter 9)

Variable: a characteristic of an entity that can assume different values. (Chapter 4)

Variance: a measure of variability, calculated as the average of the squared deviations of each score from the mean of the scores in a data set. (Chapter 4)

Wilcoxon rank-sum test: a nonparametric statistical test used to test for group differences when data are ordinal variables. (Chapter 6)

Willingness to pay: value based on the amount of money an individual would contribute for that treatment or change in disease state. (Chapter 9)

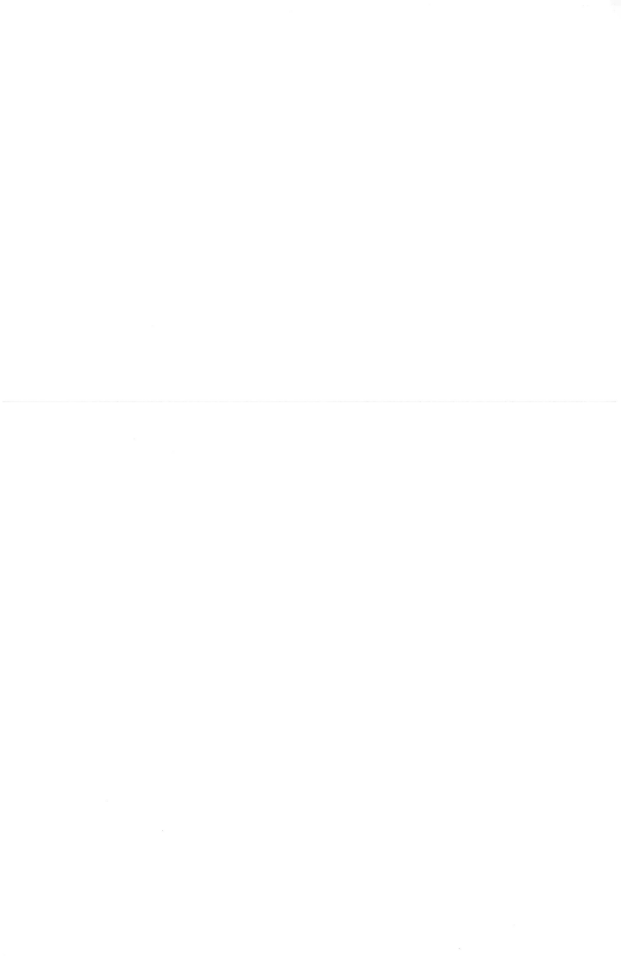

Index

Pages followed by an "f" denote figues; those followed by a "t" denote tables

359